Social Media and Public Health: Opportunities and Challenges

Social Media and Public Health: Opportunities and Challenges

Editors

Wasim Ahmed
Josep Vidal-Alaball

MDPI • Basel • Beijing • Wuhan • Barcelona • Belgrade • Manchester • Tokyo • Cluj • Tianjin

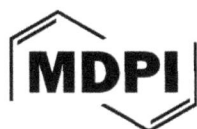

Editors
Wasim Ahmed
Stirling Management School,
Stirling University
UK

Josep Vidal-Alaball
Health Promotion in Rural Areas
Research Group, Gerència
Territorial de la Catalunya
Central, Catalan Health Institute
Spain

Editorial Office
MDPI
St. Alban-Anlage 66
4052 Basel, Switzerland

This is a reprint of articles from the Special Issue published online in the open access journal *International Journal of Environmental Research and Public Health* (ISSN 1660-4601) (available at: https://www.mdpi.com/journal/ijerph/special_issues/social_media_public_health).

For citation purposes, cite each article independently as indicated on the article page online and as indicated below:

LastName, A.A.; LastName, B.B.; LastName, C.C. Article Title. *Journal Name* **Year**, *Volume Number*, Page Range.

ISBN 978-3-0365-2349-1 (Hbk)
ISBN 978-3-0365-2350-7 (PDF)

Cover image courtesy of Josep Vidal Alaball.

© 2021 by the authors. Articles in this book are Open Access and distributed under the Creative Commons Attribution (CC BY) license, which allows users to download, copy and build upon published articles, as long as the author and publisher are properly credited, which ensures maximum dissemination and a wider impact of our publications.

The book as a whole is distributed by MDPI under the terms and conditions of the Creative Commons license CC BY-NC-ND.

Contents

About the Editors vii

Preface to "Social Media and Public Health: Opportunities and Challenges" ix

Wasim Ahmed, Josep Vidal-Alaball, Francesc Lopez Segui and Pedro A. Moreno-Sánchez
A Social Network Analysis of Tweets Related to Masks during the COVID-19 Pandemic
Reprinted from: *Int. J. Environ. Res. Public Health* **2020**, *17*, 8235, doi:10.3390/ijerph17218235 . . . 1

Yang Yang and Yingying Su
Public Voice via Social Media: Role in Cooperative Governance during Public Health Emergency
Reprinted from: *Int. J. Environ. Res. Public Health* **2020**, *17*, 6840, doi:10.3390/ijerph17186840 . . . 11

Junghwa Bahng and Chang Heon Lee
Topic Modeling for Analyzing Patients' Perceptions and Concerns of Hearing Loss on Social Q&A Sites: Incorporating Patients' Perspective
Reprinted from: *Int. J. Environ. Res. Public Health* **2020**, *17*, 6209, doi:10.3390/ijerph17176209 . . . 29

Montse Gorchs-Molist, Silvia Solà-Muñoz, Iago Enjo-Perez, Marisol Querol-Gil, David Carrera-Giraldo, Jose María Nicolàs-Arfelis, Francesc Xavier Jiménez-Fàbrega and Natalia Pérez de la Ossa
An Online Training Intervention on Prehospital Stroke Codes in Catalonia to Improve the Knowledge, Pre-Notification Compliance and Time Performance of Emergency Medical Services Professionals
Reprinted from: *Int. J. Environ. Res. Public Health* **2020**, *17*, 6183, doi:10.3390/ijerph17176183 . . . 43

Boban Melovic, Andjela Jaksic Stojanovic, Tamara Backovic Vulic, Branislav Dudic and Eleonora Benova
The Impact of Online Media on Parents' Attitudes toward Vaccination of Children—Social Marketing and Public Health
Reprinted from: *Int. J. Environ. Res. Public Health* **2020**, *17*, 5816, doi:10.3390/ijerph17165816 . . . 55

Salvatore Pirri, Valentina Lorenzoni, Gianni Andreozzi, Marta Mosca and Giuseppe Turchetti
Topic Modeling and User Network Analysis on Twitter during World Lupus Awareness Day
Reprinted from: *Int. J. Environ. Res. Public Health* **2020**, *17*, 5440, doi:10.3390/ijerph17155440 . . . 83

Carlos de las Heras-Pedrosa, Dolores Rando-Cueto, Carmen Jambrino-Maldonado and Francisco J. Paniagua-Rojano
Exploring the Social Media on the Communication Professionals in Public Health. Spanish Official Medical Colleges Case Study
Reprinted from: *Int. J. Environ. Res. Public Health* **2020**, *17*, 4859, doi:10.3390/ijerph17134859 . . . 101

Josep Vidal-Alaball, Francesc López Seguí, Josep Lluís Garcia Domingo, Gemma Flores Mateo, Gloria Sauch Valmaña, Anna Ruiz-Comellas, Francesc X Marín-Gomez and Francesc García Cuyàs
Primary Care Professionals' Acceptance of Medical Record-Based, Store and Forward Provider-to-Provider Telemedicine in Catalonia: Results of a Web-Based Survey
Reprinted from: *Int. J. Environ. Res. Public Health* **2020**, *17*, 4092, doi:10.3390/ijerph17114092 . . . 119

Francesc X Marín-Gomez, Jacobo Mendioroz Peña, Vicenç Canal Casals, Marcos Romero Mendez, Ana Darnés Surroca, Antoni Nieto Maclino and Josep Vidal-Alaball
Environmental and Patient Impact of Applying a Point-of-Care Ultrasound Model in Primary Care: Rural vs. Urban Centres
Reprinted from: *Int. J. Environ. Res. Public Health* **2020**, *17*, 3333, doi:10.3390/ijerph17093333 . . . **131**

Mengling Yan, Hongying Tan, Luxue Jia and Umair Akram
The Antecedents of Poor Doctor-Patient Relationship in Mobile Consultation: A Perspective from Computer-Mediated Communication
Reprinted from: *Int. J. Environ. Res. Public Health* **2020**, *17*, 2579, doi:10.3390/ijerph17072579 . . . **143**

Wasim Ahmed, Xavier Marin-Gomez and Josep Vidal-Alaball
Contextualising the 2019 E-Cigarette Health Scare: Insights from Twitter
Reprinted from: *Int. J. Environ. Res. Public Health* **2020**, *17*, 2236, doi:10.3390/ijerph17072236 . . . **159**

Josep Vidal-Alaball, Gemma Flores Mateo, Josep Lluís Garcia Domingo, Xavier Marín Gomez, Glòria Sauch Valmaña, Anna Ruiz-Comellas, Francesc López Seguí and Francesc García Cuyàs
Validation of a Short Questionnaire to Assess Healthcare Professionals' Perceptions of Asynchronous Telemedicine Services: The Catalan Version of the Health Optimum Telemedicine Acceptance Questionnaire
Reprinted from: *Int. J. Environ. Res. Public Health* **2020**, *17*, 2202, doi:10.3390/ijerph17072202 . . . **169**

Francesc López Seguí, Jordi Franch Parella, Xavier Gironès García, Jacobo Mendioroz Peña, Francesc García Cuyàs, Cristina Adroher Mas, Anna García-Altés and Josep Vidal-Alaball
A Cost-Minimization Analysis of a Medical Record-based, Store and Forward and Provider-to-provider Telemedicine Compared to Usual Care in Catalonia: More Agile and Efficient, Especially for Users
Reprinted from: *Int. J. Environ. Res. Public Health* **2020**, *17*, 2008, doi:10.3390/ijerph17062008 . . . **179**

Jie Zhao and Jianfei Wang
Health Advertising on Short-Video Social Media: A Study on User Attitudes Based on the Extended Technology Acceptance Model
Reprinted from: *Int. J. Environ. Res. Public Health* **2020**, *17*, 1501, doi:10.3390/ijerph17051501 . . . **189**

Francesc López Seguí, Ricardo Ander Egg Aguilar, Gabriel de Maeztu, Anna García-Altés, Francesc García Cuyàs, Sandra Walsh, Marta Sagarra Castro and Josep Vidal-Alaball
Teleconsultations between Patients and Healthcare Professionals in Primary Care in Catalonia: The Evaluation of Text Classification Algorithms Using Supervised Machine Learning
Reprinted from: *Int. J. Environ. Res. Public Health* **2020**, *17*, 1093, doi:10.3390/ijerph17031093 . . . **211**

Josep Vidal-Alaball, Jordi Franch-Parella, Francesc Lopez Seguí, Francesc Garcia Cuyàs and Jacobo Mendioroz Peña
Impact of a Telemedicine Program on the Reduction in the Emission of Atmospheric Pollutants and Journeys by Road
Reprinted from: *Int. J. Environ. Res. Public Health* **2019**, *16*, 4366, doi:10.3390/ijerph16224366 . . . **221**

Pilar Aparicio-Martinez, Alberto-Jesus Perea-Moreno, María Pilar Martinez-Jimenez, María Dolores Redel-Macías, Claudia Pagliari and Manuel Vaquero-Abellan
Social Media, Thin-Ideal, Body Dissatisfaction and Disordered Eating Attitudes: An Exploratory Analysis
Reprinted from: *Int. J. Environ. Res. Public Health* **2019**, *16*, 4177, doi:10.3390/ijerph16214177 . . . **229**

About the Editors

Wasim Ahmed is a Senior Lecturer in Digital Business (roughly equivalent to Associate Professor in the North American system). He has previously worked at the University of Sheffield, Newcastle University, and Northumbria University. He has also completed an internship at Manchester United FC producing an in-depth research report. Dr. Ahmed's research interests focus on digital health, digital sport, and digital business. Dr. Ahmed has authored many peer-reviewed academic outputs. Ahmed has had multiple media appearances, in print and broadcast, as well as news and TV show appearances.

Josep Vidal-Alaball Born in Berga, he moved to the UK in 1998, where he stayed for 9 years. In 2002, he completed a Family Medicine specialty in Devon and moved to Wales to work as a clinical researcher and professor at Cardiff University. At the end of 2006, he finished his British adventure and returned to Catalonia to work as a rural doctor, combining clinical practice with management tasks in primary care.

He has a PhD in telemedicine, currently works as a family doctor and is the Head of the Research and Innovation Unit in Primary Care of Central Catalonia, where he coordinates a team of clinical researchers focused on research and innovation in health services, mainly oriented to improve the efficiency of primary care services. He is part of the PROSAARU research group (Health Promotion in the Rural Area), where he leads the line of research on new technologies and telemedicine. He is adjunct professor of Medicine at the University of Vic - Central University of Catalonia and a member of EURIPA, the European Association of Rural Doctors, as well as a member of the assembly of the WONCA Working Group on Rural Practice (RuralWonca).

Preface to "Social Media and Public Health: Opportunities and Challenges"

We are living in an information age, with more user-generated data being generated than ever before. The rise of user-generated content derrives from the popularity of social media and other digital platforms. Social media platforms provide unfiltered public views and opinions with the ability to extract intelligence for public health purposes. This can range from using social media to track the spread of diseases to the opinion-mining of public views and opinions.

Social media and associated tehcnologies can also be drawn upon for rapid, survey-based insights into various health topics. Social media are also widely utilised by medical professionals for the purposes of sharing scholarly works, international collaboration, and engaging in policy debates and have also been drawn upon in medical emergencies and crisis situations.

This book is based on a collection of research articles that were published in a special issue of International Journal of Environmental Research and Public Health which was titled: Social Media and Public Health: Opportunitics and Challenges (First Edition). We hope that this body of work can stimulate further excellent work in this area and that organisations can find practical value in the research.

Wasim Ahmed, Josep Vidal-Alaball
Editors

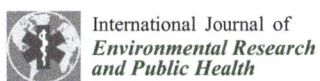

Article

A Social Network Analysis of Tweets Related to Masks during the COVID-19 Pandemic

Wasim Ahmed [1,*], Josep Vidal-Alaball [2,3], Francesc Lopez Segui [4,5] and Pedro A. Moreno-Sánchez [6]

1. Newcastle University Business School, Newcastle University, Newcastle upon Tyne NE1 4SE, UK
2. Health Promotion in Rural Areas Research Group, Gerència Territorial de la Catalunya Central, Institut Català de la Salut, 08272 Sant Fruitós de Bages, Spain; jvidal.cc.ics@gencat.cat
3. Unitat de Suport a la Recerca de la Catalunya Central, Fundació Institut Universitari per a la Recerca a l'Atenció Primària de Salut Jordi Gol i Gurina, 08272 Sant Fruitós de Bages, Spain
4. TIC Salut Social, Generalitat de Catalunya, 08005 Barcelona, Spain; francesc.lopez@cmail.cat
5. Center for Research in Health and Economics (CRES-UPF), Universitat Pompeu Fabra, 08002 Barcelona, Spain
6. School of Health Care and Social Work, Seinäjoki University of Applied Sciences, 60100 Seinäjoki, Finland; pedro.morenosanchez@seamk.fi
* Correspondence: Wasim.Ahmed@Newcastle.ac.uk; Tel.: +44-191-208-150

Received: 21 September 2020; Accepted: 4 November 2020; Published: 7 November 2020

Abstract: Background: High compliance in wearing a mask is a crucial factor for stopping the transmission of COVID-19. Since the beginning of the pandemic, social media has been a key communication channel for citizens. This study focused on analyzing content from Twitter related to masks during the COVID-19 pandemic. Methods: Twitter data were collected using the keyword "mask" from 27 June 2020 to 4 July 2020. The total number of tweets gathered were $n = 452{,}430$. A systematic random sample of 1% ($n = 4525$) of tweets was analyzed using social network analysis. NodeXL (Social Media Research Foundation, California, CA, USA) was used to identify users ranked influential by betweenness centrality and was used to identify key hashtags and content. Results: The overall shape of the network resembled a community network because there was a range of users conversing amongst each other in different clusters. It was found that a range of accounts were influential and/or mentioned within the network. These ranged from ordinary citizens, politicians, and popular culture figures. The most common theme and popular hashtags to emerge from the data encouraged the public to wear masks. Conclusion: Towards the end of June 2020, Twitter was utilized by the public to encourage others to wear masks and discussions around masks included a wide range of users.

Keywords: COVID-19; coronavirus; twitter; masks; transmission; public health

---

1. Introduction

Since emerging in China in December 2019, the beta coronavirus SARS-CoV-2 (named COVID-19) has been expanding rapidly throughout the world [1]. On 30 January 2020, the World Health Organisation (WHO) declared coronavirus COVID-19 to be a Public Health Emergency of International Concern [2]. Thereafter, in March 2020, the WHO declared COVID-19 a pandemic due to the identification of more than 118,000 cases in 114 countries [3]. Millions of people worldwide have been infected, and hundreds of thousands of people have lost their lives due to COVID-19 [4].

Different regional approaches related to the use of face masks to mitigate the transmission of COVID-19 have been developed. In East Asian countries, for example, wearing masks was ubiquitous and was performed as a hygienic habit due to past positive outcomes in 2003 during SARS.

On the contrary, in Europe and North America, the population was informed that masks were not recommended for general use [5]. The WHO states that masks can be used either for protection of healthy persons (worn to protect oneself when in contact with an infected individual) or for infection control (worn by an infected individual to prevent onward transmission) [6]. Ma et al. showed that N95 masks, medical masks, and even home-made masks could block at least 90% of the virus in aerosols [7]. From the perspective of disease spread, at the population level, wearing masks by infected individuals may be important in helping retain contagious droplets, aerosols, and particles that can infect others and contaminate surfaces [5].

The WHO notes that health workers and caregivers in clinical areas must continuously wear medical masks where there is known or suspected community transmission [3]. However, due to the lack of robust evidence in clinical trials, the WHO's recommendations about wearing masks by the general population has been ambiguous. In its interim guidance issued on 5 June 2020, the WHO advises that to effectively prevent COVID-19 transmission in areas of community transmission, governments should encourage the public to wear masks.

Universal masking, as a public health intervention, would probably intercept the transmission of COVID-19. This could especially be the case for asymptomatic infected individuals with high viral load at the early stage of the disease (suggested to be around 40–80% by Javid et al. [5]) [8]. Therefore, community-wide mask usage irrespective of symptoms may reduce the infectivity of silent asymptomatic individuals. Masks are helpful for source control of asymptomatic infectious persons but also for protecting healthy people [9]. Universal masking may become the default solution in high-risk areas with a large number of patients and without sufficient testing, where everyone can only be seen as potentially infected [10].

High compliance in wearing a mask is a crucial factor for stopping transmission. This is similar to vaccines: the more people that are vaccinated, the higher the benefit to the whole population, including those who cannot be vaccinated, such as infants or immune-compromised people [11]. Moreover, the gain is greater the earlier masks are adopted and when face masks are used to complement other measures such as social distancing [12]. Hand hygiene is a discontinuous process and sometimes difficult to practice in the community. However, wearing a mask is a continuous form of protection to stop respiratory droplets to and from others [13]. Thus, controlling harms at the source by wearing masks is at least as important as other mitigation actions such as handwashing. Universal masking would also help in removing stigmatization that could discourage symptomatic patients to wear a mask in many places, preventing any discrimination that might arise.

However, various authors have justified not wearing masks for different reasons. One of the key reasons is that there is limited evidence supported by clinical trials on the effectiveness of masks [14]. Secondly, it is claimed that prevention depends on an individual's behaviour and compliance, which has been shown to be inconsistent or inappropriate in trials, for example, people may repeatedly touch their mask [6]. It is also claimed that wearing a mask might make people feel safe and hence reduce adherence to other nonpharmaceutical measures such as hand washing and social distancing [5]. Moreover, at one stage it was also argued that because of the shortage of masks, the public should not wear them because healthcare workers would need them more and that the public buying masks could lead to major supply chain problems along with an increase in prices [15].

In this context, the aim of this study was to look at potential for Twitter to highlight public views towards universal masking. Social media is a useful platform for raising awareness of various issues and Twitter is a valuable platform for listening to public views and opinions on a range of topics in real-time. Moreover, from a public health standpoint, it is important to develop an understanding of the drivers of the discussion around masks and to gain insight into key topics of discussion.

More specifically, the research questions of this study were as follows:

1. What was the overall network shape of the discussion on Twitter?
2. What were the key hashtags?
3. Who were the most influential users?

4. Who were the most mentioned users?
5. What were the key themes of discussion that were taking place?

2. Methods

2.1. Tweet Sampling

Twitter data were collected using the keyword "mask" from 27 June 2020 21:21:21 to 4 July 2020 19:50:40 to provide coverage of about a week of data in a period when this topic was highly present in social media. The total number of tweets which were gathered (worldwide) were $n = 452{,}430$. By using the keyword "mask", tweets including words such as "masks" or "#mask" were also retrieved and included. A systematic random sample of 1% ($n = 4525$) of the tweets was extracted and analyzed using social network analysis, as described in the next section.

2.2. Social Network Analysis

The software NodeXL (Social Media Research Foundation, California, CA, USA) was used to conduct a social network analysis of the data [16]. In understanding the network graph, the results of this study build upon previous research [17,18], which has highlighted that Twitter topics may follow six network shapes and structures [19]: broadcast networks, polarized crowds, brand clusters, tight crowds, community clusters, and support networks. In the network graph provided in Figure 1, circles represent individual Twitter users and the lines between them represent connections such as mention and reply. The network graph was laid out using the Harel–Koren Fast Multiscale layout algorithm which is built into NodeXL. NodeXL uses the Search Application Processing Interface (API). Influential users were identified using NodeXL and were anonymized by providing a description of the account in line with previous research [18]. A specific subanalysis was performed for tweets that originated solely from the USA. Regional information was extracted as follows: a total of $n = 13{,}265$ tweets were extracted where users had included "USA" in their user bios and a 5% sample of tweets was extracted and analyzed in NodeXL. Individual users and/or organisations that were deemed to be not sufficiently in the "public domain" were anonymized.

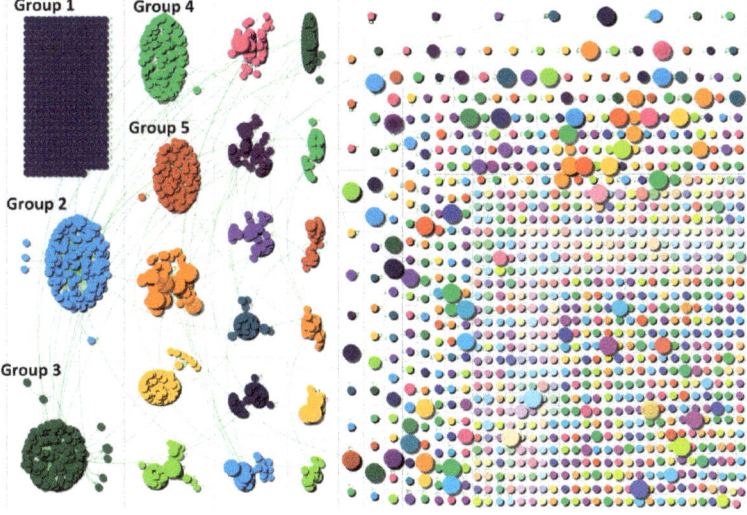

Figure 1. Network graph of masks from 27 June to 4 July.

3. Results

3.1. Top 10 Hashtags Used

Table 1 below provides an overview of the most used hashtags during this time, showing that "wearamask" (n = 34) and "maskssavelives" (n = 11) appeared among the most used hashtags.

Table 1. Top 10 hashtags.

Rank	Top Hashtags in Tweet in Entire Graph	Entire Graph Count
1	covid19	50
2	wearamask	34
3	kidlitformasks	23
4	mask	18
5	maskssavelives	15
6	マスク (Japanese for "mask")	13
7	haikyuu	11
8	hq	11
9	ビール (Japanese for "beer")	10
10	andhrapradesh	9

The hashtag "kidlitformasks" referred to authors of children's books who used this hashtag to highlight the importance of wearing masks. Twitter users also shared images from a Japanese manga series "haikyuu" and at the same time encouraged others to wear a mask using the "#haikyuu" and 'hq' hashtags, and these appeared as the 7th and 8th most popular hashtags that were used. As the discussion during this time was global in nature, there also appeared to be relevant hashtags from around the world such as "マスク" which refers to "mask" in Japanese. The word "ビール" also appeared, which is the Japanese word for "beer". This was because users conversed about a humorous mask invention which allows a user to store beer inside the mask which can be consumed. The hashtag "andhrapradesh" appeared as a popular hashtag as this referred to a state in the south-eastern coastal region of India and news reports were shared at this time related to reports about the death of a young person who was allegedly "beaten to death" by police for not wearing a mask.

3.2. Overview of Network Structure

Figure 1 is a social network graph of the discussion taking place during this time. The largest group (group 1) is an isolates group which contained users who sent tweets that did not contain mentions. Overall, the group resembled a community network shape because there were many groups of users conversing about this topic. NodeXL clustered users into different groups based on mentions. A community cluster indicated that many users were talking to each other across several groups. It was also interesting to see influential users (indicated by larger circles) scattered around the network, which indicated that the topic brought in a wide range of influential actors.

3.3. Top 10 Users Ranked by Betweeness Centrality

Table 2 highlights Twitter users that were influential during this time. The users in the network were ranked by betweenness centrality, which is a measure of centrality. These users would have acted as important bridges within the network. The follower's column refers to the amount of followers each user has. Many of the influential nodes within the network derived from ordinary citizens who became important bridges in the network. A number of popular culture figures also appeared among the most influential users within the network.

Table 2. Top 10 users ranked by betweenness centrality.

Rank	Account Type	Followers
1	Citizen	301
2	Citizen	2434
3	Citizen	3160
4	Citizen	206
5	Professor	4602
6	Citizen	2601
7	Citizen	17
8	Citizen	1002
9	Rex Chapman also known as Ice-T (American rapper)	1,786,850
10	Rex Chapman (former basketball player)	1,004,702

3.4. Top 10 Users Most Mentioned

Table 3 provides an overview of users that were most mentioned during this time which ranged from political figures, organizational accounts, and popular culture related accounts. Certain users may not have tweeted about masks but were mentioned frequently by other users. Examining the influential users from this time highlighted that the discussion had been focused in and around the United States. However, it must be noted that not all account mentions may have been relevant to medical masks, as the band Slipknot are known to wear non-medical masks.

Table 3. Top 10 users most mentioned.

Rank	Account Type	Followers
1	Donald Trump (current president of the United States)	83.8 Million
2	Joe Biden (former Vice President of the United States)	7.1 Million
3	Account Belonging to an Organization	23.1 Thousand
4	Bangtan Boys, a seven-member South Korean boy band	27.2 Million
5	Mike Pence (Vice President of the United States)	9.3 Million
6	Sarah Silverman (USA based comedian)	12.4 Million
7	Official Twitter account of YouTube	72.1 Million
8	Account Belonging to an Organisation	2.2 Thousand
9	Citizen	20.1 Thousand
10	Slipknot (an American heavy metal band from Des Moines)	2.1 Million

3.5. Content Analysis

NodeXL was used to identify the most frequently occurring co-words, as shown in Table 4. These co-related keywords provided insight into the types of discussions that may have been taking place on Twitter. Word pairs containing mentions of Twitter user handles were removed. This occurred on three occasions in group 3.

Table 4. Identifying content across clusters.

NodeXL Group	Frequent Word Pairs
1	'Wear, mask' 'wearing, mask' 'face, mask' 'f***ing, mask' 'wear, f***ing*' 'mask, public' 'stay, home'
2	's**t*, mask,' 'oh, s**t*' 'mask, really' 'really, thing' 'Wearing, mask' 'convince, y'all' 'y'all, wearing' 'Mask, hurt' 'hurt, dog' 'dog, finally'
3	'Wear, mask' 'breathing, problem' 'problem, lol' 'Lol, wear' 'mask, karen' 'f***ing*, hard' 'Hard, wear'
4	'Someone, ugly' 'ugly, personally' 'personally, mind' 'Mind, wearing' 'wearing, mask' 'mask, covers' 'Covers, half' 'half, face' 'wear, mask' 'breathing, problem'
5	'Wear, mask' 'see, someone' 'wearing, mask'

* asterisk placed by authors in expletives.

The most frequent co-related keywords were "wear" and "mask" to form the sentence "wear a mask" and, in some cases, also involved an expletive. There were also tweets related to humor. There were also co-occurring words such as "stay" and "home". Other co-occurring words which appeared across the clusters included "breathing" and "problem", which revolved around the debate of whether face masks should be mandatory as they may lead to breathing problems. In regard to this debate, Twitter users provided evidence to highlight that face masks did not cause breathing problems, whereas other users highlighted the potential for masks to cause breathing issues.

3.6. Regional Analysis of the USA

In this part of the analysis, tweets were extracted to only focus on the USA. Data were filtered by users who noted in their bios that they were from the USA.

Top Word Pairs

Table 5 provides an overview of the 5 most popular words that were used from users from the USA.

Table 5. Top 5 word pairs. Filtered by USA.

Rank	Word Pair
1	'wear, mask'
2	'wearing, mask'
3	'mask, public'
4	'face, mask'
5	'breathing, problem'

The most frequent words used together included "wear mask", "wearing mask", "mask, public", "face, mask", and "breathing problem". The first two co-words appeared to be encouraging the use of face masks and the third and fourth most used co-words appeared to be centred around general discussions around the use of masks. The fifth most used co-word appeared to relate to discussions around whether masks could cause breathing problems. Overall, there appeared to be overlaps between phrases and words used in tweets when filtering specifically for the USA, compared to analyzing tweets overall. Furthermore, content such as top hashtags and users appeared to be similar to that of the results of the analysis overall.

4. Discussion

The overall shape of the network resembled a community as there were a range of users conversing amongst each other in different clusters. When examining the most frequently used hashtags, it appeared that the most popular hashtags encouraged mask wearing among the public. It was found that a range of accounts were influential and/or mentioned, ranging from ordinary citizens, politicians, and popular culture figures. The discussion had been politicized by some users on Twitter, which led to politicians appearing as influential users within the network. Japanese hashtags also appeared within the network, which highlights the global nature of the discussions around this issue. It is important to note that some of the accounts such as the official Twitter account of YouTube might not have tweeted using the word 'mask', however, users may have shared content which contained the word 'mask' and also used the mention "@YouTube". The most common theme to emerge was the encouragement for the public to wear masks and discussions around this. Other themes were related to jokes and discussions related to whether face masks were safe for those who may have breathing problems. Our study also examined Twitter data emerging solely from the United States, which demonstrated that there was overlap in content. This could have occurred because the Twitter has the most active users in the United States.

It must be noted that Twitter discussions are constantly evolving and potentially alter on a weekly basis. A limitation of our study is that it focused specifically on the Twitter network from 27 June to the 4 July, hence our findings may not be applicable to other time periods. Future research could seek to expand time periods and examine Twitter discussions based on other locations. A further limitation is that with the 1% random sample we extracted, generic keyword and 7-day approach, we have captured some tweets coming from "temporary" discussions (for instance, beer and mask related humor in Japan). If the study had examined a longer time period, i.e., 6 months, and taken a 0.005% sample, the study would have been able to perform a much wider analysis (the masks and beer humor would not have been captured and/or captured on a lesser scale). At the same time, however, the approach adopted in this study had a better chance of capturing other issues such as conspiracy theories and/or short-lived time-based discussions. Future research could combine both approaches in the analysis. Further research could also seek to conduct a sentiment analysis of the data.

A wider limitation related to research on Twitter is the potential of 'off-topic' discussions surrounding a particular keyword or hashtag to take place. Future research could seek to eliminate irrelevant content prior to analyzing data. Twitter data can be used to study a wide range of public health topics and was recently used to study views into personal health records [20], which utilises a similar methodology to this present study. Other research has also examined disclosure of patient information [21] and COVID-19 conspiracies [22]. Future research could also seek to examine the role of influential accounts during this time.

5. Conclusions

Overall, it was found that the shape of the network resembled a community as there were a range of users conversing amongst each other in different clusters. It was found that a range of accounts were influential and/or mentioned ranging from ordinary citizens, politicians, and popular culture figures. The most common theme and popular hashtags to emerge from the data encouraged the public to wear masks. Public health authorities and influential accounts could continue to utilize social media platforms to encourage users to wear masks.

Author Contributions: Conceptualization, W.A.; data curation, W.A.; supervision, J.V.-A. and F.L.S.; writing—original draft, W.A., F.L.S. and P.A.M.-S.; writing—review and editing, W.A., J.V.-A., F.L.S. and P.A.M.-S. All authors have read and agreed to the published version of the manuscript.

Funding: This research received no external funding.

Conflicts of Interest: The authors declare no conflict of interest.

References

1. Wu, F.; Zhao, S.; Yu, B.; Chen, Y.-M.; Wang, W.; Song, Z.-G.; Hu, Y.; Tao, Z.-W.; Tian, J.-H.; Pei, Y.-Y.; et al. A new coronavirus associated with human respiratory disease in China. *Nature* **2020**, *579*, 265–269. [CrossRef] [PubMed]
2. Sohrabi, C.; Alsafi, Z.; O'Neill, N.; Khan, M.; Kerwan, A.; Al-Jabir, A.; Iosifidis, C.; Agha, R. World Health Organization declares global emergency: A review of the 2019 novel coronavirus (COVID-19). *Int. J. Surg.* **2020**, *76*, 71–76. [CrossRef]
3. WHO Director-General's Opening Remarks at the Media Briefing on COVID-19—11 March 2020. Available online: https://www.who.int/dg/speeches/detail/who-director-general-s-opening-remarks-at-the-media-briefing-on-covid-19---11-march-2020 (accessed on 15 July 2020).
4. World Health Organization. *Coronavirus Disease (COVID-19). Situation Report-176*; Publisher: Geneva, Country, 2020; Available online: https://www.who.int/docs/default-source/coronaviruse/situation-reports/20200714-covid-19-sitrep-176.pdf?sfvrsn=d01ce263_2 (accessed on 5 November 2020).
5. Javid, B.; Weekes, M.P.; Matheson, N.J. Covid-19: Should the public wear face masks? *BMJ* **2020**, *369*, m1442. [CrossRef]
6. Advice on the Use of Masks in the Community, during Home Care and in Healthcare Settings in the Context of the Novel Coronavirus (COVID-19) Outbreak. Available online: https://www.who.int/publications-detail-redirect/advice-on-the-use-of-masks-in-the-community-during-home-care-and-in-healthcare-settings-in-the-context-of-the-novel-coronavirus-(2019-ncov)-outbreak (accessed on 15 July 2020).
7. Ma, Q.; Shan, H.; Zhang, H.; Li, G.; Yang, R.; Chen, J. Potential utilities of mask-wearing and instant hand hygiene for fighting SARS-CoV-2. *J. Med. Virol.* **2020**, *92*, 1567–1571. [CrossRef]
8. Wang, G.; Zhang, Y.; Zhao, J.; Zhang, J.; Jiang, F. Mitigate the effects of home confinement on children during the COVID-19 outbreak. *Lancet* **2020**, *395*, 945–947. [CrossRef]
9. Cheng, K.K.; Lam, T.H.; Leung, C.C. Wearing face masks in the community during the COVID-19 pandemic: Altruism and solidarity. *Lancet* **2020**. [CrossRef]
10. Zhou, Z.-G.; Yue, D.-S.; Mu, C.-L.; Zhang, L. Mask is the possible key for self-isolation in COVID-19 pandemic. *J. Med. Virol.* **2020**, *92*, 1745–1746. [CrossRef]

11. Howard, J.; Huang, A.; Li, Z.; Tufekci, Z.; Zdimal, V.; van der Westhuizen, H.; von Delft, A.; Price, A.; Fridman, L.; Tang, L.; et al. Face Masks Against COVID-19: An Evidence Review. *Preprints* **2020**, 2020040203. [CrossRef]
12. Eikenberry, S.E.; Mancuso, M.; Iboi, E.; Phan, T.; Eikenberry, K.; Kuang, Y.; Kostelich, E.; Gumel, A.B. To mask or not to mask: Modeling the potential for face mask use by the general public to curtail the COVID-19 pandemic. *Infect. Dis. Model.* **2020**, *5*, 293–308. [CrossRef]
13. Cheng, V.C.-C.; Wong, S.-C.; Chuang, V.W.-M.; So, S.Y.-C.; Chen, J.H.-K.; Sridhar, S.; To, K.K.-W.; Chan, J.F.-W.; Hung, I.F.-N.; Ho, P.-L.; et al. The role of community-wide wearing of face mask for control of coronavirus disease 2019 (COVID-19) epidemic due to SARS-CoV-2. *J. Infect.* **2020**, *81*, 107–114. [CrossRef]
14. Xiao, J.; Shiu, E.Y.C.; Gao, H.; Wong, J.Y.; Fong, M.W.; Ryu, S.; Cowling, B.J. Nonpharmaceutical Measures for Pandemic Influenza in Nonhealthcare Settings—Personal Protective and Environmental Measures. *Emerg. Infect. Dis.* **2020**, *26*, 967–975. [CrossRef] [PubMed]
15. Greenhalgh, T.; Schmid, M.B.; Czypionka, T.; Bassler, D.; Gruer, L. Face masks for the public during the covid-19 crisis. *BMJ* **2020**, *369*, m1435. [CrossRef] [PubMed]
16. Ahmed, W.; Lugovic, S. Social media analytics: Analysis and visualisation of news diffusion using NodeXL. *Online Inf. Rev.* **2019**, *43*, 149–160. [CrossRef]
17. Ahmed, W.; Marin-Gomez, X.; Vidal-Alaball, J. Contextualising the 2019 E-Cigarette Health Scare: Insights from Twitter. *Int. J. Environ. Res. Public Health* **2020**, *17*, 2236. [CrossRef] [PubMed]
18. Ahmed, W.; Vidal-Alaball, J.; Downing, J.; Seguí, F.L. COVID-19 and the 5G Conspiracy Theory: Social Network Analysis of Twitter Data. *J. Med. Internet Res.* **2020**, *22*, e19458. [CrossRef] [PubMed]
19. White, D.R.; Borgatti, S.P. Betweenness centrality measures for directed graphs. *Soc. Networks* **1994**, *16*, 335–346. [CrossRef]
20. Pang, P.C.-I.; McKay, D.; Chang, S.; Chen, Q.; Zhang, X.; Cui, L. Privacy concerns of the Australian My Health Record: Implications for other large-scale opt-out personal health records. *Inf. Process. Manag.* **2020**, *57*, 102364. [CrossRef]
21. Ahmed, W.; Jagsi, R.; Gutheil, T.G.; Katz, M.S. Public Disclosure on Social Media of Identifiable Patient Information by Health Professionals: Content Analysis of Twitter Data. *J. Med. Internet Res.* **2020**, *22*, e19746. [CrossRef] [PubMed]
22. Ahmed, W.; Seguí, F.L.; Vidal-Alaball, J.; Katz, M.S. COVID-19 and the "Film Your Hospital" Conspiracy Theory: Social Network Analysis of Twitter Data (Preprint). *J. Med. Internet Res.* **2020**, *22*, 22374. [CrossRef] [PubMed]

Publisher's Note: MDPI stays neutral with regard to jurisdictional claims in published maps and institutional affiliations.

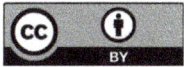

© 2020 by the authors. Licensee MDPI, Basel, Switzerland. This article is an open access article distributed under the terms and conditions of the Creative Commons Attribution (CC BY) license (http://creativecommons.org/licenses/by/4.0/).

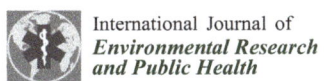

Article

Public Voice via Social Media: Role in Cooperative Governance during Public Health Emergency

Yang Yang and Yingying Su *

School of Management, Harbin Institute of Technology, Harbin 150001, China; yfield@hit.edu.cn
* Correspondence: 18b910059@stu.hit.edu.cn; Tel.: +86-188-4558-5002

Received: 31 July 2020; Accepted: 16 September 2020; Published: 18 September 2020

Abstract: With the development of the Internet, social networking sites have empowered the public to directly express their views about social issues and hence contribute to social change. As a new type of voice behavior, public voice on social media has aroused wide concern among scholars. However, why public voice is expressed and how it influences social development and betterment in times of public health emergencies remains unstudied. A key point is whether governments can take effective countermeasures when faced with public health emergencies. In such situation, public voice is of great significance in the formulation and implementation of coping policies. This qualitative study uses China's Health Code policy under COVID-19 to explore why the public performs voice behavior on social media and how this influences policy evolution and product innovation through cooperative governance. A stimulus-cognition-emotion-behavior model is established to explain public voice, indicating that it is influenced by cognitive processes and public emotions under policy stimulus. What is more, as a form of public participation in cooperative governance, public voice plays a significant role in promoting policy evolution and product innovation, and represents a useful form of cooperation with governments and enterprises to jointly maintain social stability under public health emergencies

Keywords: public voice; public health emergency; social media; policy evolution; product innovation; cooperative governance

1. Introduction

As a positive extra-role behavior, voice has attracted extensive interests from scholars and gained substantial attention in the organizational behavior literature [1–3]. Public voice is a new type of voice behavior that refers to the behavior of citizens who share opinions on social media to improve the social status quo or prevent harmful practices [4]. As a pro-social behavior, public voice is vital for advancement and betterment of society [4], and it is believed that public voice plays an important role in the cooperative governance of government and other organizations (e.g., enterprises, non-profit organizations) under a public health emergency. Considering that public participation in public administration and policy formulation is beneficial to government performance, governments attach much importance to the public's role in policy-making, especially in the areas of environmental governance, public health, and sustainable development [5–8]. In the face of extraordinary development problems, such as economic recession, public opinion in policy-making is extremely important [9]. Thus, to ensure the timeliness and efficiency of policy in the case of public health emergencies, the value of public voice, along with technical support from enterprise, should not be underestimated. In the COVID-19 epidemic, many governments have begun to cooperate with high-tech enterprises to formulate epidemic prevention and control policies such as the Health Code in China, COVIDWISE in Virginia, and Corona-Warn in Germany [10–13]. Public voice on social media has effectively promoted the evolution of epidemic control policy and tracking applications developed by enterprises, making an outstanding contribution to social stability. Thus, it is necessary to study public voice in public health emergencies in relation to the implementation of government policies and the promotion of enterprises' product innovation. Public voice is also of great significance in further realizing cooperative governance.

Voice behavior refers to the extra-role interpersonal communication behavior in which organizational members actively make constructive suggestions to the organization for the purpose of improving work or organization status quo [14]. Previous studies on voice behavior have mainly focused on employee voice and customer voice within organizations; public voice in a broader context has received little attention. The importance of employee voice and customer voice for the sustainable development of enterprises suggests that the role of public voice in social improvement should not be underestimated, and is worthy of in-depth discussion [4]. Given that public voice can have wide ranging influence in terms of social change, this research focuses on its effect on the evolution of policy implemented under public health emergencies. Public voice in public health emergencies has several important characteristics: First, the target of public voice is more extensive. The targets of employee voice and customer voice are employees inside the enterprise and customers who have cooperative relationships with the enterprise, respectively. They often offer advice to the enterprise as a single identity. However, for public voice, the target is the general public, who have dual identities as policy participants and enterprise customers. Second, under cooperative governance, multiple subjects participate in policy-making, so the targets and content of public voice are also diverse. For example, voice to a government may relate to the implementation of policy, while that to an enterprise may focus on product improvement. Third, the channels for public voice are more diverse. Employees mainly voice to supervisors face-to-face or make suggestions through the internal social networks of an enterprise, and most customer voice occurs through the virtual community created by the enterprise. As social networking sites provide a more convenient platform for people to voice their concerns and make their voices heard, the public can voice through a variety of social networking sites [4]. Finally, the effect of public voice is more significant. Public health emergencies prompt the public to respond to the policy more actively and provide timely feedback [15], which forces the governments and enterprises to absorb public opinion as soon as possible to improve policies and products. Overall, research on public voice behavior is still in its infancy. The factors driving public voice and the mechanism of its action on government policies and enterprise product innovation are unclear. The purpose of this study is to address this gap and further explore the role of public voice in promoting cooperative governance under public health emergencies.

The main contributions of this paper are threefold. First, it extends the literature on voice behavior. Most studies on voice behavior have focused on employee voice and customer voice. Under cooperative governance, the public is a participant in government policy as well as a customer of enterprises, yet the mechanisms for the influence of public voice on policy and product are not clear. This paper focuses on the dynamic role of public voice in policy-making and evolution and product innovation. Second, it constructs a dynamic model of public voice to promote policy implementation under public health emergency. Studies of public participation have mainly focused on its effect on environmental projects and decision, as public participation is seen as highly valuable and necessary to achieve the goal of environmental pollution control [8,16,17]. However, the voice behavior of the public in the formulation and evolution of policies in public health emergencies is unknown. Finally, this paper extends the literature on cooperative governance in a public health emergency and attaches more importance to the role of public voice in the process of collaborative.

This research uses China's Health Code policy under COVID-19 as an example. This is an epidemic prevention policy whose implementation relies on a health rating system developed by Alibaba, Tencent, and other firms. The system uses opaque algorithms and individuals' data, such as physical condition and contact with an infected person, to make judgments about the infection risk of system users [18]. The system then generates a QR code corresponding to this risk level that is used as a passport. Based on the evolution process of Health Code policy, this paper downloads comments about the Health Code policy to do research. This study uses the qualitative research method of grounded theory to explore the factors driving public voice and reveals the dynamic mechanism of its influence on policy formulation and product innovation. Further, this research provides support for cooperative governance involving government, enterprises, and the public under public health emergencies.

2. Literature Review

2.1. Voice Behavior

The concept of voice was first proposed by Hirchman in the field of economics. It has been further developed in the field of organizational behavior [19]. Currently, voice behavior is divided into employee voice, customer voice, and public voice. Most research on voice behavior has been in the field of organizational behavior and mainly aimed to explain employee voice within organizations. Van dyne and Lepine define employee voice behavior as a positive extra-role behavior focused on improving existing working methods and procedures through constructive suggestions; they emphasize the 'promoting' role of employee voice for the organization [14]. Van dyne et al. further expand the concept, pointing out that voice includes not only suggestions for improvement, but also concerns about the organization [20]. On this basis, Liang et al. clearly divide voice behavior into promotive voice and prohibitive voice [21]. Promotive voice refers to innovative ideas or suggestions put forward by employees to improve the overall operation of the organization, while prohibitive voice refers to employees' attention to work practices, and events and employee behaviors that are not conducive to the development of the organization [21]. Employee voice is widely considered a valuable and positive extra-role interpersonal communication behavior, a kind of organizational citizenship behavior that plays an important role in the team and organization. Scholars have conducted in-depth research on the influential factors and outcome variables of employee voice. Previous studies indicate that personal characteristics, leadership, and organizational climate can influence employee voice, which will be beneficial to organizational betterment [2,3,22–29]. Additionally, the approaches of employee voice are also optimized due to the development of the Internet [30].

With the aggravation of market competition, customer participation becomes crucial for the product and service innovation of enterprises, and enterprises have created brand virtual communities to gather customers' ideas and opinions. Research on voice behavior has also expanded from the internal voice of the organization to the field of consumer behavior. On the connotation level, Griffin and Hauser regard customer requirements as customer voice, holding the view that customers would sort their needs according to importance and convey them to enterprises [31]. Enterprises can then develop new products based on customer requirements. Lee et al. expand the connotation of customer voice and define it as a description of customers' needs and expectations or preferences and dislikes, including the pursuit of rights and interests, suggestions for new products and services, and complaints about previous use experience. Earlier definitions of customer voice are based on customer needs, but with advances in research on employee voice within organizations, scholars have begun to redefine customer voice from the perspective of role orientation. Ran and Zhou clearly define customer voice as the extra-role communication behavior in which customers actively make suggestions or express opinions to improve the status of enterprises; this kind of behavior belongs to the category of customer citizenship behavior [32]. At the dimension level, most previous studies on customer voice divide it into two categories: customer satisfaction and customer complaint [33]. With the deepening of research, scholars find that customers not only express dissatisfaction regarding product and service providers, but also express satisfaction and praise, and make their own suggestions. Therefore, with reference to the classification of employee voice by Liang et al., customer voice can be divided into promotive voice and prohibitive voice [21]. Promotive voice refers to the innovative ideas and suggestions of customers regarding improvements to the efficiency of enterprises, while prohibitive voice refers to the expression of opinions on actual and potential problems within the products, services, or management of an enterprise that are harmful to the enterprise or its customers. As the input behavior of customers to enterprises, customer voice can urge enterprises to innovate products and services to meet the needs of customers, thus improving customer satisfaction and maintaining customer loyalty. It can also help enterprises correct errors, provide solutions to problems, and improve enterprise performance [33,34].

With the rapid development of social media, people can express their views on social issues more directly and conveniently, and research on voice behavior has been further extended to a broader social life context. Public voice behavior refers to citizens sharing opinions on social media to improve their social status quo or prevent harmful practices. It is essentially a pro-social behavior [4]. Public voice channels have begun to focus on social media, because in the modern world, social media presents extensive information; people express their concern about education, security, the environment, work-life balance, and many other issues online. Moreover, the diversity and openness of social media provides a broad platform for public expression. The public can conduct online voice behavior through third-party social media and public participation is increasing. However, research on public voice based on social media is still in its infancy and is uncommon. Bhatti et al. explore the mechanism of the effect of individual moral identity and proactive personality on public promotive voice and prohibitive voice based on self-consistency theory [4].

Research on voice behavior as discussed above has several characteristics. First, the research field has shifted from intra-organization to a broader social background. Second, the voice subjects present a change trend of 'employee-customer-public'. Third, the targets of voice behavior change from organizational practice to general social phenomena. Fourth, the form of voice presents the evolution trend of "face-to-face-virtual community-social media".

2.2. Public Role in Public Policy

Citizen participation in the formulation and consultation of public policies is an important way to strengthen and support modern democracy [35]. Regarding the influence of public participation on policy, most research reveals extensive interest in environmental protection and pollution control, as public participation can help decision makers recognize public concern and demands, and handle environmental conflict in a more flexible manner [36,37]. Fu and Geng explore the influence of public participation and regulation compliance on 'green development' with panel data from 30 provinces in China from 2004 to 2014, finding that public participation can lead enterprises to improve compliance and thus promote green development [8]. Regional environmental quality (REQ) is a comprehensive indicator of emissions of waste gas, waste water, and waste solids, and its improvement requires coordination between governance and public participation. Public participation can be coordinated with governance to effectively improve REQ effectively, and further promote the optimization of environmental governance system [38]. The arrival of the Internet era has changed the method of public participation. As a branch of e-government, e-participation has been widely examined by scholars. Considering that public participation is a voluntary activity, whether the public is willing to participate is the decisive factor affecting the success of e-government platforms. Scholars consider that in addition to demographic differences, willingness to use an e-participation system is affected by system technical factors, personal incentive factors, and social capital factors. Based on the unified theory of acceptance and use of technology, planned behavior theory, social capital theory, and other information system theories, previous studies have explored the willingness of the public to use the e-community to participate in policy-making and provide strategic suggestions for governments to improve e-government platform [39,40].

2.3. Product Innovation

Product innovation is an important focus in the innovation research field and is key for enterprises to obtain sustainable competitive advantage. At present, there is no unified definition of product innovation in academia. Katila and Ahuja define it as change in design attributes—such as technology, appearance, quality, and structure—relative to the existing products of an enterprise. This is also known as technological innovation or design innovation [41]. The Organization for Economic Co-operation and Development defines product innovation as the process leading to a new or significantly improved product or service [42]. Various scholars' definitions of product innovation, identify two aspects: entity product innovation and service-related innovation. According to the different degree of innovation, product innovation can be divided into radical innovation and incremental innovation [43]. Rapid change in the external environment drives enterprise innovation; enterprises can only achieve long-term development by constantly producing more competitive products according to the needs of users. As an external innovation resource, customer voice can be regarded as a gift given by users to enterprises to help them carry out product innovation based on the collective wisdom [44–46]. Customer voice provides valuable information for enterprises, which can help product designers and engineers to understand customers' needs and preferences, and turn them into key objectives of product improvement by making targeted adjustments to products and services to meet the needs of users [47]. Further, customer voice can help enterprises identify the product attributes to which customers pay most attention and focus on product improvement and new product development [48].

2.4. Cooperative Governance

Governance refers to processes and structures in public decision making and may involve the participation of multiple agents, such as governments, corporations, and the public, with the aim of carrying out a public purpose that cannot be accomplished by single force [49]. Cooperative governance is not limited to formal government-initiated arrangements, but involves diverse kinds of multi-partner governance related to a wide range of fields [49]. For example, because of the production of pollution, enterprises take the greatest responsibility for environment contamination control. However, as it is difficult for governance goals to be achieved through the actions of a single enterprise, so governance among enterprises is indispensable [50]. With regard to cooperative governance among governments, Zhang et al. find that superior government should supervise heterogeneous local governments and increase penalties for non-cooperative parties to improve the efficiency of haze pollution control [51]. Further, cooperative governance can provide guidance for participatory governance by the public [4]. Studies of cooperative governance involving public participation have focused on environmental governance and sustainable development. When making local energy decisions, local governments should be given more autonomy and sufficient capacity to strengthen public participation. What is more, public opinion ought to be taken into consideration when developing policy [52]. Studies show that policy-making style presents convergence to the cooperation among government, public and non-profit organizations. As the government may lack the necessary resources to deal with issues, they rely on other subjects to provide support to ensure policy utility [53].

To summarize, there are several problems needing to be solved: First, research on public voice is not mature and more studies are needed to clarify its antecedents as well as its effects on policy implementation and social development. Second, it is undeniable that the public plays a crucial role in environmental governance, but the role of public voice behavior in policy-making and implementation under public health emergencies is still unclear. Third, the role played by public voice in cooperative governance and how this happens deserve exploration.

3. Data Analysis

3.1. Case Background

At the beginning of 2020, the outbreak of COVID-19 brought great impact on people's life and work. In order to contain the spread of novel coronavirus and speed up the normalization of production and life, on 7 February 2020, Yuhang first launched the Yuhang Health Code. And on 11 February 2020, Hangzhou launched the Hangzhou Health Code to implement "green code, red code, yellow code" three-color code dynamic management [18]. The implementation of this policy has aroused widespread concern of the people all over the country, and local governments have followed up and implemented a local version of code in few weeks [18]. The implementation of Health Code policy is assisted by the QR rating health code system developed by Alibaba, Tencent, or other firms. When registering, individuals should provide their names, ID numbers, phone numbers, and answer a series questions about physical health conditions and travel trajectory to get the initial rating [54]. In addition, the rating changes according to individual real-time data, which consists of individuals' travel history, directly related health information, overall medical test results, and overall risk assessment from individuals' reports, information from GPS (Global Positioning System), telecommunications supplier, consumption record, QR code usage record, etc. The system assesses individual's infection risk and generates green, yellow, or red codes according to individual's data [55]. People with green codes have a very low probability to be infected and can move around freely, while people with yellow codes have a risk to be infected to some extent and should be quarantined for a week. People with red codes are at great risk of infection and need to be quarantined for 2 weeks. During the quarantine, if people with yellow or red codes check in on the app every day, the codes will turn green at the end of quarantine periods. And if the real-time information shows that people with green codes have gone to a high-risk area or been in contact with an infected person, the code will turn yellow or red as well [10]. Up to August 2020, the Tencent Health Code covers a population of 9 hundred million people, more than 400 cities and counties, and more than 5100 villages in China, with a cumulative total of 42 billion visits [56]. With the evolution of the Health Code policy, the effective circulation of personnel from all over the country has met the needs of residents' normal life and enterprises' resumption of work and production. At present, residents only need to provide a real-time QR code generated in a mini-app embedded in Alipay (Alibaba, Hangzhou, China) or WeChat (Tencent, Shenzhen, China) to the guard, they can move around [54]. In the Health Code policy implementation process, the high-tech enterprises not only provide technical support to develop the health code system, but also participate in the formulation of policy standards and establishment of policy platforms. For example, Alibaba and Tencent have been fully involved in the formulation of national standards for the personal Health Information Code series [57,58]. Besides, during this process, the public is actively voicing on the implementation and evolution of the Health Code policy as well as improvements of health code application on social media. In the official Weibo of People's Daily, tweets about the Health Code policy get plenty of comments and followers, most of which are advice for policy implementation and system improvement. For example, the tweet about the Hangzhou Health Code has 7227 comments and 79,547 followers. The government press conference and reports about enterprises confirm the public voice does play an important role in the evolution and promotion of Health Code policy and the voice is fully considered and adopted by government and enterprises when making decisions. On the joint prevention and control conferences of COVID-19, the government spokespersons provided response to public concern and the governments also instructed local government and related enterprises to take measures to meet public voice. In addition, the enterprises responded to public voice as well. In the Government Affairs Strategy Conference, Yuepeng Qiu, vice President of Tencent, said that they had updated the system more than 50 times.

3.2. Data Collection and Analysis

This study adopts a dynamic research perspective, and takes the dynamic evolution of health codes policy as an example, focusing on exploring how public voice promoted the improvement of products by enterprises and the implementation of policies by the government under a public health emergency. The core of grounded theory emphasizes the process of collecting and analyzing original data. In the data collection stage, the researcher takes the evolution process of the Health Code policy as the time axis, and collects public comments under the official microblog of the People's Daily as the research object. Data analysis included the following stages: Firstly, open coding is used to identify phenomena, define concepts, and discover categories from the original data. Secondly, axial coding is carried out to further analyze to get the main category. Thirdly, selective coding is used to find the core category, and systematically connect it with other categories to construct a logical relationship. In the whole coding process, researchers keep supplementing the material. Finally, the selective coding is analyzed and theoretical construction is carried out, and the density, variation, and high integration of theoretical concepts are adjusted to form a theoretical framework. The qualitative analysis software Nvivo 11.0 (QSR International, Melbourne, Australia) was used for the analysis of this study.

3.2.1. Open Coding

Open coding is to analyze the original data word by word, so as to summarize the initial concepts and categories in the original data. Following the process of "tagging-conceptualization-categorization", the researchers analyzed the collected data word by word and refined the semantics of the data to obtain the corresponding concepts and categories. Examples are shown in Table 1.

Table 1. Examples of open coding.

Category	Concept	Example from Original Text
System Reliability	Filling mechanism	The above is all my own writing There will be human factors to fill in the health code all by myself
	Feedback mechanism	I never get in when call customer service consultation I didn't get any answer when I called 12345, and problems have not been dealt with after I reported to Alipay
	System fluency	Sometimes I cannot get in the system Yesterday the system crashed and it provided green code only
	Clock mechanism	Now the code is yellow. It says that the seven-day clock normally changes to green code, but I haven't been able to clock in for three days in a row. Is it a dead cycle I couldn't clock in
	Quantitative limitation	I applied early this morning and being told there were no place available today There is a quantity limit on health code, I can't apply for it
	Technical defects	There's a problem with the back-end technology
Ensure resumption of work and production	Risk control	This kind of formalism will only make Hangzhou more dangerous. Some areas do not need to be quarantined if they have proof of returning to work. Is such a perfunctory anti-epidemic measure really safe? Replacing current containment measures with health codes has serious consequences
	Daily traffic	A few days ago, Shanghai swept this health code in highway traffic, it was very fast It's really convenient to go out this way, and you don't have to worry about losing the paper material
	Quarantine	The problem is that I came back on the 2nd. The quarantine for 14 days does not count as before. It means I will be quarantined for one month Recently, cross provincial commuting is becoming crazy. There are 14 days of isolation at work and 14 days after work
	Checking routine	It's much more convenient than running around to apply material This is not only efficient to reduce the burden of screening personnel, but also can record personal travel

3.2.2. Axial Coding

The purpose of axial coding is to explore the potential logical relationship between categories and develop main categories. This study classifies different categories according to their relationship at the conceptual level, and concludes eight main categories, which are divided into three classifications. The main categories and their corresponding classifications and relations are shown in Table 2.

Table 2. Axial coding and analysis results.

Classification	Main Category	Category	Connotation
Perceived policy effectiveness	Crisis resolution	Ensure personal safety	Reduce the impact of public health emergencies on the public's personal and property safety
		Reduce public burden	Reduce the burden of public health emergencies on the public's daily life and psychology
	Social normalization	Facilitate personnel flow	Perception of the effectiveness of policy in facilitating mobility
		Ensure resumption of work and production	Perceived effectiveness of the policy in ensuring the safety and improving the efficiency of the resumption of work and production
		Promote economic recovery	Perceived effectiveness of policy in getting society back on track and restoring the economy
Public emotion	Positive emotion	Satisfaction	Emotion arises when perceived policy effectiveness lives up to expectation
	Negative emotion	Dissatisfaction	Emotion arises when perceived policy effectiveness falls short of expectation
Public voice	Policy evolution	Policy promotion	Voice proposed by the public to promote local policies nationwide
		Policy unification	Voice proposed by the public to unify local policies
		Policy normalization	Voice proposed by the public to carry out the policy under normal circumstances
	Policy implementation	Execution of grassroots organization	Implementation of government policies by grassroots workers
		Regional barriers	The problem of poor policy compatibility caused by different local policies
		User coverage	The policy is inadequate in terms of population coverage
	Product utility	System reliability	Reliability of the product system itself
		Level credibility	How reliable is the product to the user's health rating
	Potential risk	Information disclosure	There is a risk of information leakage when the product collects too much user information
		Abuse of power	There is a risk of abuse of rights when enterprises assume part of government responsibilities

3.2.3. Selective Coding

On the basis of axial coding, selective coding excavates the core category from main categories and analyzes the connection relationship among them. As shown in Figure 1, the dynamic mechanism of public voice behavior to promote policy implementation and evolution in public health emergencies is as follows: First, under the guidance of the government, enterprises participate in the development of policy and design products to assist policy implementation with advanced technologies. Second, in response to the government policy, the public will use enterprise products in their daily life and work. And through judging whether the policy can effectively solve the current problems and guide the future development of the society to form the policy effectiveness perception. Third, public's perception of the effectiveness of policies will trigger public emotions. Different perceptions of policy effectiveness can lead to positive or negative emotions. Then, emotions can induce public voice behavior, including voice for government policies and for enterprise products. Finally, the government and enterprises will give feedback to the public voice and improve the policies and products accordingly. As a new external stimulus, the improved policies and products also have an impact on the public's perception of policy effectiveness, forming a dynamic mechanism of public suggestions to promote policy evolution and product innovation, as shown in Figure 1.

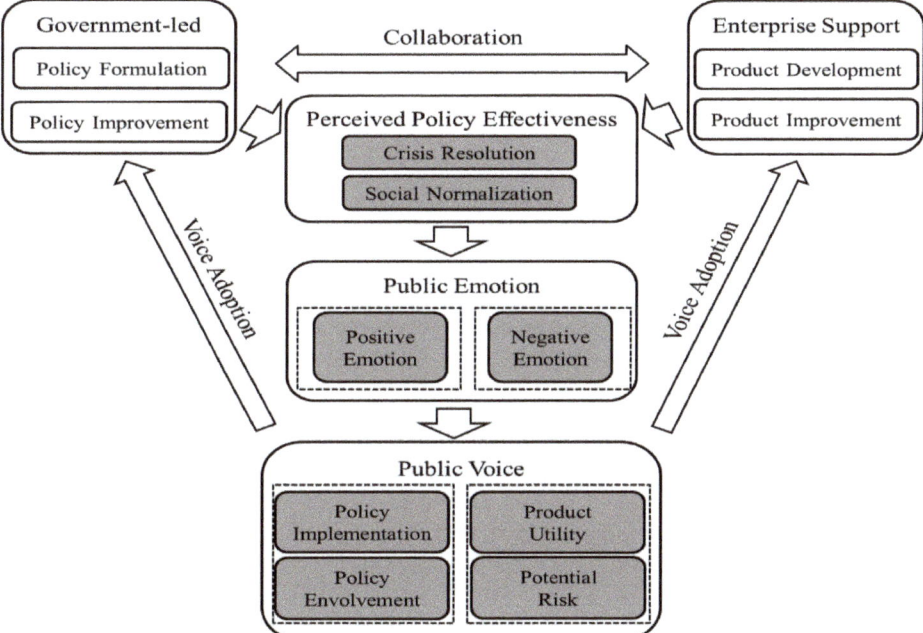

Figure 1. The model of public voice's formulation and effects. Main categories are shaded grey.

4. Results

Based on the results of grounded theory and cognitive appraisal theory of emotion, this paper constructs a driving mechanism of public voice behavior: "stimulus-cognition-emotion-behavior" model. The model shows that there are causal relationships among cognition, emotion, and behavior. According to the cognitive appraisal theory of emotion, under the stimulation of external events, the external information obtained by individuals first enters the perceptual system for compilation and processing, forming specific cognitions. Cognitions trigger the individual's emotional response, and finally produces specific behavioral tendency [59].

4.1. The Formation Process of Public Voice (Stimulus-Cognition-Emotion-Behavior)

4.1.1. Policy as the Stimulus

Public policy is the political and technical approach to solve problems, fundamentally, it is pragmatic [60]. Under the cooperative governance, the government is no longer the only decision-maker, but the main participant plays a guiding role [49]. With the advent of the new Internet era, the impact of big data, cloud computing, and other technologies on policy formulation and implementation cannot be ignored. First of all, the Internet can optimize the link of policy-making, and the process of it can be completed with the help of the Internet, thus making policy-making more efficient. Secondly, big data can provide a wider range of data sources for policy evolution. Through data mining and analysis, it can provide big data support for policy evolution, making policy formulation and implementation more reasonable. Finally, the open data system can further broaden the channels for the public to participate in policy discussions and make policy-making more democratic. Due to the immature application of big data by the government and lack of professional talents, enterprises are required to provide technical support. The technical support of enterprises is more important for the formulation of policies under public health emergencies. As public health emergencies tend to be urgent, destructive, and uncertain, putting forward higher requirements for the timeliness, scientificity, and effectiveness of policies. In this case, it is very necessary for the government to cooperate with enterprises to formulate policies. The government is responsible for policy formulation and implementation, while enterprises take technological advantages to provide products or services to assist policy implementation.

4.1.2. External Stimulus Leads to Perceived Policy Effectiveness

According to the cognitive appraisal theory of emotion, when individuals encounter the external stimuli, they will experience two-stage cognitive appraisal processes: primary appraisal and secondary appraisal. In addition, through the appraisal, people can assess the relevance of external stimuli to themselves and whether the resources they have can cope with the situation [61]. In public health emergencies, the policy launched by government-enterprise cooperation is an external stimulus for the public. Additionally, public appraisal mainly focuses on whether the policy can achieve policy purpose and effectively solve specific public problems, that is, perceived policy effectiveness. Under the policy stimulation, the public will use the cognitive system to make evolution of it [62]. The perception of policy effectiveness reflects the individual's judgment of the correlation between the policy and himself and is an important way for policy to act on public behavior. A high level of perceived policy effectiveness indicates that the public believes the policy is beneficial to their daily life, while on the contrary, they consider that the policy has no significant positive impact or may pose a threat. Policy is the action route or method to guide the current and future decision-making, and its role should not be limited to solving the current problems, but also should be instructive for future development of society [63]. According to the results of analysis, the policy effectiveness in public health emergency includes crisis resolution and social normalization. In the case of public health emergencies, the first problem to be solved by policies is to reduce the adverse impact of emergencies, that is crisis resolution. On the premise that the crisis is under control, policies should also have effects of accelerating the social normalization and promoting economic recovery, that is, the social normalization function. Taking the Health Code policy as an example, if the public thinks that the Health Code policy cannot effectively control the spread of COVID-19, or cannot speed up work resumption, the public's perceived effectiveness of Health Code policy will be low. Otherwise, the perception will be high.

4.1.3. Perceived Policy Effectiveness Arouses Public Emotion

Emotions are the products of an individual's appraisal of the person–environment relationship and of great diagnostic value to help an individual identify what is important under a specific situation. Additionally, emotions vary with the change of appraisals [61]. The public's emotional response to policy is formed on the basis of perceived policy effectiveness. According to the cognitive appraisal theory of emotion, emotion intuitively shows the public's evolution of external stimulus perception, and its core is evaluative cognition. Almost everything will stimulate people to produce emotion, no matter if it happens or not [62]. However, emotion cannot be aroused by external stimulus directly; the appraisal process of relationship between person–environment is necessary to evoke emotion. When individuals are in a certain situation, they will evaluate it, be satisfied or dissatisfied, beneficial or harmful, and make corresponding emotional reactions [59]. If perceived policy effectiveness is high, the public will have a positive emotion, or vice versa. Taking the Health Code policy as an example, different perceptions of public policy effectiveness will stimulate different emotions. When the public perceive that the Health Code policy can effectively control the spread of COVID-19 or accelerate economic recovery, they will generate positive emotions. Otherwise, they will hold negative emotions. Examples of comments about Health Code policy are as follows.

Comment 1: As I am from Hubei province, I didn't go back to my hometown, so I couldn't enter the market for 20 days. After having the health code, I entered the market for the first time without being stopped. It is easy to use and it's really convenient, give it a thumb up!

Comment 2: I'm in Fuyang, and I'm not even allowed to go to my husband's hometown in the countryside. I haven't left Fuyang for nearly a month. I haven't even gone to downtown or move around Fuyang. What the hell is this code? I don't understand. I'm so angry!

4.1.4. Public Emotion Stimulates Public Voice

According to the cognitive appraisal theory of emotion, the cognition and appraisal of external environment will stimulate special emotions. Then, the emotion will motivate coping behaviors to prevent harm or to improve the prospects for benefit [64]. Public voice behavior is generated under the influence of public emotions. According to cognitive appraisal theory of emotion, emotional response will lead to an individual's specific behavior tendency to regulate the emotion (emotion-focused coping) or change for the better the problem (problem-focused coping) [61]. On the basis of the public perceived policy effectiveness, the emotional reaction is finally transformed into the driving force to improve the effectiveness of the policy, which urges the public to put forward a constructive voice or point out the problems existing in the policies and products. When the public believe the policy can effectively defuse the current crisis and benefit future development, they will hold positive emotions and employ behaviors that can maximize the policy benefits. However, when the public think that there are some defects in the process of policy implementation undermining the policy effectiveness, they will generate negative emotions and take actions to reduce potential harm. After analysis, it is found that public voice can be divided into two dimensions: policy voice and product voice. According to the content of voice, policy voice can be divided into policy evolution and policy implementation. Policy evolution voice is promotive voice and usually occurs when the public is in positive emotion, referring to the public's suggestions on the promotion and unification of policies across the nation. Policy implementation voice refers to the voice made by the public for the actual implementation process of policies. In a public health emergency, policy implementation voice is mainly in the form of pointing out defects in the process of policy implementation, and it usually happens when the public is in negative emotion. Public voice on products can be divided into product utility and potential risk. Product utility voice refers to the public's suggestions on improving product efficiency and it includes both promotive voice as well as prohibitive voice. While potential risk voice is prohibitive voice, referring to the public's concern about the negative effects caused by enterprise's products. The examples of the Health Code policy are shown below.

Comment 3: Now in many provinces, the biggest problem is that people are not allowed to enter the community! Not even people with health codes! This is too unreasonable! If a policy is made, it is to be implemented. What good is policy if the implementation problem at the grassroots level is not solved?

Comment 4: The Health Code really gives me a great convenience in my life. It's easy to go out with it. I hope it can be promoted nationwide.

In conclusion, the formation process of public voice behavior conforms to the "stimulus-cognition-emotion-behavior" model of cognitive appraisal theory of emotion. Policy stimulus leads to the public's cognition of the effectiveness of policy, which arouses public emotion response and further leads to public voice behavior.

4.2. The Dynamic Process of Public Voice on Policy Evolution

The formation and evolution of policy is a dynamic and continuous process. Previous studies have paid more attention to the impact of public participation in the policy-making stage [65,66]. However, this study finds that after policies are made, public voice also has a great impact on the evolution and implementation of policies. Based on the results of grounded analysis, this paper divides the process of policy evolution into three stages: policy formation, policy promotion, and policy optimization, and constructs a dynamic mechanism of public voice to promote policy evolution and product innovation, as shown in Figure 2.

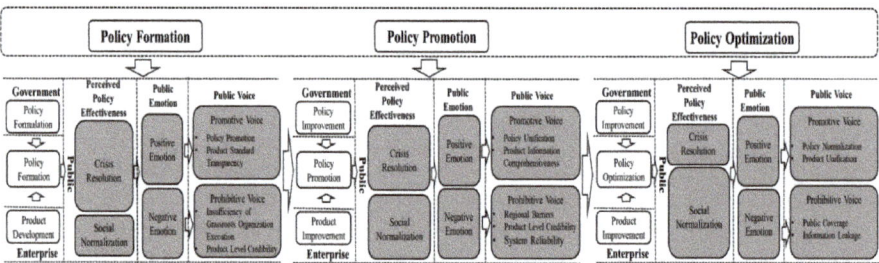

Figure 2. Model of the dynamic effect of public voice behavior on policy, results of grounded theory are shaded grey.

4.2.1. Policy Formation Stage

The policy is formed in accordance with the rigorous policy-making process in order to solve specific public problems. As the output of the political system, the main function of policy is to solve social public problems effectively. As public health emergencies often pose a major threat to social security and public order, as well as the safety of citizens' lives and property, the policy under public health emergencies aims to resolve the crisis state timely and effectively and restore the normal life order as soon as possible [15]. As an external stimulus, the formation of policies will lead to the public's perceived policy effectiveness. At this stage, citizens' cognition of policy effectiveness mainly focuses on crisis resolution. Whether the policy can effectively alleviate the adverse impact of public health emergencies is an important factor affecting public emotion. When policy is implemented, the public will form the perception of whether the policy can resolve the crisis effectively. When perceived policy effectiveness is high, the public will have positive emotion and tend to conduct promotive voice. As the construction of national emergency management system follows the basic principles of "ability-standard" and "center of gravity down", the local government is in the front line when dealing with public health emergencies and bears the main responsibility. Therefore, the policies under public health emergencies are often formulated by the local government, and the superior government selectively promotes the policies according to the evolution of the applicability. So the public will suggest to promote policy across the country if they think the policy is effective enough. Besides, the public will provide promotive voice to improve product utility in a state of positive emotion. When the public perceive the policy is not effective enough, they will have negative emotion and tend to conduct a prohibitive voice. Public health emergencies prevent policy-making from following a strictly procedural process. The government needs to complete the implementation of the policy in a limited time, and it is difficult to guarantee the implementation of the grassroots administrative staff in a short time [15]. Therefore, the prohibitive voice mainly focuses on pointing out the problems existing in the implementation of the policy at the grassroots level. In the policy formation stage, as the implementation of enterprise's product auxiliary policy, the public's requirements for its effectiveness are more stringent. Therefore, the public will be more active in pointing out problems in the use of products.

4.2.2. Policy Promotion Stage

Through the evolution and adoption of public voice, the government improves the policy and policy evolution enters the policy promotion stage. As a new external stimulus, the improved policy continues to act on public cognition. More than that, the focus of perceived policy effectiveness begins to shift from crisis resolution to social normalization. Under the control of the government, the grassroots implementation has been further improved, and the effectiveness of policies to solve current problems (i.e., crisis resolution effectiveness) has been effectively played. However, the effects of policies cannot limit to provide methods to solve the current problems, but also play a guiding role in the future development of society [63]. Public health emergencies make society change from normal state to emergency state, which has a great impact on public life and work [15]. Therefore, on the basis of effective resolution of the crisis, whether the policy can further promote the recovery of social normality has been widely concerned by the public. Under the influence of public emotion caused by the cognition of policy utility, voice behavior emerges. In the stage of policy promotion, public promotive voice is policy unification. Government policy-making under public health emergencies emphasizes the local government's ability of 'territorial management'. However, with the promotion of local policies across the country, the problem of compatibility between policies begins to emerge. The inconsistency of policies in different regions will bring many inconveniences to the public. Therefore, in order to improve the effectiveness of policies, the public suggests that policies should be unified across the country. At this stage, with policy promotion, the audience range of the product is constantly expanding, the public's attention to the product utility is also increased. Improvement suggestions to enhance the effectiveness are still the focus of voice. However, in addition to the utility of the product, the public also began to pay attention to the use experience of the product, pointing out the problems of the system in the use process.

4.2.3. Policy Optimization Stage

Under the influence of public voice, the government and enterprises constantly improve the policies and products, and the policy evolution enters the optimization stage. At this time, with the public health emergency in the rehabilitation stage, the effectiveness of the policy has been played out to a greater extent; the public urgently need to return to normal life and work state, so the focus of perceived policy effectiveness is social normalization. Public voice is still affected by the emotional response based on cognition, and the content of public voice has changed further. Considering the adverse impact of public health emergencies, with the purpose of preventing the recurrence of the public health emergency, the public suggest that the policy should be normalized. Policy normalization can predict the occurrence of public health emergencies in the early stage and minimize the loss. In addition, the public begin to pay attention to the coverage of the policy, pointing out that the omission of the population covered by the policy may have a negative impact on the fairness. With regards to the products of enterprises, the public voice focuses on the risks of long-term use of products. Products are tools for enterprises to participate in cooperative governance and used to supply policy implementation. With the help of products, enterprises take part of the responsibilities originally belonging to the government, which will cause public concern.

To sum up, public voice plays an important role in the evolution of policies. First, public opinion provides the widest source of information for policy feedback. Public health emergencies require the government to formulate effective policies in the shortest time based on the least information and resources, and the effectiveness of the policies is uncertain [15]. The public voice gives quick feedback to the policy, which provides the basis for the government to evaluate the effectiveness of the policy. Second, the public voice expresses the public interest demands and promotes the policy to be more democratic and efficient [67]. In order to gain more and more public support in the process of policy-making, public voice is an important consideration for the government in the process of formulating and implementing policies. Finally, public voice behavior also plays an important role in product improvement and innovation. It can be seen from the analysis, that in the policy of government enterprise cooperation, due to the particularity of the product, the public's requirements are more stringent. Voice for product improvement aims at making it more suitable to assist policy implementation, and it will provide an important reference for enterprise product innovation.

5. Conclusions

This study reveals the driving mechanism of public voice behavior and enriches the literature on voice behavior. First, based on the results of qualitative research, this paper employs the cognitive appraisal theory of emotion to explain the process of formation of public voice behavior under public health emergencies, via the stimulus-cognition-emotion-behavior model. Unlike voice within an organization, public voice on social media is a kind of self-motivated behavior free from the pressure of peers and organizational climate [4]. What is more, as the purpose of public voice is to improve social status quo, the cognitive appraisal theory of emotion is eminently suitable for explaining the formation of public voice behavior. As an external stimulus, a policy will have an impact on the public's cognitive processes, and prompt them to evaluate whether the policy can resolve a current issue and play a guiding role in the future development of society. When the public perceives the policy to be highly effective, they will have positive emotions; otherwise, they will have negative emotions. Take the Health Code policy as an example, if the public think that the policy can effectively contain the spread of the novel coronavirus and speed up the resumption of the normal activities, they will experience positive emotions, and vice versa. In accordance with the cognitive appraisal theory of emotion, emotional response will stimulate behavioral tendencies. The public's positive emotions will lead them to employ a promotive voice to expand the effectiveness and coverage of the policy, whereas the public has the tendency to use prohibitive voice to reduce the possible negative effects of a policy when they are not satisfied with its effectiveness. This result is consistent with previous studies that make a clear distinction between promotive voice and prohibitive voice, where the former is positive in tone and the later negative [68]. In this study, members of the public feeling positive emotions will voice to promote a policy and establish uniform standards throughout the nation, whereas those experiencing negative emotions will identify deficiencies such as implementation at the grassroots level. Second, this study clarifies the objects and types of public voice. Compared with employee voice and customer voice, the coverage of public voice is more extensive. Thus, for different problems, the objects of public voice are also different, which require separate analysis in each situation. Under this circumstance, the objects of public voice include two main bodies involved in policy-making: governments and enterprises. For the Health Code policy, the objects of public voice are the government, Alibaba, and Tencent. With regard to voice type, there is some similarity with the other two kinds of voice—public voice can also be divided into promotive voice and prohibitive voice. Finally, through qualitative research, this paper has attempted to reveal the role of public voice in policy evolution and product innovation, clarifying the promoting effect of public voice on societal improvement. The study emphasizes the importance of public voice via social media, suggesting that both government and enterprises ought to attach more significance to public voice when making decisions.

Taking China's Health Code policy under COVID-19 as an example, this paper has constructed a dynamic mechanism for the effects of public voice on policy evolution. The study focused on the promotion of public voice for policy improvement and evolution in the late stages of policy-making. Public opinion contains information about demands and aspirations which is very valuable for decision makers. To absorb more public opinions and take into account public aspirations or priorities before policy formulation, previous research has paid much attention to the impact of public opinions at the pre-policy-making stage [65,66]. No studies have examined the impact of public voice on policy after its implementation. The development of social media not only provides a wider source of information for the public, but also builds a more convenient platform for the public to voice their opinions at any stage of policy formulation or implementation, thus having effect on policy. This study shows that after a policy is implemented, public voice is still of great value for policy evolution. However, this study divides policy evolution into three stages: policy formation, policy promotion, and policy optimization. It introduces changes in public policy utility perception and public voice content at different stages, and constructs the dynamic mechanism of the effect of public advice on policy improvement based on the government's adoption of public advice to promote policy evolution and implementation.

To some extent, this study provides support for cooperative governance research. Cooperative governance has different connotations in different situations, and there are also some differences among participants. The formulation and evolution of policies under public health emergencies is an important practice of cooperative governance. Faced with a public health emergency, the government, enterprises, and citizens should form an open overall system to jointly govern social public affairs. The government, enterprises, and individuals play their own roles, participate and cooperate with each other to effectively reduce the negative impacts of a crisis and maintain the stable development of society. In this process, governments, enterprises, and the public are in a more equal position, and multi-agent participation is truly realized. Faced with COVID-19, Yaowen Wang, deputy director of Shenzhen Municipal Government Service Data Management Bureau, said the epidemic situation was a great challenge to the government's governance ability and level. In addition, the fundamental problem was laid in whether the whole society could be quickly mobilized and organized to participate in the prevention and control in a short period of time. As an organ of power, the government is responsible for the formulation and implementation of policies. Enterprises participate in the formulation of policies, and provide products and services with technical advantages to assist with policy implementation. As for the public, in addition to regulating their own behaviors under the guidance of policies, they also provide feedback and voice on policies and enterprises' products and services. Take China's Health Code policy as an example, the government is responsible for the formulation and implementation of the policy. Alibaba and Tencent are committed to the development and updating of the health code system and participate in the formulation of the policy standards. The public need to move around in strict accordance with the policy guidelines and actively provide voice. Under a public health emergency, public voice is an important way for public to participate in cooperative governance. It provides real-time feedback for policy, helping government and enterprises to make decisions as quickly as possible and set aside more time to fight against emergencies. Further, public voice can facilitate the promotion of effective policy, improving prevention efficiency. As a universal way of participating in cooperative governance, public voice via social media deserves more attention in the future.

Although this research makes several contributions, there are still some limitations. First, we studied the influence of public voice only on policy evolution and specific product innovation. As public voice is social-oriented, it will affect almost all social affairs and phenomena. Future research can explore the influence of public voice behavior in other respects. Second, this study revealed the generative mechanism of public voice behavior from the perspective of emotional cognition. As a self-oriented behavior, public voice may be triggered by other internal processes. Future research could explore the antecedents of public voice from different perspectives. Third, this study was conducted under a public health emergency, COVID-19. As public emergencies take several forms, the results differ in different situations. Future research might examine public voice in other contexts. Fourth, although many countries and regions have formulated corresponding policies in the context of public health emergencies, results from the study of China's Health Code policy under COVID-19 may not be fully applicable to other nations, and future research should be conducted in different cultural contexts.

Author Contributions: Y.Y. conceived the idea of this study, Y.S. collected and analyzed data and wrote this paper. All authors have read and agreed to the published version of the manuscript.

Funding: This research was funded by the National Natural Science Foundation of China, grant number 71972062; the National Natural Science Foundation of China, grant number 71872058; the Fundamental Research Funds for the Central Universities, grant number HIT.HSS.201842.

Conflicts of Interest: The authors declare no conflict of interest.

References

1. Li, C.W.; Liang, J.; Farh, J.L. Speaking up when water is murky: An uncertainty-based model linking perceived organizational politics to employee voice. *J. Manag.* **2020**, *46*, 443–469. [CrossRef]
2. James, R.D.; Ethan, R.B. Leadership behavior and employee voice: Is the door really open? *Acad. Manag. J.* **2007**, *50*, 869–884.
3. Walumbwa, F.O.; Schaubroeck, J. Leader personality traits and employee voice behavior: Mediating roles of ethical leadership and work group psychological safety. *J. Appl. Psychol.* **2009**, *94*, 1275–1286. [CrossRef]
4. Bhatti, Z.A.; Arain, G.A.; Akram, M.S.; Fang, Y.H.; Yasin, H.M. Constructive voice behavior for social change on social networking sites: A reflection of moral identity. *Technol. Forecast. Soc. Chang.* **2020**, *157*, 120101. [CrossRef]
5. Beeri, I.; Uster, A.; Vigoda-Gadot, E. Does performance management relate to good governance? A study of its relationship with citizens' satisfaction with and trust in Israeli local government. *Public Perform. Manag. Rev.* **2019**, *42*, 241–279. [CrossRef]
6. Tritter, J.Q.; McCallum, A. The snakes and ladders of user involvement: Moving beyond Arnstein. *Health Policy* **2006**, *76*, 156–168. [CrossRef]
7. Stephan, H.; Davies, A.R. Public participation, engagement, and climate change adaptation: A review of the research literature. *Wiley Interdiscip. Rev. Clim. Chang.* **2020**, *11*. [CrossRef]
8. Fu, J.; Geng, Y. Public participation, regulatory compliance and green development in China based on provincial panel data. *J. Clean. Prod.* **2019**, *230*, 1344–1353. [CrossRef]
9. Alex, J.H.; Liang, M. Citizen Participation, Perceived Public Service Performance, and Trust in Government: Evidence from Health Policy Reforms in Hong Kong. *Public Perform. Manag. Rev.* **2020**. [CrossRef]
10. How China Is Using QR Code Apps to Contain Covid-19. Available online: https://technode.com/2020/02/25/how-china-is-using-qr-code-apps-to-contain-covid-19/ (accessed on 25 February 2020).
11. Coronavirus Tracing Apps Launching in 3 More States. Available online: https://www.foxnews.com/health/coronavirus-tracing-apps-launching-more-states (accessed on 14 August 2020).
12. Germany's R-Rate Spikes Above 1 Ahead of Tracing App Rollout. Available online: https://news.yahoo.com/germanys-r-rate-spikes-above-175850444.html (accessed on 15 June 2020).
13. French Lawmakers Endorse the Country's Virus Tracing App. Available online: https://news.yahoo.com/frances-virus-tracing-app-ready-121639411.html (accessed on 27 May 2020).
14. Van Dyne, L.; Lepine, J.A. Helping and voice extra-role behaviors: Evidence of construct and predictive validity. *Acad. Manag. J.* **1998**, *41*, 108–119.
15. Ali, F. (Ed.) *Handbook of Crisis and Emergency Management*; Marcel Dekker: New York, NY, USA, 2001.
16. Wu, J.; Xu, M.; Zhang, P. The impacts of governmental performance assessment policy and citizen participation on improving environmental performance across Chinese provinces. *J. Clean. Prod.* **2018**, *184*, 227–238. [CrossRef]
17. De'Arman, K.J. Is Public Participation Public Inclusion? The Role of Comments in US Forest Service Decision-Making. *Environ. Manag.* **2020**, *66*, 91–104. [CrossRef] [PubMed]
18. China Voices. How Alibaba Built China's Health Code. Available online: https://technode.com/2020/04/07/china-voices-how-alibaba-built-chinas-health-code/ (accessed on 7 April 2020).
19. Hirschman, A.O. *Exit, Voice and Loyalty: Responses to Decline in Firms, Organizations and States*; Harvard University Press: Cambridge, MA, USA, 1970.
20. Van Dyne, L.; Ang, S.; Botero, I.C. Conceptualizing employee silence and employee voice as multidimensional constructs. *J. Manag. Stud.* **2003**, *40*, 1359–1392. [CrossRef]
21. Liang, J.; Farh, C.I.C.; Farh, J.L. Psychological antecedents of promotive and prohibitive voice: A two-wave examination. *Acad. Manag. J.* **2012**, *55*, 71–92. [CrossRef]

22. LePine, J.A.; Van Dyne, L. Voice and cooperative behavior as contrasting forms of contextual performance: Evidence of differential relationships with big five personality characteristics and cognitive ability. *J. Appl. Psychol.* **2001**, *86*, 326–336. [CrossRef]
23. Avery, D.R. Personality as a predictor of the value of voice. *J. Psychol.* **2003**, *137*, 435–446. [CrossRef]
24. Premeaux, S.F.; Bedeian, A.G. Breaking the silence: The moderating effects of selfmonitoring in predicting speaking up in the workplace. *J. Manag. Stud.* **2003**, *40*, 1537–1562. [CrossRef]
25. Dutton, J.E.; Ashford, S.J.; Lawrence, K.A.; Rubino, K.M. Red light, green light: Making sense of the organizational context for issue selling. *Organ. Sci.* **2002**, *13*, 355–369. [CrossRef]
26. Ashford, S.J.; Rothbard, N.P.; Piderit, S.K.; Dutton, J.E. Out on a limb: The role of context and impression management in selling gender-equity issues. *Adm. Sci. Q.* **1998**, *43*, 23–57. [CrossRef]
27. Morrison, E.W.; Milliken, F.J. Organizational silence: A barrier to change and development in a pluralistic world. *AMR* **2000**, *25*, 706–725. [CrossRef]
28. Edmondson, A.C. Psychological safety and learning behavior in work teams. *Adm. Sci.* **1999**, *44*, 350–383. [CrossRef]
29. Argyris, C.; Schon, D. *Organizational Learning*; Addison-Wesley: Reading, MA, USA, 1978.
30. Holland, P.; Cooper, B.K.; Hecker, R. Use of social media at work: A new form of employee voice? *Int. J. Hum. Resour. Man.* **2016**, *27*, 2621–2634. [CrossRef]
31. Griffin, A.; Hauser, J.R. The voice of the customer. *Mark. Sci.* **1993**, *12*, 1–27. [CrossRef]
32. Ran, Y.; Zhou, H. Customer–company identification as the enabler of customer voice behavior: How does it happen? *Front. Psychol.* **2020**, *11*, 777. [CrossRef] [PubMed]
33. Assaf, A.G.; Josiassen, A.; Cvelbar, K.; Linda, L.W. The effects of customer voice on hotel performance. *Int. J. Hosp. Manag.* **2015**, *44*, 77–83. [CrossRef]
34. Anderson, E.W.; Mittal, V. Strengthening the satisfaction-profit chain. *J. Serv. Res.* **2000**, *3*, 107–120. [CrossRef]
35. Kipenis, L.; Askounis, D. Assessing e-participation via user's satisfaction measurement: The case of OurSpace platform. *Ann. Oper. Res.* **2015**, *247*, 599–615. [CrossRef]
36. Johnson, T. Environmentalism and NIMBYism in China: Promoting a rules-based approach to public participation. *Env. Polit.* **2010**, *19*, 430–448. [CrossRef]
37. Fung, A. Varieties of participation in complex governance. *Public Adm. Rev.* **2006**, *66*, 66–75. [CrossRef]
38. Wu, L.H.; Ma, T.S.; Bian, Y.C.; Li, S.J.; Yi, Z.Q. Improvement of regional environmental quality: Government environmental governance and public participation. *Sci. Total Environ.* **2020**, *717*, 137265. [CrossRef]
39. Schmidthuber, L.; Hilgers, D.; Gegenhuber, T.; Etzelstorfer, S. The emergence of local open government: Determinants of citizen participation in online service reporting. *Gov. Inf. Q.* **2017**, *34*, 457–469. [CrossRef]
40. Naranjo-Zolotov, M.; Oliveira, T.; Cruz-Jesus, F.; Martins, J.; Goncalves, R.; Branco, F.; Xavier, N. Examining social capital and individual motivators to explain the adoption of online citizen participation. *Future Gener. Comput. Syst.* **2019**, *92*, 302–311. [CrossRef]
41. Katila, R.; Ahuja, G. Something old, something new: A longitudinal study of search behavior and new product introduction. *Acad. Manag. J.* **2002**, *45*, 1183–1194.
42. OECD. *Oslo Manual, Guidelines for Collecting and Interpreting Innovation Data*, 3rd ed.; OECD: Paris, France, 2005.
43. Henderson, R.M.; Clark, K.B. Architectural innovations: The reconfiguration of existing systems and failure of established firms. *Adm. Sci. Q.* **1990**, *35*, 9–30. [CrossRef]
44. Gangi, P.M.D.; Wasko, M. Steal my idea! Organizational adoption of user innovations from a user innovation community: A case study of Dell IdeaStorm. *Decis. Support Syst.* **2009**, *48*, 303–312. [CrossRef]
45. Barlow, J.; Moller, C. *A Complaint Is a Gift: Recovering Customer Loyalty When Things Go Wrong*; Berrett-Koehler Publishers: Oakland, CA, USA, 2008.
46. Lichtenthaler, U. Open innovation: Past research, current debates, and future directions. *Acad. Manag. Perspect.* **2011**, *25*, 75–93.
47. Aguwa, C.C.; Monplaisir, L.; Turgut, O. Voice of the customer: Customer satisfaction ratio based analysis. *Expert Syst. Appl.* **2012**, *39*, 10112–10119. [CrossRef]
48. Woodruff, R.B. Customer value: The next source for competitive advantage. *J. Acad. Mark. Sci.* **1997**, *25*, 139–153. [CrossRef]
49. Balogh, S. An integrative framework for cooperative governance. *J. Public Adm. Res. Theory* **2012**, *22*, 1–30.

50. Luo, M.; Fan, R.D.; Zhang, Y.Q.; Zhu, C.P. Environmental governance cooperative behavior among enterprises with reputation effect based on complex networks evolutionary game model. *Int. J. Environ. Res. Public Health* **2020**, *17*, 1535. [CrossRef]
51. Zhang, M.; Li, H.; Xue, L.; Wang, W.W. Using three-sided dynamic game model to study regional cooperative governance of haze pollution in China from a government heterogeneity perspective. *Sci. Total Environ.* **2019**, *694*, 135559. [CrossRef] [PubMed]
52. Schmid, B.; Meister, T.; Klagge, B.; Seidl, I. Energy Cooperatives and Municipalities in Local Energy Governance Arrangements in Switzerland and Germany. *J. Environ. Dev.* **2019**, *29*. [CrossRef]
53. Papadopoulos, Y. Cooperative forms of governance: Problems of democratic accountability in complex environments. *EJPR* **2003**, *42*, 473–501. [CrossRef]
54. Hangzhou Proposes More Expansive Health Code System. Available online: https://technode.com/2020/05/26/hangzhou-proposes-more-expansive-health-code-system/ (accessed on 26 May 2020).
55. We Read the Technical Standards for China's 'Health Code.' Here's What We Learned. Available online: https://technode.com/2020/07/10/we-read-the-technical-standards-for-chinas-health-code-heres-what-we-learned/ (accessed on 20 July 2020).
56. Tencent Health Code Upgrade "City Code" Has Launched for 100 Days, Covering 1 Billion Users. Available online: https://tech.huanqiu.com/article/3yIIexxK7LV (accessed on 19 May 2020). (In Chinese).
57. The National Health Code Standard, Which Tencent Participated in Developing, Was Officially Released. Available online: https://tech.huanqiu.com/article/3y39Vrg8RdA (accessed on 30 April 2020). (In Chinese).
58. The National Standard of Personal Health Code Was Released, and Alibaba Participated in the Formulation. Available online: https://tech.huanqiu.com/article/3y4MsE43uy7 (accessed on 2 May 2020). (In Chinese).
59. Lazarus, R.S.; Folkman, S. *Stress, Appraisal, and Coping*; Springer: New York, NY, USA, 1984.
60. Lascoumes, P.; Patrick, L.G. Introduction: Understanding public policy through its instruments—From the nature of instruments to the sociology of public policy instrumentation. *Governance* **2010**, *20*, 1–21. [CrossRef]
61. Folkman, S.; Lazarus, R.S. If it changes it must be a process: Study of emotion and coping during three stages of a college examination. *J. Pers. Soc. Psychol.* **1985**, *48*, 150–170. [CrossRef] [PubMed]
62. Smith, C.A.; Lazarus, R.S. Emotion and Adaptation. In *Handbook of Personality Theory and Research*; Guilford: New Haven, CT, USA, 1990.
63. Tableman, B. How Governmental Policy is Made. *Best Pract. Briefs* **2005**, *34*, 1–7.
64. Folkman, S. Dynamics of a stressful encounter: Cognitive appraisal, coping, and encounter outcomes. *J. Pers. Soc. Psychol.* **1986**, *50*, 992–1003. [CrossRef]
65. Lane, M.; Ross, H.; Dale, A.P.; Rickson, R.E. Sacred land, mineral wealth, and biodiversity at Coronation Hill, Northern Australia: Indigenous knowledge and SIA. *Impact Assess. Proj. Apprais.* **2003**, *2*, 89–98. [CrossRef]
66. Lockie, S.; Franetovich, M.; Sharma, S.; Rolfe, J. Democratisation versus engagement? Social and economic impact assessment and community participation in the coal mining industry of the Bowen Basin, Australia. *Impact Assess. Proj. Apprais.* **2008**, *26*, 177–188. [CrossRef]
67. Roberts, N. Public Deliberation in an Age of Direct Citizen Participation. *Am. Rev. Public Adm.* **2016**, *34*, 315–353. [CrossRef]
68. Arain, G.A.; Hameed, I.; Crawshaw, J.R. Servant leadership and follower voice: The roles of follower felt responsibility for constructive change and avoidance-approach motivation. *Eur. J. Work Organ. Psychol.* **2019**, *28*, 555–565. [CrossRef]

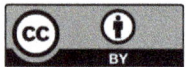

© 2020 by the authors. Licensee MDPI, Basel, Switzerland. This article is an open access article distributed under the terms and conditions of the Creative Commons Attribution (CC BY) license (http://creativecommons.org/licenses/by/4.0/).

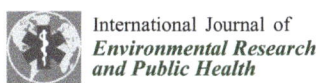

Article

Topic Modeling for Analyzing Patients' Perceptions and Concerns of Hearing Loss on Social Q&A Sites: Incorporating Patients' Perspective

Junghwa Bahng [1,*] and Chang Heon Lee [2,*]

1. Department of Audiology and Speech Language Pathology, Hallym University of Graduate Studies, HUGS Center for Hearing and Speech Research, Seoul 06157, Korea
2. College of Business and Economics, United Arab Emirates University, Al Ain 15551, UAE
* Correspondence: bahng.jh@hallym.ac.kr (J.B.); changlee@uaeu.ac.ae (C.H.L.)

Received: 27 June 2020; Accepted: 24 August 2020; Published: 27 August 2020

Abstract: Hearing loss is the most common human sensory deficit, affecting normal communication. Recently, patients with hearing loss or at risk of hearing loss are increasingly turning to the online health community for health information and support. Information on health-related topics exchanged on the Internet is a useful resource to examine patients' informational needs. The ability to understand the patients' perspectives on hearing loss is critical for health professionals to develop a patient-centered intervention. In this paper, we apply Latent Dirichlet Allocation (LDA) on electronic patient-authored questions on social question-and-answer (Q&A) sites to identify patients' perceptions, concerns, and needs on hearing loss. Our results reveal 21 topics, which are both representative and meaningful, and mostly correspond to sub-fields established in hearing science research. The latent topics are classified into five themes, which include "sudden hearing loss", "tinnitus", "noise-induced hearing loss", "hearing aids", "dizziness", "curiosity about hearing loss", "otitis media" and "complications of disease". Our topic analysis of patients' questions on the topic of hearing loss allows achieving a thorough understanding of patients' perspectives, thereby leading to better development of the patient-centered intervention.

Keywords: hearing loss; latent topic; LDA; topic modeling; social Q&A

---

1. Introduction

Hearing loss is the most common human sensory deficit, affecting normal communication. Hearing loss is a multifactorial disorder caused by both genetic and environmental factors [1]. According to recent reports from the World Health Organization (WHO) [2], the global prevalence of hearing loss has increased rapidly over the last decade. The WHO estimated that, in 2018, 6.1% of the world's population or 466 million people experienced some degree of hearing loss. Furthermore, it is expected that the number of people with hearing loss will rise to 900 million by 2050 [2]. Hearing loss can negatively affect the quality of life as it has adverse effects on communication performance as well as emotional and social functions [3,4]. Thus, understanding the patients' perspective of their hearing loss is an essential step toward patient improvement.

Developing adequate healthcare and public health promotion interventions requires not only an in-depth knowledge of diseases and traits, but also a comprehensive understanding of patients' perceptions, misconceptions, concerns, and needs about the diseases. Clinical and behavioral interventions are more effective when seeking to improve outcomes that are central to patients' experiences and perspectives [5]. A review of prior literature showed that patient-centered interventions are responsive to patients' needs and thus, patients are encouraged to actively participate in the research process, especially regarding the identification of salient issues and concerns. By recognizing the importance of patient engagement, scholars have increasingly paid attention to electronic patient-authored texts as sources of valuable information [6].

With the advances in Internet and communication technologies, healthcare professionals and patients can easily communicate about patient-provided data. In addition, patients not only can easily generate and share their health data and concerns with others, but also look for relevant medical information from peers who have experienced a similar diagnosis, set of symptoms or treatments. Fox and Duggan [7] investigated the use of online resources and found that 72% of Internet users used the Internet to search for health-related information, and 39% of these online health seekers looked for health information related to their own health or medical situation [7]. Research about health communication has demonstrated that health information exchanged on the Internet is a useful resource to examine patients' perceptions, concerns, and needs. Among Internet-based platforms, community-based question-and-answer forums are increasingly becoming popular as a medium for exchanging health information [8,9].

It is not surprising that patients with hearing loss or hearing difficulties use social media channels and social Q&A, such as Yahoo! Answers in English, Baidu Knows in Chinese, and Naver Knowledge-IN in Korean, to exchange information to address their concerns about hearing problems. Prior research has demonstrated that a collection of questions that patients post on social Q&A provides not only interesting but also important information to health professionals [9–11]. Topic analysis of patients' questions on the topic of hearing loss allows for achieving a thorough understanding of patients' perspectives, thereby leading to better development of the patient-centered intervention.

In this paper, we investigate the electronic patient-authored questions on social Q&A sites by applying the natural language analytics. This study adopts a multi-component semantic and computational linguistics method to discover and analyze themes or topics from hearing loss-related health conversations in the social Q&A sphere. Computational linguistics analysis is suitable to process unstructured textual data and identify hidden patterns in the data. Notably, a probabilistic topic modeling is applied to answer our research questions—topic prevalence, topic correlation, and topic evolution: what are hearing loss-related topics being asked or communicated in the social Q&A sphere? What are the prevalent topics in the hearing loss health community? How are those topics interrelated?

First, to the best of our knowledge, no prior studies have examined questions and conversations on social media Q&A as a viable source of understanding patients' prevalent concerns on hearing loss. By applying LDA topic modeling for text analysis techniques on electronic patient-authored hearing loss questions, our present study extracts latent topics and their dominant words, which might provide useful insights for understanding patients' perspectives and concerns on hearing loss. Second, our results reveal that patients post about the relationship between hearing loss and other diseases such as otitis media, tinnitus, and chronic kidney disease. These topic relations between categories have implications for the development of a patient-centered intervention. Lastly, our present research demonstrates evidence that topic model analysis techniques applied to electronic patient-authored questions are effective in studying patient-focused engagement strategy. The extant literature on hearing loss indicates that survey-based methods have been a primary study design to assess patients' concerns and perceptions about hearing loss and related issues. Using this traditional engagement strategy is costly to capture and analyze a massive volume of patients' concerns. Data analytics on patient-authored texts on social Q&A have the potential to improve patient-centered outcome research.

2. Related Literature

2.1. Hearing Loss

Hearing loss is the most common sensory deficit. Among 432 million people with hearing loss, 93% of them are adults, and 54% of them are male—over 5% of the world's population have hearing loss. Furthermore, it is estimated that the number of people with hearing loss will rise to over 900 million by 2050. Untreated hearing loss can negatively affect individuals' communication performance and thus the quality of life in individuals and their families. Hearing loss can be reduced speech understanding, declined acoustic information, and impaired localization of sound sources [12]. Hearing loss is associated with comorbidities such as social isolation, loneliness [13], depression [14–16], balance problem [17], acoustic neuroma(vestibular schwannoma), multiple sclerosis, cardiovascular disease [18], and diabetes [19,20]. Recently, a growing body of research has shown that hearing loss and dementia are related [21–24]. Hearing loss in later life is one of the factors that play an important role in decreasing cognitive ability and developing dementia.

Hearing loss can be caused by damage to any portion of the peripheral and central auditory systems. The main causes of sensorineural hearing loss are degenerative processes associated with aging, genetic mutations, noise exposure, exposure to therapeutic drugs that have ototoxic side effects, and chronic conditions [25]. The most common cause of hearing loss is aging [17]. Age-related hearing loss, generally referred to as presbycusis, typically arises from gradual changes in the inner ear, affecting the sum of sensory, neural, and metabolic causes. Additionally, other factors such as ear diseases and the effects of noise exposure may affect people at all ages and stages in life [26]. Noise-induced hearing loss is caused by loud noise exposure for more extended periods. It has been suggested that more than 12% of the global population is at risk for hearing loss from noise [27]. The WHO estimates that one-third of all cases of hearing loss can be attributed to noise exposure.

Several options are available for hearing loss, ranging from medical treatment to listening devices such as hearing aids and cochlear implants. Treatment depends on the cause and severity of hearing loss. For age-related and noise-induced hearing loss, hearing cannot be treated, but hearing can be restored after using hearing aids or cochlear implantation [25].

2.2. Social Q&A Community

Social Q&A is an online question-and-answer platform enabled by Internet and Web technologies. It is a community-driven platform that allows online users to exchange information by asking questions and providing answers [28,29]. It is open to the public, where interested parties submit questions to be answered by other fellow online users around the world. Over the last decade, social Q&A has gained popularity, and the number of visits to the top Q&A sites such as Yahoo! Answers has increased dramatically [30]. For example, Yahoo! Answer includes more than 300 million questions and 90 million unique users worldwide as of 2012 since the service launched in 2005 [10]. Another popular social Q&A site launched in 2006, Wiki Answers, has 17 million answers posted. Questions and answers on topics ranging from education to diet become a source of rich experience and opinion for anyone with similar concerns or problems. Naver is the largest online platform in South Korea, referred to as the "Google of South Korea", and Naver provides the Social Q&A platform, Knowledge-iN. Users can post any topics on Knowledge-iN, and professionals or people who know the issues make comments and provide information and solutions, in content-centered platforms, and then users select the most valuable answers, and respondents earn awards or points.

2.3. Social Q&A Log Analysis

According to the Pew Internet and American Life Project data, more than 70% of Internet users use the Internet to search for health or medical information [7]. Increased use of such online platforms such as social Q&A sites leads to the generation of unprecedented volumes of information about symptoms, treatments, and health directly from patients, which is generally referred to as electronic patient-authored text [6,31]. As the volume of potentially valuable patient-authored text on social Q&A is growing, more researchers have paid attention to identifying the potential of online data sharing platforms for education and health service. Online patient narratives are a reliable data source for detecting disease trends and identifying medical terms [31]. Moreover, novel insights into patients' treatment decisions and drug-treatment effects were discovered on PatientsLikeMe [32].

A review of the literature on the electronic patient-authored text on the social Q&A community indicates that the existing research streams can be divided into content-centered (e.g., question and answer narratives) and user-centered (e.g., questioners, answerer, and the community) studies. The content-centered studies have mainly focused on three areas: (1) detection of diverse types of health-related questions and answers [9,33,34]; (2) identification of medical concepts in the patient-authored text [31]; and (3) evaluation of the quality of questions and answers with a distinct set of criteria [35,36].

The first type of research has examined electronic patient-authored questions and answers from social Q&A sites to detect health-related hot topics [33,34,37]. Lu et al. (2013) applied text clustering techniques to detect disease topics such as lung cancer, breast cancer, and diabetes, and related symptoms, medical tests, drugs, procedures, and complications. Sadah et al. [33] identified a set of popular topics and associated sentiments based on the patients' demographics. The second type has focused on identifying medically relevant terms and mapping words from the patient-authored text to medical concepts [9,31]. A language gap between patients and health care professionals is known to hinder effective communication between the two groups, so identifying and bridging the vocabulary gap is crucial [31]. Park et al. [8] applied the named entity recognition method to identify medical terms in their collected diabetes dataset and then map the identified terms to the formal medical vocabularies in the Unified Medical Language Systems (UMLS). Lastly, with concerns about the quality of both health-related questions and answers, researchers have proposed a diverse set of quality criteria and empirically examined them [36,38]. Harper et al. [37] employed supervised machine learning algorithms to distinguish information and conversational intent questions automatically. Their findings show evidence that conversational questions yield a lower archival value than informational questions.

3. Methods

Our approach carries our semantic and linguistic analysis to reveal the health characteristics of patients' questions in online textual questions containing hearing loss-related words. The present study consists of three phases: data collection, topic discovery, and topic extraction. Figure 1 shows the overall procedure of the research analysis.

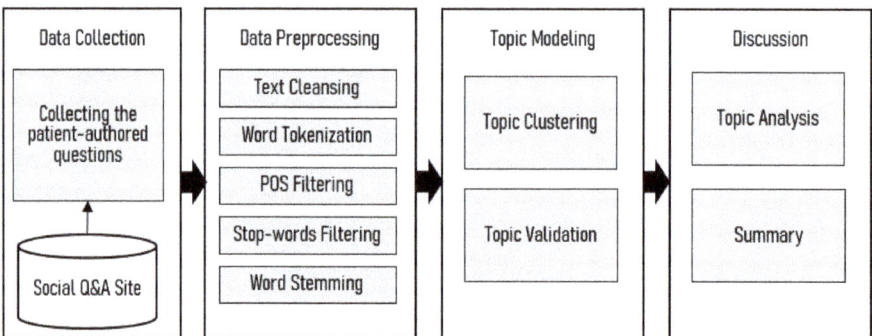

Figure 1. Overall research flow.

3.1. Data Collection

Electronic patient-authored texts on the topic of hearing loss were collected from the social Q&A, namely Naver Knowledge-iN. Launched in 2002, Naver Knowledge-iN is the largest social Q&A community platform in South Korea, where online users can post and share questions related to various topics ranging from insurance policy to medical treatment. Health topics are popular among the questioners. To collect research data, we developed a software program to access and gather the questions posted from 2009 to 2019 on Naver Knowledge-iN. We collected 68,327 questions using the key word of "hearing loss". Repeated or duplicated questions posted were excluded. In addition, questions were excluded if a question contained less than 10 words. As a result, our final sample dataset consists of 65,842 questions that were analyzed for this study.

3.2. Topic Discovery via Latent Dirichlet Allocation (LDA)

To discover the topics from the collected textual questions, we utilized a topic modeling approach that clusters the semantically associated words with "hearing loss" into subtopics. Topic modeling has been widely applied in health and medical domains such as extracting relevant clinical concepts from patient health records [31], discovering health topics in social media [11,39,40] identifying emerging patterns of clinical events [41], and detecting new disease breakout [42]. Among diverse topic modeling techniques, Latent Dirichlet Allocation (LDA) [43] has gained popularity as a tool for automatic text summarization and visualization. In this study, we apply the LDA model to extract topics from the collected corpus.

The automatic text analysis method is usually divided into supervised and unsupervised methods. The unsupervised method does not classify the text content in advance but reduces the dimension of the text through statistical probability inference and explains the text as a whole by means of the reduced dimension theme. The LDA model is an unsupervised machine learning method that uses a bag-of-words representation method. It utilized a latent variable *topic* between observed variables *document* and *word* to explain the semantic topic distribution of documents. The LDA modeling approach considers each document to be presented as a random mixture over latent topics, where each topic is characterized by a probability distribution over words.

LDA is a generative probabilistic model that assigns sets of words collected from documents to be explained by unobserved topic groups that explain why some parts of the data are similar. Each document consists of a small number of different topics, and each word's generation is attributional to one of the topics of the document. The plate diagram of the LDA model is shown in Figure 2, which helps to explain the components of the LDA model.

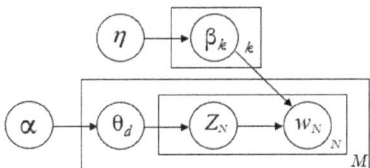

Figure 2. Plate model representation of Latent Dirichlet Allocation (LDA).

LDA assumes that documents and the words within them are derived from a generative probabilistic model [43]. Here, k is the number of topics. M is the number of documents and N is the number of words within the document. Given a corpus D consisting of M documents, with documents having N_d having ($d \in 1, \ldots, M$), LDA models D according the followings.

- The number of words N is represented by the vector w as a *bag-of-words*.
- The model parameter θ_d represents topic proportions for the documents, which is a random variable drawn from a Dirichlet (α) prior with parameter α
- For each topic, the model parameter β_k is the multinomial distribution of words and is drawn from the prior Dirichlet distribution using the parameter η.
- For each word in the document, the topic of the word z_{ij} is a random variable drawn from a multinomial (θ_d) distribution. Thus, z_{ij} is the topic that generates w_{ij} having the j th word in the i th document.

$$P(\theta, z | w, \alpha, \beta) = \frac{P(\theta, z, w | \alpha, \beta)}{P(w | \alpha, \beta)} \quad (1)$$

3.3. Topic Extraction

The topic extraction is the final step of understanding and understanding the topics found. The meaning of the topic is determined by analyzing the most likely terms along with the most likely related documents. First, a thorough investigation was performed on the relevant documents to verify that the initial interpretation based on word probability was meaningful. Second, the two researchers independently interpret and label 21 topics, and each topic is classified into one of five theme categories, except for minor word differences.

4. Results

The LDA topic extraction results concerning the first question reveal similar dimensions to those addressed in the literature on hearing loss. The twenty-one topics resulting from the LDA computation are shown in Table 1. The lists of words that make up a particular topic are displayed below the topic title for each theme. The finding suggests that the identified themes not only resembled the categorization of hearing loss diagnosis and treatments but also cover issues on topics relating to hearing loss.

We then examined the extracted 21 topics and merged similar topics. Finally, the topics were classified into five themes, which were "sudden hearing loss", "tinnitus", "noise-induced hearing loss", "hearing aids", "dizziness", "curiosity about hearing loss", "otitis media" and "complications of disease". Topics and words with probabilities for each topic are shown in Table 1.

Theme 1. Sudden Hearing Loss. *Four of the identified topics, namely Topics 3, 13, 17, and 22, pertain to sudden sensorineural hearing loss, commonly known as "sudden deafness", so the main theme derived from the four topics is labelled as sudden hearing loss. Specifically, this theme addresses causes, diagnosis, medication treatments, prescriptions, and effects associated with both sudden hearing loss.*

Topic 3 contains the words related to the medication treatments of sudden sensorineural hearing loss: "steroid", "injection", "treatment", "drug", "prescription", "shot", and "sudden deafness". We found that, based on the selected keywords, the main concern is related to steroid use for the treatment of sudden deafness. Steroids taken orally or given by injection are commonly used to treat patients who experience sudden deafness. Topic 3 shows evidence that people with sudden hearing loss post questions to learn more about the effectiveness of treatment with steroid drugs and direct injections into their ears.

Topic 13 reflects diagnosis and test related to sudden hearing loss with keywords specifically "diagnosis", "cause", "hospital", "test", "result", "nose", and "infection". It is evident that patients who have been diagnosed with sudden deafness recently posted questions about what causes sudden deafness.

Topic 17 and 21 represent prescriptions and side effects, respectively. Terms such as "side effect", "treatment", "prescription", "drug", "worry", and "recovery" explain that patients with sudden deafness express concerns about the side effects of steroid and hearing recovery. A greater portion of patients diagnosed with sudden deafness have expressed concerns about the side effects of steroid use and have posted questions about whether their steroid treatment is appropriate in terms of frequency and dosage.

Theme 2. Tinnitus. *Four of the identified topics, namely Topics 1, 6, 15, and 19, pertain to tinnitus, so the central theme derived from the four topics is labeled as tinnitus. Specifically, the tinnitus theme addresses symptoms, causes, and treatments associated with both tinnitus and hearing loss.*

Table 1. The most probable keywords in the topic of LDA with 21 topics.

Topic No.	Topic Label	Keywords	Theme Category
1	Tinnitus Symptoms	ringing, buzzing, tinnitus, sound, hear, constant, continue, hissing, severe, ear	Tinnitus
2	Loud Music	loud, music, earphone, listen, eardrum, affect, damage, cause, headset, longtime	Noise-induced Hearing Loss
3	Steroids for Sudden Deafness	steroid, injection, treatment, drug, pill, prescription, shot, sudden, deafness, effect	Sudden Hearing Loss
4	Symptoms of Otitis Media	symptoms, otitis media, pain, headache, sore throat, infection, deafen, today, morning,	Otitis Media
5	Hearing Test Results	diagnosis, treatment, cure, curious, communication, hospital, learning, disability, quality, doubt	General Inquiry
6	Tinnitus Symptoms	tinnitus, loud, noise, hear, sleep, night, worse, stress, ear, feel, tired	Tinnitus
7	Complications	complication, cause, chronic, diabetes, anemia, cancer, thyroid, hepatitis, kidney, disease	Complications
8	Degree of Disability	handicap, disability, degree, disabled, support, experience, hearing, aids, cochlear, implant	Hearing Aids
9	Dizziness	dizzy, cause, awake, morning, severe, pain, balance, nausea, sudden	Dizziness
10	Otitis Media Treatments	surgery, hospital, medication, otitis media, medicine, doctor, condition, after, hearing, test	Otitis Media
11	Cochlear Implant	cochlear, implant, surgery, cost, normal, restore, wear, test, support, wonder	Hearing Aids
12	Health Screening	health, screening, increase, urine, test, radiation, surgery, complication, infection, hospital,	Complications
13	Diagnosis of Sudden Deafness	sudden, loss, diagnosis, cause, hospital, test, results, nose, ear, infection, damage	Sudden Hearing Loss
14	Headache	headache, stress, frequent, dizziness, symptom, discomfort, ménière, disease, nerve, brain	Dizziness
15	Tinnitus Treatments	tinnitus, treatment, hospital, recommend, food, symptoms, effects, audiologist, pain, doctor	Tinnitus
16	Hearing Aids Recommendation	Hearing, aids, recommend, brand, place, good, hospital, uncomfortable, price, impaired	Hearing aids
17	Treatment and Side Effects	treatment, sudden deafness, medicine, right, ear, left, test, normal, restore	Sudden Hearing Loss
18	Shooting	shooting, military, gun, explosion, damage, hospital, degree, diagnosis, protection, accident	Noise-induced Hearing Loss
19	Causes of Tinnitus	tinnitus, infection, drug, earwax, loud, noise, stress, medication, cause, sick	Tinnitus
20	General Inquiry	stress, headache, serious, nerve, exercise, job, worry, cause, diet, decibel	General Inquiry
21	Treatment and Side Effects	side effect, steroid, drug, virus, hours, memory, worry, recovery	Sudden Hearing Loss

Topic 1 and 6 represent issues of hearing loss, with tinnitus symptoms and problems due to tinnitus such as "ringing", "buzzing", "sound", "loud", "noise", "sleep", "hissing", "night", "severe", and "stress". Interestingly, the keywords identified in the two topics show that questioners or patients in social Q&A detail their hearing problems with specific vibrations and sounds (e.g., "ringing", "buzzing" and "hissing"), and specify a level of severity when posting a tinnitus symptom. Tinnitus, commonly referred to as buzzing in the ears, is "often accompanied by hearing loss but not everyone with hearing loss experiences tinnitus" [44]. However, the results indicate that a significantly greater portion of patients who experience tinnitus are involved in the hearing loss topic. Additionally, patients seem to be more stressed at night due to tinnitus and worry that severe or persistent tinnitus is a sign of going deaf.

Topic 15 shows the keywords involved in treatments of tinnitus. This included words such as "treatment", "hospital", "doctor", "food", "audiologist", "pain", and "doctor". The topic results show that patients are in search of diverse tinnitus treatments, and specifically seek for good hospitals or doctors, and alternative treatments for tinnitus. We also found that, based on the selected keywords, effective food is a frequently occurring word, implying that tinnitus patients also search for foods to help reduce tinnitus.

Topic 19 represents a cause of tinnitus with keywords specifically including "infection", "drug", "earwax", "noise", "stress", and "medication". The topic results show that people want to understand what causes tinnitus. Patients who are suffering from tinnitus want to know more about whether their recent illness, such as ear infection, ear wax, or stress, causes tinnitus. Additionally, patients with tinnitus post inquiries about the relationship between tinnitus and hearing loss, and particularly ask whether tinnitus can lead to hearing loss. Most importantly, the results show that many patients with hearing loss post questions whether exposure to loud noise causes tinnitus.

Theme 3. Noise-Induced Hearing Loss. *Topic 2 contains terms such as "loud", "music", "earphone", "headset", "cause", "damage", referred to as "noise-induced hearing loss". These words imply that users want to ask about the relationship between listening to loud music through earphones or headsets with a personal listening device and hearing loss. In addition, people want to know how long listening to music is safe for not getting hearing loss per day.*

The authors can observe the terms "shooting", "military", "gun", "explosion", "compensation", "degree", and "diagnosis", "hospital" in Topic 18. These terms imply that people who are exposed to excessive and continuous noise wonder and get the information whether and how they can get any compensation with their degree of hearing loss. Notably, South Korea has adopted a conscription system. Noise-induced hearing loss is a severe disease in the military because military personnel remain in a noisy environment for the completion of their missions. Thus, the prevalence of hearing loss and tinnitus in the military is higher than the general public [45].

Theme 4. Hearing Aids. *Topics 8, 11, and 16 were identified as hearing aids. Hearing aids are the most popular option of treating hearing loss for improving speech understanding. Topic 8 contains the words, "hearing aids", "cochlear implant", "handicap degree", "disabled", and "support". In South Korea, the registered disabled person with hearing loss gets the subsidy of their hearing aid expense every five years. People with hearing loss or their family members want to know whether their hearing loss degree gets financial support.*

In Topic 11, the authors also observe the term "cochlear implant" and "surgery". In a person with severe to profound hearing loss, hearing aids do not give many benefits. So, instead of hearing aids, cochlear implantation can help to improve speech understanding to people with severe to profound hearing loss. People want to ask about alternative interventions, such as cochlear implantation surgery, other than hearing aids.

Topic 16 consists of the keywords: "hearing aids", "recommend", "brand", "hospital", and "price". Those keywords indicate that patients post questions by asking for a specific recommendation for an excellent hearing aid with a reasonable price in social Q&A.

Theme 5. Otitis media. *Topics 4 and 10 include the terms related to hearing loss with symptoms of otitis media, such as "pain", "sore throat", "infection", "deafen", "headache" and "eardrum". Otitis media is an infection of the middle ear, and it is one of the most common disease in children [46]. The symptoms of otitis media are sore throat, night restlessness, fever, and ear pain [47].*

Topic 10 also contains keywords related to the treatment of otitis media, "hospital", "surgery", "medication", "test", "after". The results indicate that people asked about hearing loss after taking medication or undergoing surgery for otitis media. The term "hospital", "after", and "doctor" imply that, right after visiting doctors, users ask questions about otitis media treatment, such as drugs and surgery. Mild hearing loss can come with otitis media, and usually, hearing loss recovers after otitis media is cured. However, if otitis media occurs repeatedly, it causes permanent hearing loss [48].

Theme 6. Dizziness. Topic 9 contains the words "dizzy", "cause", "headache", "awake", "morning", "severe" and "sudden" referred to as "dizziness". Topic 14 also contains the keywords "headache", "stress", and "dizziness" referred to as "dizziness". One of the most common cause of dizziness is problems of the inner ear. The vestibular system, which is responsible for balance, is located within the inner ear with the auditory system. There are many diseases that affect dizziness and hearing loss, including severe cold, and bacterial or virus infections of the inner ear. In particular, Ménière's disease is a disorder of the inner ear that leads to dizziness and sudden hearing loss. The affected ear may lead to progressive and/or permanent hearing loss [49]. Other symptoms of Ménière's disease are tinnitus, migraines, and nausea. Ménière's disease is very hard to diagnose due to the fact that not all of the symptoms are shown at the early stage [50]. These words relating to topic 9 may represent the symptoms of Ménière's disease.

Theme 7. Curiosity or general inquiry about hearing loss. Topics 5 and 20 contain a higher number of words relating to hearing loss itself. The authors could observe that users want to know about assessment results, such as the units (decibel) which are used for describing hearing loss. Additionally, the terms such as "stress", "nerve", "headache", "worry" imply that users ask about their symptoms relating to hearing loss.

The terms "treatment", "hospital", "communication" "learning" imply that people went to the hospital to have assessments of their hearing, but they did not fully understand their hearing loss and how to treat their hearing loss. In social Q&A, they want to get the information about their hearing loss.

Theme 8: Complications of disease. Topic 7 and 12 represent the terms "chronic", "anemia", "cancer", "thyroid", "hepatitis", "kidney" and "disease". All the diseases in topic 12 are related to hearing loss. Hearing loss is a side effect of some chemotherapy drugs [51–54]. Additionally, anemia, iron deficiency, and thyroid hormone deficiency lead to hearing loss [55–58]. The hepatitis virus B and C are very strong risk factors of sudden sensorineural hearing loss [59]. Hearing loss is linked to chronic kidney disease [60], too. In social Q&A, patients or their family members seek the information about different complications leading to a hearing loss.

5. Discussion

Hearing loss subtopics indicated that users posted about the relationship between hearing loss and hearing loss-related disease. The themes of sudden deafness, noise-induced hearing loss, and otitis media, and related complications of diseases are covered by hearing loss-related disease. Sudden deafness and otitis media themes show that users searched for social Q&A about the cause of diseases, treatment options, and side effects of the medicine. These topics confirmed that people are not well-informed about their medications. Notably, sudden deafness is considered an otologic emergency. Patients with sudden deafness can recover from the hearing loss problem if they receive appropriate treatments promptly. Prior studies reported that treatment within seven days of the onset of sudden deafness is effective for better hearing recovery [61]. The standard gold treatment of sudden deafness is oral high-dose corticosteroids [62]. Our findings reveal that users want to get the information and are worried about the side effect of the steroids, which means that patients did not get the information about their treatment and medicine.

In the theme complications, we found several keywords are related to diseases, including diabetes, anemia, cancer, thyroid, hepatitis, and kidney disease. The medications for these diseases have side effects that can cause hearing loss. Based on our findings, health providers, such as physicians, did not give enough information about treatment and medicine. Lee et al. [63] indicated that the average real consultation time for outpatients was 4.2 min in Korea, and patient satisfaction was too low regarding consultations. This consultation time is not long enough to ask questions about their treatments. The physicians need to ensure that they have enough consultation time for effective communication.

On the other hand, noise-induced hearing loss is a slow-occurring hearing loss. In subtopics of noise-induced hearing loss, users post about the causes of hearing loss, such as loud noise exposure and the usage of listening devices with headphones. People wonder how much loud noise exposure causes hearing loss. Exposure to noise increases the risk of tinnitus, as well. Noise-induced hearing loss is the only preventable loss, so education on the usage of a safe listening device is necessary [64]. For preventing noise-induced hearing loss, people are advised to avoid listening to loud music or noise above 85 dB (A) for no longer than 1 h. People need to avoid listening to music because it increases the volume when they listen to it under noisy circumstances. Interestingly, in these subtopics, we found keywords related to the military. Military personnel exposed to significant impulse noise. For this reason, in social Q&A, many people seek information about the relationship between hearing loss and military noise. The hearing conservation program needs to be developed adequately to ensure the health of military personnel in Korea.

Next, users posted the relationship between hearing loss and symptoms of hearing loss, tinnitus, and dizziness. The highest subtopics are related to tinnitus. Tinnitus is a symptom associated with ear disease, including hearing loss, but tinnitus does not cause hearing loss. More than 50 million people, with an estimated prevalence of 10–15% in adults, reported that they experienced tinnitus in the U.S. [65]. The keywords related to hearing loss indicated that people want to know about the cause of tinnitus, medicines, and difficulties caused by tinnitus. The findings show that people want to find a way to cure tinnitus. However, the treatment of tinnitus focuses on minimizing the impact and burden of tinnitus rather than the "cure" of tinnitus [65]. There are several rehabilitation methods for relieving tinnitus, such as counseling and sound therapy. Additionally, there are applications that patients can use to alleviate their tinnitus. Health providers need to inform the options of tinnitus relief.

Tinnitus is a symptom that people feel chronically, while dizziness is a symptom that people feel acutely. Our results reveal several keywords related to the symptoms of Ménière's disease. Ménière's disease is a disorder of the inner ear that leads to dizziness and sudden hearing loss. The affected ear may lead to progressive or permanent hearing loss [49]. Other distinct symptoms of Ménière's disease include tinnitus, migraines, and nausea. Ménière's disease is hard to diagnose because not all of the signs are shown at the early stage [50]. The patients who feel dizziness need to visit the Ear, Nose and Throat (ENT) doctor and check their conditions.

Lastly, people want to search for information about the treatment options of hearing loss, such as hearing aids and cochlear implants. Hearing aid usage is the most common treatment to reduce the adverse effects, including communication difficulties and cognitive decline, caused by hearing loss [66]. In addition, the use of hearing aids improves productive time use, quality of life, economic circumstances and mental health for listeners with hearing loss [67]. In our results, people searched for information on hearing aid benefits or the specification of hearing aids. Additionally, they searched about brands of hearing aids and reasonable prices for hearing aids. They also asked for recommendations regarding good hearing aid centers. Since the national insurance subsidizes all or part of the cost of purchasing hearing aids or cochlear implants for hearing impairments in Korea, users search the information about disability degree and national insurance benefit. This information should be provided to websites so that those who want to use hearing aids can accurately check the price and specifications of hearing aids and get national insurance benefits.

6. Conclusions

Hearing loss is the most frequently occurring human sensory deficit and has many different causes. Hearing loss is also known to be related to many other health issues. Analyzing patient-authored questions can be a useful approach to better understand patients' perceptions, concerns and needs. Traditional surveys are limited to small sample sizes. However, social Q&A offers a new environment for patients to easily share various opinions and medical experiences, so a large volume of patient-authored data can accumulate. Exploring how patients with hearing loss use social questions and answers to find health information not only helps to identify a set of critical topics and issues for various types of research but also improves communication between patients and healthcare professionals. To the best of our knowledge, this is the first analysis of patient-authored contents on the topic of hearing loss from the social Q&A community, and these results provide valuable methodological and content insights.

This study provides a computational linguistic approach to perform an in-depth analysis using patient-authored data from sizeable online data sets. Our framework decodes public health views from hearing loss-related questions, which can be useful for developing adequate healthcare and public health promotion interventions. Our results reveal that those characterized topics ranging from sudden deafness to hearing aids are both representative and meaningful, and mostly correspond to sub-fields established in hearing science research.

Author Contributions: Conceptualization, J.B. and C.H.L.; Data curation, C.H.L.; Formal analysis, J.B. and C.H.L.; Funding acquisition, J.B. and C.H.L.; Investigation, J.B.; Project administration, J.B.; Software, C.H.L.; Supervision, J.B.; Writing—original draft, J.B. and C.H.L.; Writing—review & editing, J.B. and C.H.L. All authors have read and agreed to the published version of the manuscript.

Funding: This work was supported by the Ministry of Education of the Republic of Korea and the National Research Foundation of Korea (NRF-2019S1A5A2A01039904). This research was partially funded by the UAE University, grant number G00002617 (Funding No. 31B088).

Conflicts of Interest: The authors declare no conflict of interest.

References

1. Willems, P.J. Genetic causes of hearing loss. *N. Engl. J. Med.* **2000**, *342*, 1101–1109. [CrossRef]
2. World Health Organization. Deafness and Hearing Loss. Available online: https://www.who.int/news-room/fact-sheets/detail/deafness-and-hearing-loss (accessed on 10 March 2020).
3. Dalton, D.S.; Cruickshanks, K.J.; Klein, B.E.; Klein, R.; Wiley, T.L.; Nondahl, D.M. The impact of hearing loss on quality of life in older adults. *Gerontologist* **2003**, *43*, 661–668. [CrossRef]
4. Seidman, M.D.; Standring, R.T. Noise and quality of life. *Int. J. Environ. Res. Public Health* **2010**, *7*, 3730–3738. [CrossRef]
5. Iezzoni, L.I.; O'Day, B.L.; Killeen, M.; Harker, H. Communicating about health care: Observations from persons who are deaf or hard of hearing. *Ann. Intern. Med.* **2004**, *140*, 356–362. [CrossRef]
6. Dreisbach, C.; Koleck, T.A.; Bourne, P.E.; Bakken, S. A systematic review of natural language processing and text mining of symptoms from electronic patient-authored text data. *Int. J. Med. Inform.* **2019**, *125*, 37–46. [CrossRef]
7. Fox, S.; Duggan, M. Health online 2013. *Health* **2013**, *2013*, 1–55.
8. Oh, S.; Yi, Y.J.; Worrall, A. Quality of health answers in social Q&A. *Proc. Am. Soc. Inf. Sci. Technol.* **2012**, *49*, 1–6.
9. Park, M.S.; He, Z.; Chen, Z.; Oh, S.; Bian, J. Consumers' use of UMLS concepts on social media: Diabetes-related textual data analysis in blog and social Q&A sites. *JMIR Med. Inform.* **2016**, *4*, e41. [PubMed]
10. Zhang, J.; Chen, Y.; Zhao, Y.; Wolfram, D.; Ma, F. Public health and social media: A study of Zika virus-related posts on Yahoo! Answers. *J. Assoc. Inf. Sci. Technol.* **2019**, *71*, 282–299. [CrossRef]
11. Jones, J.; Pradhan, M.; Hosseini, M.; Kulanthaivel, A.; Hosseini, M. Novel Approach to Cluster Patient-Generated Data Into Actionable Topics: Case Study of a Web-Based Breast Cancer Forum. *JMIR Med. Inform.* **2018**, *6*, e45. [CrossRef]
12. Divenyi, P.L.; Stark, P.B.; Haupt, K.M. Decline of speech understanding and auditory thresholds in the elderly. *J. Acoust. Soc. Am.* **2005**, *118*, 1089–1100. [CrossRef] [PubMed]

13. Sung, Y.K.; Li, L.; Blake, C.; Betz, J.; Lin, F.R. Association of Hearing Loss and Loneliness in Older Adults. *J. Aging Health* **2016**, *28*, 979–994. [CrossRef]
14. Donovan, N.J.; Okereke, O.I.; Vannini, P.; Amariglio, R.E.; Rentz, D.M.; Marshall, G.A.; Johnson, K.A.; Sperling, R.A. Association of Higher Cortical Amyloid Burden With Loneliness in Cognitively Normal Older Adults. *Jama Psychiatry* **2016**, *73*, 1230–1237. [CrossRef] [PubMed]
15. Mener, D.J.; Betz, J.; Genther, D.J.; Chen, D.; Lin, F.R. Hearing loss and depression in older adults. *J. Am. Geriatr. Soc.* **2013**, *61*, 1627–1629. [CrossRef] [PubMed]
16. Hsu, W.T.; Hsu, C.C.; Wen, M.H.; Lin, H.C.; Tsai, H.T.; Su, P.; Sun, C.T.; Lin, C.L.; Hsu, C.Y.; Chang, K.H.; et al. Increased risk of depression in patients with acquired sensory hearing loss: A 12-year follow-up study. *Medicine* **2016**, *95*, e5312. [CrossRef]
17. Lin, F.R.; Ferrucci, L. Hearing loss and falls among older adults in the United States. *Arch. Intern. Med.* **2012**, *172*, 369–371. [CrossRef]
18. Friedland, D.R.; Cederberg, C.; Tarima, S. Audiometric pattern as a predictor of cardiovascular status: Development of a model for assessment of risk. *Laryngoscope* **2009**, *119*, 473–486. [CrossRef]
19. Kim, M.-B.; Zhang, Y.; Chang, Y.; Ryu, S.; Choi, Y.; Kwon, M.-J.; Moon, I.J.; Deal, J.A.; Lin, F.R.; Guallar, E. Diabetes mellitus and the incidence of hearing loss: A cohort study. *Int. J. Epidemiol.* **2016**, *46*, 717–726. [CrossRef]
20. Bainbridge, K.E.; Hoffman, H.J.; Cowie, C.C. Diabetes and hearing impairment in the United States: Audiometric evidence from the National Health and Nutrition Examination Survey, 1999 to 2004. *Ann. Intern. Med.* **2008**, *149*, 1–10. [CrossRef]
21. Gurgel, R.K.; Ward, P.D.; Schwartz, S.; Norton, M.C.; Foster, N.L.; Tschanz, J.T. Relationship of hearing loss and dementia: A prospective, population-based study. *Otol. Neurotol.* **2014**, *35*, 775–781. [CrossRef]
22. Fritze, T.; Teipel, S.; Ovari, A.; Kilimann, I.; Witt, G.; Doblhammer, G. Hearing Impairment Affects Dementia Incidence. An Analysis Based on Longitudinal Health Claims Data in Germany. *PLoS ONE* **2016**, *11*, e0156876. [CrossRef] [PubMed]
23. Wayne, R.V.; Johnsrude, I.S. A review of causal mechanisms underlying the link between age-related hearing loss and cognitive decline. *Ageing Res. Rev.* **2015**, *23*, 154–166. [CrossRef] [PubMed]
24. Lin, F.R.; Metter, E.J.; O'Brien, R.J.; Resnick, S.M.; Zonderman, A.B.; Ferrucci, L. Archives of Neurology. *Arch. Neurol.* **2011**, *68*, 214–220. [CrossRef] [PubMed]
25. Cunningham, L.L.; Tucci, D.L. Hearing Loss in Adults. *N. Engl. J. Med.* **2017**, *377*, 2465–2473. [CrossRef] [PubMed]
26. Rabinowitz, P.M. Noise-induced hearing loss. *Am. Fam. Physician* **2000**, *61*, 2749–2756, 2759–2760.
27. Le, T.N.; Straatman, L.V.; Lea, J.; Westerberg, B. Current insights in noise-induced hearing loss: A literature review of the underlying mechanism, pathophysiology, asymmetry, and management options. *J. Otolaryngol. Head Neck Surg.* **2017**, *46*, 41. [CrossRef]
28. Oh, S. The characteristics and motivations of health answerers for sharing information, knowledge, and experiences in online environments. *J. Am. Soc. Inf. Sci. Technol.* **2012**, *63*, 543–557. [CrossRef]
29. Gazan, R. Social Q&A. *J. Am. Soc. Inf. Sci. Technol.* **2011**, *62*, 2301–2312.
30. Rosenbaum, H.; Shachaf, P. A structuration approach to online communities of practice: The case of Q&A communities. *J. Am. Soc. Inf. Sci. Technol.* **2010**, *61*, 1933–1944.
31. MacLean, D.L.; Heer, J. Identifying medical terms in patient-authored text: A crowdsourcing-based approach. *J. Am. Med. Inform. Assoc.* **2013**, *20*, 1120–1127. [CrossRef]
32. Wicks, P.; Massagli, M.; Frost, J.; Brownstein, C.; Okun, S.; Vaughan, T.; Bradley, R.; Heywood, J. Sharing health data for better outcomes on PatientsLikeMe. *J. Med. Internet Res.* **2010**, *12*, e19. [CrossRef] [PubMed]
33. Foufi, V.; Timakum, T.; Gaudet-Blavignac, C.; Lovis, C.; Song, M. Mining of textual health information from Reddit: Analysis of chronic diseases with extracted entities and their relations. *J. Med. Internet Res.* **2019**, *21*, e12876. [CrossRef] [PubMed]
34. Sadah, S.A.; Shahbazi, M.; Wiley, M.T.; Hristidis, V. Demographic-Based Content Analysis of Web-Based Health-Related Social Media. *J. Med. Internet Res.* **2016**, *18*, e148. [CrossRef]
35. Bae, B.J.; Yi, Y.J. What answers do questioners want on social Q&A? User preferences of answers about STDs. *Internet Res.* **2017**. [CrossRef]
36. Oh, S.; Worrall, A. Health answer quality evaluation by librarians, nurses, and users in social Q&A. *Libr. Inf. Sci. Res.* **2013**, *35*, 288–298.

37. Lu, Y.; Zhang, P.; Liu, J.; Li, J.; Deng, S. Health-related hot topic detection in online communities using text clustering. *PLoS ONE* **2013**, *8*, e56221. [CrossRef]
38. Harper, F.M.; Moy, D.; Konstan, J.A. Facts or friends? Distinguishing informational and conversational questions in social Q&A sites. In Proceedings of the Sigchi Conference on Human Factors in Computing Systems, Boston, MA, USA, 4–9 April 2009; pp. 759–768.
39. Paul, M.J.; Dredze, M. Discovering health topics in social media using topic models. *PLoS ONE* **2014**, *9*, e103408. [CrossRef]
40. Ghosh, D.; Guha, R. What are we 'tweeting'about obesity? Mapping tweets with topic modeling and Geographic Information System. *Cartogr. Geogr. Inf. Sci.* **2013**, *40*, 90–102. [CrossRef]
41. Chandola, V.; Sukumar, S.R.; Schryver, J.C. Knowledge discovery from massive healthcare claims data. In Proceedings of the 19th ACM SIGKDD International Conference on Knowledge Discovery and Data Mining, Chicago, IL, USA, 11–13 August 2013; pp. 1312–1320.
42. Charles-Smith, L.E.; Reynolds, T.L.; Cameron, M.A.; Conway, M.; Lau, E.H.; Olsen, J.M.; Pavlin, J.A.; Shigematsu, M.; Streichert, L.C.; Suda, K.J. Using social media for actionable disease surveillance and outbreak management: A systematic literature review. *PLoS ONE* **2015**, *10*, e0139701. [CrossRef]
43. Blei, D.M.; Ng, A.Y.; Jordan, M.I. Latent dirichlet allocation. *J. Mach. Learn. Res.* **2003**, *3*, 993–1022.
44. Husain, F.T.; Medina, R.E.; Davis, C.W.; Szymko-Bennett, Y.; Simonyan, K.; Pajor, N.M.; Horwitz, B. Neuroanatomical changes due to hearing loss and chronic tinnitus: A combined VBM and DTI study. *Brain Res.* **2011**, *1369*, 74–88. [CrossRef] [PubMed]
45. Yong, J.S.; Wang, D.Y. Impact of noise on hearing in the military. *Mil. Med. Res.* **2015**, *2*, 6. [CrossRef] [PubMed]
46. Zielhuis, G.A.; Rach, G.H.; van den Bosch, A.; van den Broek, P. The prevalence of otitis media with effusion: A critical review of the literature. *Clin. Otolaryngol. Allied Sci.* **1990**, *15*, 283–288. [CrossRef]
47. Kontiokari, T.; Koivunen, P.; Niemela, M.; Pokka, T.; Uhari, M. Symptoms of acute otitis media. *Pediatric Infect. Dis. J.* **1998**, *17*, 676–679. [CrossRef]
48. Gravel, J.S.; Wallace, I.F.; Ruben, R.J. Auditory consequences of early mild hearing loss associated with otitis media. *Acta Oto-Laryngol.* **1996**, *116*, 219–221. [CrossRef] [PubMed]
49. Sarna, B.; Abouzari, M.; Lin, H.W.; Djalilian, H.R. A hypothetical proposal for association between migraine and Meniere's disease. *Med. Hypotheses* **2020**, *134*, 109430. [CrossRef]
50. Sajjadi, H.; Paparella, M.M. Meniere's disease. *Lancet* **2008**, *372*, 406–414. [CrossRef]
51. Hirose, Y.; Simon, J.A.; Ou, H.C. Hair cell toxicity in anti-cancer drugs: Evaluating an anti-cancer drug library for independent and synergistic toxic effects on hair cells using the zebrafish lateral line. *J. Assoc. Res. Otolaryngol.* **2011**, *12*, 719–728. [CrossRef]
52. Ding, D.; Allman, B.L.; Salvi, R. Review: Ototoxic characteristics of platinum antitumor drugs. *Anat. Rec. Adv. Integr. Anat. Evol. Biol.* **2012**, *295*, 1851–1867. [CrossRef]
53. Vermorken, J.B.; Remenar, E.; van Herpen, C.; Gorlia, T.; Mesia, R.; Degardin, M.; Stewart, J.S.; Jelic, S.; Betka, J.; Preiss, J.H.; et al. Cisplatin, fluorouracil, and docetaxel in unresectable head and neck cancer. *N. Engl. J. Med.* **2007**, *357*, 1695–1704. [CrossRef]
54. Oldenburg, J.; Gietema, J.A. The Sound of Silence: A Proxy for Platinum Toxicity. *J. Clin. Oncol.* **2016**, *34*, 2687–2689. [CrossRef] [PubMed]
55. Shih, J.-H.; Li, I.; Pan, K.-T.; Wang, C.-H.; Chen, H.-C.; Fann, L.-Y.; Tseng, J.-H.; Kao, L.-T.; Health, P. Association between Anemia and Auditory Threshold Shifts in the US Population: National Health and Nutrition Examination Survey. *Int. J. Environ. Res. Public Health* **2020**, *17*, 3916. [CrossRef] [PubMed]
56. Chung, S.D.; Chen, P.Y.; Lin, H.C.; Hung, S.H. Sudden sensorineural hearing loss associated with iron-deficiency anemia: A population-based study. *JAMA Otolaryngol. Head Neck Surg.* **2014**, *140*, 417–422. [CrossRef] [PubMed]
57. Ben-Tovim, R.; Zohar, Y.; Zohiar, S.; Laurian, N.; Laurian, L. Auditory brain stem response in experimentally induced hypothyroidism in albino rats. *Laryngoscope* **1985**, *95*, 982–986. [CrossRef] [PubMed]
58. Vanasse, M.; Fischer, C.; Berthezene, F.; Roux, Y.; Volman, G.; Mornex, R. Normal brainstem auditory evoked potentials in adult hypothyroidism. *Laryngoscope* **1989**, *99*, 302–306. [CrossRef]
59. Chen, H.-C.; Chung, C.-H.; Wang, C.-H.; Lin, J.-C.; Chang, W.-K.; Lin, F.-H.; Tsao, C.-H.; Wu, Y.-F.; Chien, W.-C. Increased risk of sudden sensorineural hearing loss in patients with hepatitis virus infection. *PLoS ONE* **2017**, *12*, e0175266. [CrossRef]

60. Vilayur, E.; Gopinath, B.; Harris, D.C.; Burlutsky, G.; McMahon, C.M.; Mitchell, P. The association between reduced GFR and hearing loss: A cross-sectional population-based study. *Am. J. Kidney Dis.* **2010**, *56*, 661–669. [CrossRef]
61. Chen, W.T.; Lee, J.W.; Yuan, C.H.; Chen, R.F. Oral steroid treatment for idiopathic sudden sensorineural hearing loss. *Saudi Med. J.* **2015**, *36*, 291. [CrossRef]
62. Chandrasekhar, S.S.; Surgery, N. Updates on methods to treat sudden hearing loss. *Oper. Tech. Otolaryngol. -Head Neck Surg.* **2003**, *14*, 288–292. [CrossRef]
63. Lee, C.H.; Lim, H.; Kim, Y.; Park, A.H.; Park, E.-C.; Kang, J.-G. Analysis of appropriate outpatient consultation time for clinical departments. *Health Policy Manag.* **2014**, *24*, 254–260. [CrossRef]
64. You, S.; Kwak, C.; Han, W.; Health, P. Use of Personal Listening Devices and Knowledge/Attitude for Greater Hearing Conservation in College Students: Data Analysis and Regression Model Based on 1009 Respondents. *Int. J. Environ. Res. Public Health* **2020**, *17*, 2934. [CrossRef] [PubMed]
65. Tunkel, D.E.; Bauer, C.A.; Sun, G.H.; Rosenfeld, R.M.; Chandrasekhar, S.S.; Cunningham Jr, E.R.; Archer, S.M.; Blakley, B.W.; Carter, J.M.; Granieri, E.C. Clinical practice guideline: Tinnitus. *Otolaryngol. Head Neck Surg.* **2014**, *151*, S1–S40. [CrossRef] [PubMed]
66. Arlinger, S. Negative consequences of uncorrected hearing loss—A review. *Int. J. Audiol.* **2003**, *42* (Suppl. 2), 2S17–2S20. [CrossRef] [PubMed]
67. Spreckley, M.; Macleod, D.; González Trampe, B.; Smith, A.; Kuper, H.; Health, P. Impact of Hearing Aids on Poverty, Quality of Life and Mental Health in Guatemala: Results of a before and after Study. *Int. J. Environ. Res. Public Health* **2020**, *17*, 3470. [CrossRef] [PubMed]

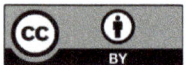

© 2020 by the authors. Licensee MDPI, Basel, Switzerland. This article is an open access article distributed under the terms and conditions of the Creative Commons Attribution (CC BY) license (http://creativecommons.org/licenses/by/4.0/).

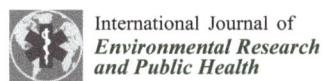

Article

An Online Training Intervention on Prehospital Stroke Codes in Catalonia to Improve the Knowledge, Pre-Notification Compliance and Time Performance of Emergency Medical Services Professionals

Montse Gorchs-Molist [1,2,*], Silvia Solà-Muñoz [1], Iago Enjo-Perez [2,*], Marisol Querol-Gil [1], David Carrera-Giraldo [3], Jose María Nicolàs-Arfelis [2], Francesc Xavier Jiménez-Fàbrega [1,2] and Natalia Pérez de la Ossa [4]

1. Catalonian Emergency Medical System, 08908 L'Hospitalet de Llobregat, Spain; silviasola@gencat.cat (S.S.-M.); marisol.querol@gmail.com (M.Q.-G.); francescxavierjimenez@gencat.cat (F.X.J.-F.)
2. School of Medicine and Healthcare Sciences, University of Barcelona, 08036 Barcelona, Spain; nicolas@ub.edu
3. Departament of Neurosurgery, University Hospital Doctor Negrín, 35010 Las Palmas de Gran Canarias, Spain; david__carrera@hotmail.com
4. Departament of Neurology, University Hospital Germans Trias i Pujol, 08916 Badalona, Spain; natperezossa@gmail.com
* Correspondence: montsegorchs@ub.edu (M.G.-M.); enjo@ub.edu (I.E.-P.)

Received: 31 July 2020; Accepted: 17 August 2020; Published: 26 August 2020

Abstract: Strokes are a time-dependent medical emergency. The training of emergency medical service (EMS) professionals is essential to ensure the activation of stroke codes with pre-notification, as well as a rapid transfer to achieve early therapy. New assessment scales for the detection of patients with suspected large vessel occlusion ensures earlier access to endovascular therapy. The aim of this study was to evaluate the impact on an online training intervention focused on the Rapid Arterial oCclusion Evaluation (RACE) scoring of EMS professionals based on the prehospital stroke code in Catalonia from 2014 to 2018 in a pre–post intervention study. All Catalonian EMS professionals and the clinical records from primary stroke patients were included. The Kirkpatrick model guided the evaluation of the intervention. Data were collected on the knowledge on stroke recognition and management, pre-notification compliance, activated stroke codes and time performance of EMS professionals. Knowledge improved significatively in most items and across all categories, reaching a global achievement of 82%. Pre-notification compliance also improved significantly and remained high in the long-term. Increasingly higher notification of RACE scores were recorded from 60% at baseline to 96.3% in 2018, and increased on-site clinical care time and global time were also observed. Therefore, the online training intervention was effective for increasing EMS professionals' knowledge and pre-notification compliance upon stroke code activation, and the wide adoption of a new prehospital scale for the assessment of stroke severity (i.e., the RACE scale) was achieved.

Keywords: stroke; prehospital emergency care; training; stroke code; large vessel occlusion; prehospital scales

1. Introduction

Strokes are a time-dependent medical emergency, in which treatment delay negatively influences patient prognosis [1]. For acute ischemic stroke patients with an evolution of less than 4.5 h of evolution, fibrinolysis therapy improves prognosis [2], yet its benefits are limited for the subgroup of patients with large vessel occlusion (LVO) [3]. These patients benefit the most from endovascular thrombectomy, with a therapeutic window of up to 24 h from stroke onset according to multimodal neuroimaging criteria, at an adequate specialized tertiary hospital, which doubles their chances of clinical improvement [4]. For this reason, in recent years, stroke code (SC) systems have been developed to rapidly identify patients with acute stroke, allowing agile transfers to a specialized center [5,6]. This rapid assessment of acute stroke patients is paramount to obtaining the maximum benefits from reperfusion therapies. Thus, emergency medical services (EMS) are essential [7], not only for identifying stroke patients, but also for identifying a subgroup of patients with suspected large vessel occlusion (LVO), who would benefit the most from endovascular treatment [8]. The traditional prehospital assessment scales were developed to detect the typical symptoms of stroke patients [9]. Since then, several new scales for the specific detection of LVO patients have been designed, but few have been validated prospectively in prehospital care [10]. Implementing these new prehospital diagnostic tools as part of SCs is a priority to ensure familiarity with the protocol and to achieve current therapeutic standards [11]. Giving pre-notification of patients to the receiving center is also important to ensure allocation of in-hospital resources and to accelerate diagnostic and therapeutic decision-making through a minimum set of clinical data [12]. Additionally, international guidelines also emphasized the need to prioritize specific training in SCs, diagnostic tools and pre-notification systems for EMS professionals [13–15]. Following these recommendations, our group developed the Rapid Arterial oCclusion Evaluation (RACE) [16] scale for prehospital assessment of patients with a suspected LVO stroke (Figure S1). The RACE scale was validated in 2014, and international guidelines endorsed the RACE scale as a valid tool alongside others [17,18]. For implementation by EMS professionals, an online training intervention (OTI) was designed to update their knowledge on acute stroke recognition and the SC activation circuit, as well as to train them on the administration of the RACE scale.

The aim of this study was to evaluate the impact on an OTI focused on the RACE scoring for EMS professionals based on prehospital SCs in Catalonia from 2014 to 2018.

2. Materials and Methods

We performed a pre–post intervention study from January 2014 to December 2018 in the Catalonian EMS (prehospital care). This EMS provides care for 7.5 million people, employing more than 4000 professionals, and it activated approximately eight daily SCs before 2014. For this study, we included data from both EMS professionals and stroke patients. All EMS professionals (i.e., emergency technicians, nurses, and physicians) were invited to participate, and all of those who accepted were included, as no exclusion criteria were considered. A non-probabilistic sampling method was used. All clinical records of patients older than 18 years old and classified as primary acute stroke patients upon activation of SCs by the dispatch center were included. Records of patients who were being transferred between hospital settings were excluded.

2.1. Online Training Intervention

An online training intervention (OTI) was developed to provide 6 h of training through a learning management system (i.e., Moodle). The programme comprised four modules: Three theoretical modules that addressed the (a) signs and symptoms of a stroke, (b) stroke treatment, and (c) prehospital management of stroke, including the administration of prehospital scales and SC protocol; the final module was practical, and was introduced to address the application of the RACE scale using five clinical scenarios. The contents and evaluation methods considered the recommendations of the Cerebrovascular Disease Master Plan in Catalonia to attain content validity. Additionally, international recommendations from the European and American Stroke Organizations were incorporated into the curriculum. A pilot test was performed with an interprofessional group of 30 individuals that included neurologists and EMS professionals (i.e., physicians, nurses, and emergency technicians) between March and April 2014. The training was accredited by the regional council for the continuous education of healthcare professionals.

The OTI was administered progressively according to the Catalonian healthcare regions. All professionals from the same region participated in the course simultaneously for a 30-day period with on-demand access to the training platform. Fourteen replications of the training program were necessary to cover all regions and professionals. The training was completed by 2830 EMS professionals from May to September 2014. All EMS professionals were supported by forum interactions with the faculty, and additional resources were provided. A collaboration network was established by developing a Facebook group, a Twitter account (@escalaRACE), and a website (www.racescale.org).

2.2. Assessment of the Online Training Programme

The variables measuring the effectiveness of the OTI with regard to prehospital SCs were categorized using Kirkpatrick's [19,20] model of training evaluation as follows:

- Kirkpatrick level 1 (reaction): A satisfaction survey (Supplementary material S2) was administered at the end of the training using a five-point Likert scale based on five dimensions. Satisfaction of the aims of the training, the available materials, the RACE scale usefulness in clinical practice, and the faculty, as well as the overall satisfaction regarding the perceived increased in knowledge or competency, were addressed.
- Kirkpatrick level 2 (learning): A knowledge-related multiple-choice questionnaire about knowledge was administered prior to and 3 months after the intervention (Supplementary material S3). A set of 24 questions were used, most of which (i.e., 10) were related to the identification of signs and symptoms of a stroke, as well as available treatment options. Eight questions explored respondents' knowledge on the SC protocol, prehospital management, and prehospital assessment scales for stroke patients. A final set of six questions were used to analyze the decision-making on acute stroke medical emergencies in clinical scenarios.
- Kirkpatrick level 3 (behavior): The transfer to clinical practice was measured by compliance rates with the EMS prenotification system (i.e., Minimum Data Set register). We observed the notification of the patient's identification number, the time of the onset of symptoms, anticoagulant treatment, glycaemia, systolic and diastolic blood pressure, and RACE scores.
- Kirkpatrick level 4 (results): The impact of the intervention on prehospital SC was assessed by determining the number of activated codes and the changes in prehospital care times. The observed times were: (a) The alert time, that is, the period between the start and the end of a call; (b) the activation time, that is, the time from the start of a call to the allocation of clinical resources; (c) the response time, that is, the period from resource allocation to the arrival of the EMS team; (d) the care time, that is, the time from the arrival at the place of care to the start of the transfer; (e) the transfer time, that is, the period from the start of the transfer to the arrival at the receiving center; and (f) a global time was also registered.

2.3. Data Collection

This study was performed at five time-points: (a) Baseline (first quarter of 2014 (Q1)), (b) training intervention (second (Q2) and third quarter (Q3) of 2014), (c) immediate follow-up (fourth quarter of 2014 (Q4)), (d) follow-up after 1–2 years (2015–2016), and (e) follow-up after 3–4 years (2017–2018). The period between 2014 Q1 (baseline) and Q4 (immediate follow-up) was used to pilot the training intervention (March to April 2014); and to train the EMS professionals (May to September 2014).

Data from EMS professionals were obtained on the same learning management system (i.e., Moodle) on which the course was provided. Socio-demographics were obtained at the beginning of the intervention (i.e., 2014 Q2 and Q3). Data on Kirkpatrick level 1 was recorded at the end of the intervention (i.e., 2014 Q2 and Q3). Kirkpatrick level 2 data were obtained at the beginning of the intervention (i.e., 2014 Q2 and Q3), and 3 months after the end of the training (2014 Q4). Data on all results from Kirkpatrick levels 3 and 4 were obtained through the Informatic System for Emergency Management (SITREM®) register between 2014 and 2018 (all periods except the intervention, that is,

2014 Q2 and Q3). This register prospectively records information about all Catalonian EMS activity, including details on SC activation, patients, time of call, first time of care, and arrival at the receiving hospital. From September 2014, RACE scores were also included in the register.

The data were processed in compliance with the European Data Protection Regulation 2016/679. The study was approved by the Clinical Research Ethics Committee of the University Hospital Germans Trias i Pujol (Badalona, Spain) with identification code PI-15-030.

2.4. Statistical Analysis

The results are expressed in means and standard deviations (SDs) for quantitative variables, and absolute frequencies and percentages for qualitative variables.

The Student's *t*-test was used for the comparative analysis of paired data. A *p*-value of <0.05 was considered statistically significant. Data were analyzed with the statistical software program SPSS version 24.0 (SPSS Inc.; Chicago, IL, USA).

3. Results

A total of 2830 EMS professionals undertook the training programme, and 69.5% completed the baseline questionnaire while 53.2% answered the three-month follow-up (Figure 1). The majority were males (76.7%) with a mean age of 35.8 years (SD = 6.3) and more than 10 years of experience in EMS (45.4%). Emergency medical technicians accounted for 90.3% of the staff, followed by nurses (6.4%) and then physicians (3.2%). Most of them worked as care providers (98.3%) and only 1.7% did so in the dispatch center. Meanwhile, 65% had received previous training on strokes. The satisfaction survey (Kirkpatrick level 1) at the end of the training was completed by 2668 (94.3%), scoring at least 4 out of 5 in all items.

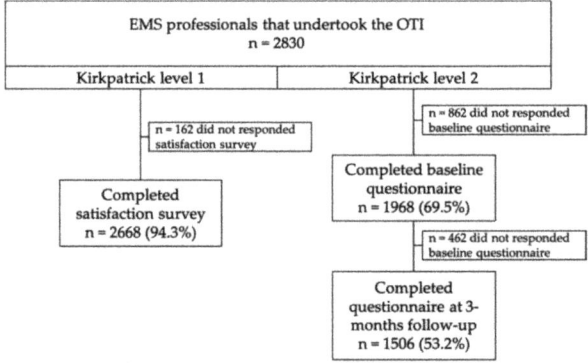

Figure 1. Flowchart of emergency medical services (EMS) professionals' participation.

3.1. Learning Assessment (Kirkpatrick Level 2)

After the OTI, there was a significant increase in 80% of the questions related to the recognition of the signs and symptoms of a stroke (Table 1), especially for those addressing location-specific signs, as well as the treatment. Two generic questions about strokes were non-significant but scored high prior to the training. The questions regarding SCs, prehospital management, and prehospital stroke assessment increased significantly, with most scores above 85%. Changes were observed in stroke recognition, with improved identification in 5/6 of the clinical scenarios.

Table 1. Differences in the responses to the knowledge multiple-choice test.

Topics	Baseline (n = 1968) (% Correct)	After Training (n = 1506) (% Correct)	p-Value (* <0.05)
Signs and symptoms of a stroke	1960 (99.6)	1500 (99.7)	0.97
Ischemic stroke etiology	1934 (98.3)	1483 (98.5)	0.645
Hemorrhagic stroke etiology	1891 (96.1)	1491 (99.1)	<0.001 *
Left hemisphere stroke signs/symptoms	1029 (5.2)	925 (61.4)	<0.001 *
Right hemispheres stroke signs/symptoms	267 (13.7)	615 (40.9)	<0.001 *
Transient ischemic attack definition	1272 (64.6)	1024 (68.0)	0.038 *
Brainstem stroke signs/symptoms	1245 (63.2)	1240 (82.3)	<0.001 *
Window for thrombolysis	689 (35.0)	774 (51.4)	<0.001 *
Endovascular indications	974 (49.5)	1022 (67.9)	<0.001 *
Benefits of stroke treatment	1027 (52.2)	1209 (80.3)	<0.001 *
Aim of the stroke code	1833 (93.1)	1446 (96.0)	<0.001 *
Target age for the stroke code	1510 (76.7)	1430 (95.0)	<0.001 *
Time criteria from onset to code activation	1247 (63.3)	1322 (87.8)	<0.001 *
Criteria for activation of the stoke code	1251 (63.6)	1341 (89.1)	<0.001 *
Recognition of comorbidity scales	403 (40.1)	906 (60.2)	<0.001 *
Recognition of stroke diagnostic scales	1186 (50.3)	1393 (92.5)	<0.001 *
RAPID [1] scale recognition	1033 (52.5)	1236 (82.1)	<0.001 *
RANCOM [2] scale recognition	1616 (82.1)	1390 (92.3)	<0.001 *
Hypertension and nausea	1298 (65.9)	961 (63.8)	0.189
Transient ischemic attack	1534 (77.9)	1277 (84.8)	<0.001 *
90 years. 5 h start of symptoms	1515 (77.0)	1364 (90.6)	<0.001 *
Treatment with anticoagulants	1560 (79.3)	1288 (85.5)	<0.001 *
Awakening stroke	1644 (83.5)	1430 (95.0)	<0.001 *
RANCOM [2] scale	1309 (66.5)	1145 (76.0)	<0.001 *

[1] The smile, raise the arm, talk, stroke, call 911 fast mnemotechnic (i.e., RAPID) is a Catalan stroke assessment tool, equivalent to the FAST mnemotechnic in English-speaking countries. [2] Rankin Comorbidity (i.e., RANCOM) is a Catalan comorbidity scale for prehospital assessment of stroke patients. * $p < 0.05$.

3.2. Transfer to the Clinical Setting (Kirkpatrick Level 3)

The Minimum Data Set (MDS) records available in the SITREM® register were analyzed for 17,135 patients in the study period (Table 2). Immediately after the training, we found a significant increase in the registration of patient identification (ID) codes, glycaemia, systolic and diastolic blood pressure (SBP/DBP), and RACE scores, yet notification of the time of the onset of symptoms decreased. For the 2015–2016 follow-up, only the patient ID and RACE records continued to increase, in contrast to the time of symptom onset (TSO), SBP and DBP. There were significant differences for all items in the 2017–2018 follow-up period: All items increased (i.e., TSO, glycaemia, ID, SBP, DBP, and RACE notification), and the frequency of anticoagulant treatment notification decreased. Overall, 71.5% of the items increased from baseline to the last follow-up. Only the registration of TSO and the notification of anticoagulant treatment diminished consistently over time.

Compliance with the RACE scale upon SC activation increased continuously over time. Starting from 60.9% immediately after training, compliance rose to over 85% by the 2017–2018 follow-up, reaching a 96.3% compliance level in 2018.

Table 2. Differences in the pre-notification items from the Minimum Data Set register over time.

Item	Baseline (2014)		Immediately after Training (2014 Q4)			1–2 Years after Training (2015–2016)			1–2 Years after Training (2015–2016)	3–4 Years after Training (2017–2018)	
	n = 834		n = 965			n = 7261			n = 7261	n = 8075	
	n (%)		n (%)	p-Value		n (%)		p-Value	n (%)	n (%)	p-Value
Patient identification no.	460 (55.2%)		632 (65.5%)	<0.001 *		4998 (68.8%)		0.036 *	4998 (68.8%)	6904 (85.5%)	<0.001 *
Time from onset of symptoms	714 (85.6%)		759 (78.7%)	<0.001 *		5305 (73.1%)		<0.001 *	5305 (73.1%)	6211 (76.9%)	<0.001 *
Anticoagulant therapy	704 (84.4%)		809 (83.8%)	0.738		6237 (85.9%)		0.086	6237 (85.9%)	6327 (78.3%)	<0.001 *
Glycaemia	246 (29.5%)		672 (69.6%)	<0.001 *		4922 (67.8%)		0.247	4922 (67.8%)	6524 (80.8%)	<0.001 *
Systolic blood pressure	255 (30.6%)		711 (73.7%)	<0.001 *		5043 (69.5%)		0.009 *	5043 (69.5%)	7007 (86.8%)	<0.001 *
Diastolic blood pressure	254 (30.5%)		711 (73.7%)	<0.001 *		5044 (69.5%)		0.007 *	5044 (69.5%)	6516 (80.7%)	<0.001 *
RACE scores	—		588 (60.9%)			5165 (71.1%)		<0.001 *	5165 (71.1%)	7350 (91.0)	<0.001 *

RACE, Rapid Arterial oCclusion Evaluation; * $p < 0.05$.

3.3. Impact on Prehospital Stroke Code (Kirkpatrick Level 4)

3.3.1. Stroke Code Activation

Activation of SCs increased over time. At baseline (2014 Q1), 9.2 codes were activated daily (n = 834), which increased immediately after training (2014 Q4) to 10.7 (n = 965), maintaining at 9.9 in both 2015 (n = 2635) and 2016 (n = 3635). In 2017, 10.6 codes were initiated (n = 3888), which reached a daily maximum of 11.4 (n = 4187) in 2018.

3.3.2. Time Performance in Stroke Code

The main differences in time performance were the overall time of prehospital care (Table 3), which increased from 48.9 to 53.6 min ($p = 0.015$). This extra time was mostly due to increased on-site clinical care time ($p = 0.034$) prior to transfer to hospital, which increased from 21.5 to 24.3 min. However, there were no changes in activation, alert, response, or transfer times.

Table 3. Differences in time performance over time.

Item	Baseline (2014 Q1) n = 834 Mean (SD)	Immediately after Training (2014 Q4) n = 965 Mean (SD)	1–2 Years after Training (2015–2016) n = 7261 Mean (SD)	3–4 Years after Training (2017–2018) n = 8075 Mean (SD)	95%CI of the Difference	p-Value
Alert time [1]	3.10 (6.7)	2.96 (5.6)	2.90 (5.8)	3.13 (6.1)	−0.25 to 0.56	0.877
Activation time [2]	4.78 (7.1)	4.97 (6.7)	4.86 (7.0)	5.35 (7.6)	−1.64 to 0.73	0.053
Response time [3]	8.08 (4.9)	8.68 (5.3)	8.57 (5.6)	8.70 (6.0)	−0.34 to 1.23	0.083
Clinical care time [4]	21.51 (8.4)	21.87 (8.3)	22.24 (8.9)	24.32 (8.9)	0.75 to 3.27	0.034 *
Transfer time [5]	12.29 (10.1)	13.11 (10.6)	12.73 (10.3)	12.86 (11.2)	−1.51 to 1.66	0.402
Overall time [6]	48.9 (19.9)	51.60 (19.5)	51.52 (19.6)	53.62 (20.0)	1.04 to 5.33	0.015 *

[1] Alert time: The time between the start and the end of a call at the dispatch center. [2] Activation time: The time from the start of a call to the allocation of clinical resources at the dispatch center. [3] Response time: The period from the resource allocation to the arrival of the EMS team at point of care. [4] Clinical care time: The time from the arrival of the EMS team at the point of care to the start of transfer; on-site care is provided. [5] Transfer time: The time of transportation from the point of care to arrival at the receiving center. [6] Overall time: The sum of all previous times. CI, confidence interval; SD standard deviation. * $p < 0.05$.

4. Discussion

Time is brain when dealing with acute stroke patients. International Stroke Organizations advocate for the development of specific training programs for healthcare professionals, as those who have not been trained specifically on strokes contribute to delay patients' access to adequate therapy [21]. On the other hand, the Stroke Alliance for Europe advocates for a systematic approach to continuous education in EMS as one of their 12 quality care indicators on strokes [22].

In this study, the OTI was well-received, scoring high in satisfaction (Kirkpatrick level 1). It was associated with a knowledge gain for all categories (Kirkpatrick level 2), as observed in similar studies with EMS professionals [23–25]. Participants accurately identified the signs and symptoms of a stroke and became aware of the differences between hemorrhagic and ischemic strokes. On the other hand, very few improvements were observed in recognizing transient ischemic attacks. Despite most EMS professionals (65%) having had previous education on strokes, a lot of heterogeneity was found at baseline for the recognition of very specific signs and symptoms. This training improved their competency, which is consistent with the improvements in knowledge observed by Hsieh et al. [23] in Taiwan, where 48% had previously received training. The window for thrombolytic therapy was only identified by a third of the participants, and half signaled the indications for endovascular treatment. However, these items might be very specific, which could explain the low number of correct answers in our case, or why a similar study in Dubai [24], received no correct responses for these questions. It should be noted that while diagnostic and comorbidity scales determine the activation of the SCs, only 50.3% and 40.1%, respectively, were familiarized with them, which is similar to the finding of DiBiasio in Rhode Island [25]. An integrative review [26] on the impact of training programs on strokes found that only 1 of 21 courses was taught online. In that single UK-based study (RESPONSE [27]), there was a greater improvement in knowledge compared to our findings (95.6% vs. 82%), while the response rates varied (39% vs. 54%). These differences could be explained by the fact that our study managed to include a greater percentage of EMS professionals and that the context of the education was different. Most professionals in RESPONSE were paramedics (55%), who had received 2–5 years of university training (Paramedic Sciences), in contrast to our 90.3% participation of emergency technicians, who had received a 2-year non-university qualification. This could also explain some of the very low scores at baseline when recognizing specific stroke signs and symptoms.

Improving pre-notification systems in SCs is essential for ensuring the allocation of in-hospital resources and for accelerating communication between EMS teams and receiving hospitals [28]. We observed a progressive improvement in the compliance with the pre-notification register in 80% of the items, increasing from an overall 53% compliance score in 2014 to a 73% in 2015–2016, and 83% in 2017–2018 (Kirkpatrick level 3). This increment was greater than in another study performed in the USA [29] that achieved an increase from 60.9% to 77.3%; the last peak of 10% increase in our case could have been due to the start of RACECAT, a clinical trial focused on different transfer approaches for stroke patients. Pre-notifications systems have also been found effective in improving in-hospital times for therapy access [30,31]. We observed fewer notifications of TSO, which could be explained by the presence of more cases of awakening strokes in the last period (2017–2018).

New specific scales for LVO patients have been created, but most are still uncommon in EMS [32–34]. Our group developed and validated the RACE scale [12] in 2014, which has received endorsement by international guidelines [35–37]. We documented a great compliance with the prehospital assessment of LVO patients with the RACE scale, starting at 61% immediately after training (Kirkpatrick level 3), up to 71% at the 1- to 2-year follow-up, and 91% in the 3- to 4-year follow-up. During the last year (i.e., 2018) compliance reached 96.3%, which is similar to that found in a study in Ohio (USA) [38] that reached 100% compliance in recoding RACE scores. The results of studies using other scales for LVO recognition are varied; for example, an Australian study [39] reached 88% notification, while another study involving multiple EMS agencies involved only provided data in 53% of the cases. In our study, support from the EMS directorate and continuous education department, as well as the inclusion of the RACE scores in the EMS clinical register (i.e., SITREM®), were paramount to achieving these positive long-term results.

Acute strokes are a time-dependent medical emergency where time between the onset of symptoms and treatment is essential. We recorded changes in prehospital care time as overall prehospital care time, which increased by 4.7 min (Kirkpatrick level 4). Additionally, on-site clinical care time increased by 2.8 min. A UK study, PASTA [40], showed an increase in time from assessment to thrombolysis by 8.5 min after a specific training programme for paramedics. Another UK project [41] focused on training at the dispatch center revealed a non-significant 2.8 min reduction in the time between alert activation to the arrival of the ambulance. The benefits of patient assessment using the RACE and the obtained pre-registration data (i.e., vital signs, assessment of stroke severity, and RACE scores) could outweigh the slight increase in the overall prehospital care time.

However, this study has some limitations. First, it was limited to the prehospital setting. Second, the correlation between the RACE score at prehospital assessment and endovascular therapy effectiveness remains unknown. Finally, we have no data on the prognosis and evolution of the stroke patients (i.e., final diagnosis, false positives or negatives, stroke mimics, and reperfusion therapy rates). Future studies should seek to include further in-hospital clinical variables.

5. Conclusions

An interprofessional OTI on strokes in the Catalonian EMS was effective in increasing the participants' knowledge on cerebrovascular medical emergencies. Both strengths and areas for improvement were detected for future training opportunities. This study had a positive long-term impact on prehospital compliance with the pre-notification system upon SC activation. This training intervention permitted the wide adoption of a new prehospital scale for the assessment of stroke severity (i.e., the RACE scale), reaching high notification compliance.

These results encouraged the Catalonian EMS to maintain this training intervention in their continuous education program, which, starting back in 2015, is delivered twice a year.

Supplementary Materials: The following are available online at http://www.mdpi.com/1660-4601/17/17/6183/s1, Figure S1: Summary table RACE Scale and Instructions to evaluate the RACE scale, S2: satisfaction survey, S3: knowledge-related multiple-choice questionnaire.

Author Contributions: Conceptualization, N.P.d.l.O. and F.X.J.-F.; methodology, M.G.-M., S.S.-M. and I.E.-P.; validation, M.G.-M., S.S.-M. and J.M.N.-A.; formal analysis, M.G.-M. and S.S.-M.; investigation, M.G.-M., D.C.-G. and M.Q.-G.; resources, N.P.; data curation, M.G.-M., S.S.-M. and I.E.-P.; writing—original draft preparation, M.G.-M. and I.E.-P.; writing—review and editing, I.E.-P. and S.S.-M.; visualization, M.G.-M.; supervision, N.P.d.l.O. and F.X.J.-F.; project administration, N.P.d.l.O. and F.X.J.-F.; funding acquisition, N.P.d.l.O. All authors have read and agreed to the published version of the manuscript.

Funding: This research was funded by the Spanish Ministry of Health, Instituto de Salud Carlos III (Fondo de Investigación En Salud), grant number PI13/02041.

Conflicts of Interest: The authors declare no conflict of interest. The funders had no role in the design of the study; in the collection, analyses, or interpretation of the data; in the writing of the manuscript, or in the decision to publish the results.

References

1. Stroke Unit Trialists' Collaboration. Organised inpatient (stroke unit) care for stroke. *Cochrane Database. Syst. Rev.* **2013**, *2013*, CD000197. [CrossRef]
2. Emberson, J.; Lees, K.R.; Lyden, P.; Blackwell, L.; Albers, G.; Bluhmki, E.; Brott, T.; Cohen, G.; Davis, S.; Donnan, G.; et al. Effect of treatment delay, age, and stroke severity on the effects of intravenous thrombolysis with alteplase for acute ischemic stroke: A meta-analysis of individual patient data from randomized trials. *Lancet* **2014**, *384*, 1929–1935. [CrossRef]
3. Goyal, M.; Menon, B.K.; van Zwam, W.H.; Dippel, D.; Mitchell, P.J.; Demchuk, A.M.; Dávalos, A.; Majoie, C.H.; van der Lugt, A.; de Miquel, M.A.; et al. Endovascular thrombectomy after large-vessel ischaemic stroke: A meta-analysis of individual patient data from five randomised trials. *Lancet* **2016**, *387*, 1723–1731. [CrossRef]
4. XLin, Y.; Schulze, V.; Brockmeyer, M.; Parco, C.; Karathanos, A.; Heinen, Y.; Gliem, M.; Hartung, H.P.; Antoch, G.; Jander, S.; et al. Endovascular Thrombectomy as a Means to Improve Survival in Acute Ischemic Stroke: A Meta-analysis. *JAMA Neurol.* **2019**, 6–10. [CrossRef]
5. De Luca, A.; Toni, D.; Lauria, L.; Sacchetti, M.L.; Giorgi Rossi, P.; Ferri, M.; Puca, E.; Prencipe, M.; Guasticchi, G.; The "IMPLementazione Percorso Clinico Assistenziale ICtus Acuto (IMPLICA) Study Group". An emergency clinical pathway for stroke patients—Results of a cluster randomized trial (isrctn41456865). *BMC Health Serv. Res.* **2009**, *9*, 1–10. [CrossRef]
6. Baldereschi, M.; Piccardi, B.; Di Carlo, A.; Lucente, G.; Guidetti, D.; Consoli, D.; Toni, D.; Sacchetti, M.L.; Polizzi, B.M.; Inzitari, D.; et al. Relevance of Prehospital Stroke Code Activation for Acute Treatment Measures in Stroke Care: A Review. *Cerebrovasc. Dis.* **2012**, *10*, 182–190. [CrossRef]
7. Crocco, T.J.; Grotta, J.C.; Jauch, E.C.; Kasner, S.E.; Kothari, R.U.; Larmon, B.R.; Saver, J.L.; Sayre, M.R.; Davis, S.M. EMS management of acute stroke—Prehospital triage (resource document to NAEMSP position statement). *Prehospital Emerg. Care* **2007**, *11*, 313–317. [CrossRef]
8. Powers, W.J.; Derdeyn, C.P.; Biller, J.; Coffey, C.S.; Hoh, B.L.; Jauch, E.C.; Johnston, K.C.; Johnston, S.C.; Khalessi, A.A.; Kidwellet, C.S.; et al. 2015 American Heart Association/American Stroke Association Focused Update of the 2013 Guidelines for the Early Management of Patients with Acute Ischemic Stroke Regarding Endovascular Treatment: A Guideline for Healthcare Professionals from the American Heart Association/American Stroke Association. *Stroke* **2015**, *46*, 3020–3035. [CrossRef]

9. Zhelev, Z.; Walker, G.; Henschke, N.; Fridhandler, J.; Yip, S. Prehospital stroke scales as screening tools for early identification of stroke and transient ischemic attack. *Cochrane Database Syst. Rev.* **2019**, *4*, CD011427. [CrossRef]
10. Smith, E.E.; Kent, D.M.; Bulsara, K.R.; Leung, L.Y.; Lichtman, J.H.; Reeve, M.J.; Towfighi, A.; Whiteley, W.N.; Zahuranec, D.B. Accuracy of prediction instruments for diagnosing large vessel occlusion in individuals with suspected stroke: A systematic review for the 2018 guidelines for the early management of patients with acute ischemic stroke. *Stroke* **2018**, *49*, e111–e122. [CrossRef]
11. Turc, G.; Bhogal, P.; Fischer, U.; Khatri, P.; Lobotesis, K.; Mazighi, M.; Schellinger, P.D.; Toni, D.; de Vries, J.; White, P.; et al. European Stroke Organisation (ESO)—European Society for Minimally Invasive Neurological Therapy (ESMINT) Guidelines on Mechanical Thrombectomy in Acute Ischaemic StrokeEndorsed by Stroke Alliance for Europe (SAFE). *Eur. Stroke J.* **2019**, *4*, 6–12. [CrossRef] [PubMed]
12. Lin, C.B.; Peterson, E.D.; Smith, E.E.; Saver, J.L.; Liang, L.; Xian, Y.; Olson, M.D.; Shah, B.R.; Hernandez, A.F.; Schwamm, L.H.; et al. Emergency medical service hospital prenotification is associated with improved evaluation and treatment of acute ischemic stroke. *Circ. Cardiovasc. Qual. Outcomes* **2012**, *5*, 514–522. [CrossRef] [PubMed]
13. Jauch, E.C.; Saver, J.L.; Chair, V.; Adams, H.P.; Bruno, A.; Connors, J.; Demaerschalk, B.M.; Khatri, P.; McMullan, P.W.; Qureshi, A.I.; et al. AHA/ASA Guidelines for the Early Management of Patients With Acute Ischemic Stroke A Guideline for Healthcare Professionals From the American Heart Association/American Stroke Association. *Am. Hear. Assoc Stroke Counc.* **2013**, *44*, 870–947. [CrossRef]
14. Kobayashi, A.; Czlonkowska, A.; Ford, G.A.; Fonseca, A.C.; Luijckx, G.J.; Korv, J.; Pérez de la Ossa, N.; Price, C.; Russell, D.; Tsiskaridze, A.; et al. European Academy of Neurology and European Stroke Organization consensus statement and practical guidance for pre-hospital management of stroke. *Eur. J. Neurol.* **2018**, *25*, 425–433. [CrossRef]
15. Boulanger, J.M.; Lindsay, M.P.; Gubitz, G.; Smith, E.E.; Stotts, G.; Foley, N.; Bhogal, S.; Boyle, K.; Braun, L.; Goddard, T.; et al. Canadian Stroke Best Practice Recommendations for Acute Stroke Management: Prehospital, Emergency Department, and Acute Inpatient Stroke Care, 6th Edition, Update 2018. *Int. J. Stroke* **2018**, *13*, 949–984. [CrossRef]
16. De La Ossa, N.P.; Carrera, D.; Gorchs, M.; Querol, M.; Millán, M.; Gomis, M.; Dorado, L.; López-Cancio, E.; Hernández-Pérez, M.; Chicharro, V.; et al. Design and validation of a prehospital stroke scale to predict large arterial occlusion: The rapid arterial occlusion evaluation scale. *Stroke* **2014**, *45*, 87–91. [CrossRef]
17. Pride, G.L.; Fraser, J.F.; Gupta, R.; Alberts, M.J.; Rutledge, J.N.; Fowler, R.; Ansari, S.A.; Abruzzo, T.; Albani, B.; Arthur, A.; et al. Prehospital care delivery and triage of stroke with emergent large vessel occlusion (ELVO): Report of the Standards and Guidelines Committee of the Society of Neurointerventional Surgery. *J. Neurointerv. Surg.* **2017**, *9*, 802–812. [CrossRef]
18. Fiehler, J.; Cognard, C.; Gallitelli, M.; Jansen, O.; Kobayashi, A.; Heinrich, P.; Mattle, H.P.; Keith, W.; Muir, K.W.; Mikael Mazighi, M.; et al. European Recommendations on Organisation of Interventional Care in Acute Stroke (EROICAS). *Int. J. Stroke* **2016**, *11*, 701–716. [CrossRef]
19. Ruiz, J.G.; Mintzer, M.J.; Leipzig, R.M. The impact of e-learning in medical education. *Acad Med.* **2006**, *81*, 207–212. [CrossRef]
20. Kirkpatrick, D.L. *Evaluating Training Programs. The Four Levels*; Berrett-Koehler: Philadelphia, PA, USA, 1998.
21. Acker, J.E.; Pancioli, A.M.; Crocco, T.J.; Eckstein, M.K.; Jauch, E.C.; Larrabee, H.; Meltzer, N.M.; Mergendahl, W.C.; Munn, J.W.; Prentiss, S.M.; et al. Implementation strategies for emergency medical services within stroke systems of care: A policy statement from the American Heart Association/American Stroke Association expert panel on emergency medical services systems and the stroke council. *Stroke* **2007**, *38*, 3097–3115. [CrossRef]
22. King's College London. The Burden of Stroke in Europe. London. 2017. Available online: http://www.strokeeurope.eu/downloads/TheBurdenOfStrokeInEuropeReport.pdf (accessed on 29 October 2018).
23. Hsieh, H.-C.; Hsieh, C.-Y.; Lin, C.-H.; Sung, P.-S.; Li, C.-Y.; Chi, C.-H.; Chen, C.H. Development of an Educational Program for Staffs of Emergency Medical Service to Improve Their Awareness of Stroke within 3 Hours of Symptom Onset: A Pilot Study. *Acta Neurol. Taiwan* **2013**, *22*, 4–12. [PubMed]
24. Shire, F.; Kasim, Z.; Alrukn, S.; Khan, M. Stroke awareness among Dubai emergency medical service staff and impact of an educational intervention. *BMC Res. Notes* **2017**, *10*, 255. [CrossRef] [PubMed]

25. DiBiasio, E.L.; Jayaraman, M.V.; Oliver, L.; Paolucci, G.; Clark, M.; Watkins, C.; DeLisi, K.; Wilks, A.; Yaghi, S.; Morgan Hemendinger, M.; et al. Emergency medical systems education may improve knowledge of pre-hospital stroke triage protocols. *J. Neurointerv. Surg.* **2020**, *12*, 370–373. [CrossRef] [PubMed]
26. Jones, S.P.; Miller, C.; Gibson, J.M.E.; Cook, J.; Price, C.; Watkins, C.L. The impact of education and training interventions for nurses and other health care staff involved in the delivery of stroke care: An integrative review. *Nurse Educ. Today* **2017**. [CrossRef]
27. Jones, S.; McLoughlin, A.; Watkins, C. Acute stroke management: An online course. *J. Paramed. Pract.* **2011**, *3*, 322–327. [CrossRef]
28. Oostema, J.A.; Nasiri, M.; Chassee, T.; Reeves, M.J. The quality of prehospital ischemic stroke care: Compliance with guidelines and impact on in-hospital stroke response. *J. Stroke Cerebrovasc. Dis.* **2014**, *23*, 2773–2779. [CrossRef]
29. Oostema, J.A.; Chassee, T.; Baer, W.; Edberg, A.; Reeves, M.J. Brief Educational Intervention Improves Emergency Medical Services Stroke Recognition. *Stroke* **2019**, *50*, 1193–1200. [CrossRef]
30. Bae, H.J.; Kim, D.H.; Yoo, N.T.; Choi, J.H.; Huh, J.T.; Cha, J.K.; Kim, S.K.; Choi, J.S.; Kim, J.W. Prehospital notification from the emergency medical service reduces the transfer and intra-hospital processing times for acute stroke patients. *J. Clin. Neurol.* **2010**, *6*, 138–142. [CrossRef]
31. Mckinney, J.S.; Mylavarapu, K.; Lane, J.; Roberts, V.; Ohman-Strickland, P.; Merlin, M.A. Hospital prenotification of stroke patients by emergency medical services improves stroke time targets. *J. Stroke Cerebrovasc. Dis.* **2013**, *22*. [CrossRef]
32. Teleb, M.S.; Ver Hage, A.; Carter, J.; Jayaraman, M.V.; McTaggart, R.A. Stroke vision, aphasia, neglect (VAN) assessment-a novel emergent large vessel occlusion screening tool: Pilot study and comparison with current clinical severity indices. *J. Neurointerv. Surg.* **2017**, *9*, 122–126. [CrossRef]
33. Schlemm, L.; Ebinger, M.; Nolte, C.H.; Endres, M. Impact of prehospital triage scales to detect large vessel occlusion on resource utilization and time to treatment. *Stroke* **2018**, *49*, 439–446. [CrossRef]
34. Noorian, A.R.; Sanossian, N.; Shkirkova, K.; Liebeskind, D.S.; Eckstein, M.; Stratton, S.J.; Pratt, F.D.; Conwit, R.; Chatfield, F.; Sharma, L.K.; et al. Los Angeles Motor Scale to identify large vessel occlusion: Prehospital validation and comparison with other screens. *Stroke* **2018**, *49*, 565–572. [CrossRef]
35. American Heart Association. American Heart Association Mission Lifeline: Stroke Severity-Based Stroke Triage Algorithm for EMS. 2018. Available online: https://www.heart.org/HEARTORG/Professional/MissionLifelineHomePage/MissionLifeline-Stroke_UCM_491623_SubHomePage.jsp (accessed on 26 December 2019).
36. Ahmed, N.; Steiner, T.; Caso, V.; Wahlgren, N. ESO-KSU session participants. Recommendations from the ESO-Karolinska Stroke Update Conference, Stockholm, 13–15 November 2016. *Eur Stroke J.* **2017**, *2*, 95–102. [CrossRef] [PubMed]
37. Powers, W.J.; Rabinstein, A.A.; Ackerson, T.; Adeoye, O.M.; Bambakidis, N.C.; Becker, K.; Biller, J.; Brown, M.; Demaerschalk, B.M.; Hoh, B.; et al. Guidelines for the Early Management of Patients with Acute Ischemic Stroke: 2019 Update to the 2018 Guidelines for the Early Management of Acute Ischemic Stroke: A Guideline for Healthcare Professionals From the American Heart Association/American Stroke Association. *Stroke* **2019**, *50*, 344–418. [CrossRef]
38. Jumaa, M.A.; Castonguay, A.C.; Salahuddin, H.; Shawver, J.; Saju, L.; Burgess, R.; Kung, V.; Slawski, D.E.; Tietjen, G.; Parquette, B.; et al. Long-term implementation of a prehospital severity scale for EMS triage of acute stroke: A real-world experience. *J. NeuroIntervent. Surg.* **2020**, *12*, 19–24. [CrossRef]
39. Bray, J.E.; Martin, J.; Cooper, G.; Barger, B.; Bernard, S.; Bladin, C. An interventional study to improve paramedic diagnosis of stroke. *Prehosp. Emerg. Care* **2005**, *9*, 297–302. [CrossRef] [PubMed]
40. Price, C.I.; Shaw, L.; Dodd, P.; Exley, C.; Flynn, D.; Francis, R.; Islam, S.; Javanbakht, M.; Lakey, R.; Lally, J.; et al. Paramedic Acute Stroke Treatment Assessment (PASTA): Study protocol for a randomised controlled trial. *Trials* **2019**, *20*, 121. [CrossRef] [PubMed]
41. Watkins, C.L.; Leathley, M.J.; Jones, S.P.; Ford, G.A.; Quinn, T.; Chris, J.; Sutton, C.J. Training emergency services' dispatchers to recognise stroke: An interrupted time-series analysis. *BMC Health Serv. Res.* **2013**, *13*, 318. [CrossRef] [PubMed]

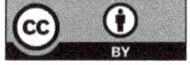 © 2020 by the authors. Licensee MDPI, Basel, Switzerland. This article is an open access article distributed under the terms and conditions of the Creative Commons Attribution (CC BY) license (http://creativecommons.org/licenses/by/4.0/).

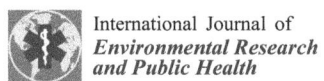 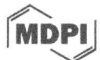

Article

The Impact of Online Media on Parents' Attitudes toward Vaccination of Children—Social Marketing and Public Health

Boban Melovic [1], Andjela Jaksic Stojanovic [2], Tamara Backovic Vulic [1], Branislav Dudic [3,4,*] and Eleonora Benova [3]

1. Faculty of Economics, University of Montenegro, 81000 Podgorica, Montenegro; bobanm@ucg.ac.me (B.M.); tassabacc@ucg.ac.me (T.B.V.)
2. Faculty of Culture and Tourism, University of Donja Gorica, 81000 Podgorica, Montenegro; andjela.jaksic@unimediteran.net
3. Faculty of Management, Comenius University in Bratislava, 82005 Bratislava, Slovakia; eleonora.benova@fm.uniba.sk
4. Faculty of Economics and Engineering Management, University Business Academy, 21000 Novi Sad, Serbia
* Correspondence: branislav.dudic@fm.uniba.sk

Received: 11 July 2020; Accepted: 6 August 2020; Published: 11 August 2020

Abstract: The aim of this paper was to investigate the level of influence of online media on the parents' attitudes toward vaccination of children in three countries of the Western Balkans—Montenegro, Serbia, and Bosnia and Herzegovina, in order to use the potentials of this form of communication effectively and efficiently. Online media are a critical factor of influence on the formation of attitudes in many areas of modern society, which is why their proper use plays an important role in strengthening vaccine confidence and which may further contribute to improvement of public health. On the other side, having in mind the fact that communication is an integral part of marketing, it is clear that social marketing has an extremely important role regarding the analyzed topic, especially because of the fact that social marketing activities tend to change or maintain people's behavior for the benefit of individuals and society as a whole. For the purpose of this research, a conceptual model was developed. Quantitative research was conducted online in the first quarter of 2020 using the survey method. Statistical analysis was applied to data collected from 1593 parents in the analyzed countries. The relevance of the hypotheses was tested using standard statistical tests, ANOVA test, eta coefficient, and logistic regression. The research showed that all analyzed variables from the model have a significant impact on the parents' attitudes toward the vaccination of children and that they correlate with the degree of trust in vaccines. The results also approved that online media have a significant influence on the formation of parents' attitudes toward the vaccination of children (obtained values of eta coefficient $\eta^2 = 0.216$, $\eta^2 = 0.18$, $\eta^2 = 0.167$, $\eta^2 = 0.090$, reliability Cronbach's Alpha 0.892), which confirms the importance of the use of social marketing in order to direct communication properly and to strengthen the level of trust in vaccines. Additionally, the results of logistic regression showed that the following groups of parents are particularly vulnerable to the influence of online media on attitudes toward vaccines: women, parents of younger age ("millennials"), and parents who are in common law marriage, as well as parents who have more children. In addition, the results showed that there is no statistically significant difference in the attitudes of parents in the observed countries ($\eta^2 = 0.000$, F = 0.85). Based on the results of the research, the authors suggest that decision makers should pay more attention to modern forms of online communication and social marketing in order to use their potential for improvement of public health, as well as avoid the harmful impact that certain forms of communication may have on the formation of attitudes and loss of confidence in vaccines. The findings provide an important contribution for public health policy makers to identify and understand properly the impact of online media and social marketing and thus to better adapt their initiatives to changes in modern society.

Keywords: online media; social media; vaccination; social marketing; public health

1. Introduction

Today, people may find a lot of different information regarding public health online. Research studies have shown that online sources represent a well-established and important site of health-related information seeking behavior [1,2], and, moreover, have a significant role in shaping health behaviors [3]. For example, one in three adults in the United States tries to diagnose a medical condition online [4]. Online sources have thus become the primary source of information in the 21st century, which is especially present in the field of medicine and public health. Through online information, almost everyone has access to numerous information with just few clicks. In other words, online media represent a critical factor of influence toward attitudes in different areas, which is why the proper use of this form of communication also plays an important role in improvement of public health. However, online sources also contain misinformation that may negatively affect attitudes and behavior and, as such, may have extremely harmful effects on public health [5]. In addition, health misinformation, which is against established medical understanding [6], may be widely distributed in order to reach a large population in a short time in the digital age [7]. This is extremely important because previous studies have shown that many parents mostly receive vaccination information through online sources [8].

Although vaccination is considered to be the most effective and cost-effective way of preventing the contraction of an infectious disease [9,10], there are numerous controversies about vaccines. First of all, it is important to point out that vaccination is recognized as an integral part of public health policies and each country implements vaccination requirements in order to achieve satisfactory vaccination coverage. Avoidance of vaccination by parents directly leads to a lower vaccination rate among their children, increasing the social risk of infection [11]. In line with the above, a large number of previous studies have focused on the benefits of vaccinating children [12,13], which further positively reflects on strengthening trust in vaccines. Thus, researchers in many countries have emphasized the cost-effectiveness of vaccination in preventing disease [14–16] and this issue is especially important in less developed countries. Despite the trend of increasing vaccination rates around the world, many factors may influence the formation of negative attitudes, especially in developing countries, such as the countries of the Western Balkans region. Namely, these countries, most often, have a lower level of development of the health system and public health policy, which further reflects the influence of online media on the formation of attitudes and level of trust in vaccines, which is one of the motives of this research. This problem is faced not only by developing countries but also by developed countries. The issues related to vaccines are increasingly politicized today. An international study on attitudes towards vaccination has shown that, although overall confidence in vaccines is positive, it is the lowest in the European region [17].

Although there is a certain number of studies on trust in vaccines [18–20], it is often pointed out that there is a lack of such research, especially in less developed countries, which is why this issue continues to cause a lot of controversy. Namely, despite the scientific consensus that vaccines are safe and effective, there are still unconfirmed claims that doubt their safety [21]. In line with the above, some research studies show that public confidence in vaccines is increasingly lost, and there are more and more people who are beginning to question the safety of vaccines, changing the recommended vaccination schemes, or even rejecting vaccination [22–24]. This problem is especially pointed out when it comes to less developed countries, such as most of the countries of the Western Balkans. In recent years, vaccines have been "notorious" in these countries. This especially refers to the measles-mumps-rubella (MMR) vaccine because of its potential association with autism [25]. This creates a dilemma among parents whether to vaccinate their children or not, not only when it comes to this but also to other vaccines. The confirmation for this statement is the fact that there is a large number of cases that the pediatrician informed the health inspector that the parents refused to vaccinate or revaccinate the child. In order to increase the number of vaccinated children, the countries of the Western Balkans often prescribe penalties. Thus, for example, parents in Montenegro, although in a dilemma, are obliged to vaccinate their children against ten infectious diseases, and, if they do not do so, they must pay a fine which is prescribed by the Law on Protection of the Population from Infectious Diseases [26]. However, there is another indirect sanction for parents who do not vaccinate their children. Namely, an unvaccinated child cannot be enrolled in a kinder garden or school, and the parents should provide medical certificates in order to confirm that the child is vaccinated. However, according to the latest data of the Institute of Public Health from the February 2020, 8000 children in Montenegro of ages from three to five did not receive mandatory vaccines [27]. In the past two years, the Directorate for Inspection Affairs has filed over 177 misdemeanor charges against parents who did not vaccinate their children according to the compulsory immunization calendar, while courts imposed 150 fines worth of 15,000 euros in total while the other 27 parents received a reprimand [28]. The situation is similar in other countries of the Western Balkans, especially in Serbia and Bosnia and Herzegovina, which are included in this research. All this leads to the conclusion that a large number of parents have a dilemma about vaccination and that they have distrust in vaccines, which is why they often do the research about vaccines for themselves in order to make a decision. Distrust in vaccines served as one of the motives for this study.

So, in many countries, health experts state that there is a trend of mistrust when it comes to vaccines, and thus a refusal to use them. The World Health Organization (WHO) has included this trend in one of the 10 threats to world health in 2019 [29]. At the same time, it should have in mind that a number of studies highlight the negative aspects of vaccination, which are very often the result of media influence. A health scare, or panic created by the media in relation to health issues, has been shown to increase people's need for information and for people to begin to question traditional sources of information as trustworthy [30]. Furthermore, research shows that vaccination rates vary depending on the use of the mass media [31], especially online media, which is the dominant form of communication in most countries. In line with the above, some studies have shown that more and more parents are searching for vaccination information on various online sources [8].

As previously pointed out, online media are a critical factor of influence on the formation of attitudes in many areas of modern society, which is why their proper use plays an important role in increasing trust in vaccines, and thus improving public health. Online media include various forms, such as medical websites, social networks, portals, blogs, forums, etc., and research shows that some of them like social media have the capacity to influence and shape public opinion regarding vaccination in a viral manner—both positively and negatively [32]. In this context, it is extremely important to analyze online media as a part of marketing communication and social marketing, which also has an important role in the improvement of public health. Namely, social marketing is an approach used to develop activities aimed at changing or maintaining people's behavior for the benefit of individuals and society as a whole. Social marketing, through its various forms and strategies, plays a significant role in the field of medicine and public health [33]. In this way, social marketing influences parents' attitudes and better understanding of online media and marketing communications and decision makers as an important factor in strengthening trust in vaccines and improving public health. More specifically, it is very important that both parents and decision-makers understand social marketing, as well as to understand how particular forms of marketing communication, such as online media, influence perceptions, and attitudes about vaccination of children [31], which is one of the motives of this research. This is because, as mentioned above, despite the existence of numerous studies that explain the benefits of vaccination, there are still many conflicting views on pro-vaccine and anti-vaccine [34], especially having in mind more intensive use of online media and marketing campaigns in modern age. Research studies show that anti-vaccine articles are more likely to be shared, commented on, and reacted to online than pro-vaccine messages [35]. Online anti-vaccine messages may lead parents to question the safety of vaccine, distrust health professionals, and seek non-medical vaccine exemptions [36,37]. Regarding this matter, several studies have been conducted in order to analyze how online information influence parents' attitudes and decisions about vaccination. Some studies have focused on specific vaccines, while others have been general [8]. According to one of the studies, "the most recent statistics available show 16% of seekers searched online for vaccination information and 70% say what they found affected by their treatment decisions" [38].

In line with the above, research studies around the world show that media exposure may significantly facilitate a change in parents' behavior [21,39], which is especially important when it comes to using online media. This would contribute to the strengthening of trust in vaccines, as well as to the improvement of public health, through adequate online communication and various forms of social marketing. It should have in mind that, in addition to the positive effects, online media may also use groups to get people to oppose vaccination, raising skepticism about the scientific evidences regarding the risks and benefits of vaccines [40]. Online media, especially web pages against vaccination, are widely spread on Internet [41] and, in many countries, may be more compelling sources of information than vaccination sources [42]. People have been shown to be more responsive to personal stories than statistics [43], which means that online vaccine sources and their personal stories may create a stronger emotional response for readers than official health online sites with statistics and arguments.

Thus, media in general and specially the online media, have significantly contributed to widespread public distrust of vaccines in many countries around the world [44], and countries in our region are no exception. In fact, the dissemination of negative information about immunizations has been increased by the progress of certain forms of online resources, such as individual social networks (Facebook and Twitter) [44,45]. Since 2013, the World Economic Forum has cited mass digital misinformation among the major threats to our society [46]. Recent studies emphasize that the spread of misinformation is the result of a paradigm shift in content consumption caused by the advent of social media. In fact, the platforms of particular forms of online media, such as Facebook or Twitter, have created a direct path for users to produce and consume content, changing the way people inform themselves [32,47,48] and form attitudes. It is often discussed that online media, and especially social media, have important role in creating hesitancy [10] and fear in parents and encouraging them to avoid vaccination. Many of these fears come from information that parents find online and many of these sources not only propagate unproven claims regarding vaccines but may also undermine the physician-family relationship by challenging parents' trust in the medical professionals [49].

On the other hand, many parents from many countries who have decided not to vaccinate their children have done their own (online) research. Research studies show that parents seeking for information about vaccine risk will find more online sources that are against the vaccine, compared to parents seeking information about the benefits of vaccines [50]. This means that it is likely that parents who are worried about vaccination will find online sources to confirm their fears. So, today the information is widely spread through different forms of online marketing especially social media and networks. For example, a quick Facebook search provided more anti-vaccination groups from around the world. Anti-vaccine content exists in many of the vaccine-related top Google search results [42,51]. By doing a Google search on the key term "vaccine refusal", 3,340,000 results could be found [8]. It may be concluded that despite all the advantages of vaccination, there is still a strong resistance in form of anti-vaccine movements, which are on the one side the result of mistrust, and on the other of the strong influence of the media. It is important to emphasize that vaccine-related misinformation, which is often spread via the Internet by vaccine groups [51], may be the most commonly distributed health-related misinformation [52].

Relying on the results of previous research and the observed literary gap, the authors wanted to conduct a study that would target the impact of online media on parents' attitudes towards vaccination of children, as well as the impact of other characteristics (gender, age, country of origin, etc.), in order to direct social marketing activities to strengthening trust in vaccines, thus improving public health. So, in order to discover, identify and understand the relationship between online media and parents' attitudes toward children's vaccination, especially from the country of respondents' origin (Montenegro, Serbia, and Bosnia and Herzegovina), this paper tends to fill the gap compared to previous studies. Therefore, the aim of the paper was to investigate the level of influence that online media, as a form of marketing communication, have on the formation of parents' attitudes toward the vaccination of children, that is trust in vaccines in analyzed countries of the Western Balkans region, as well as a role of social marketing in strengthening trust in vaccines and improvement of public health.

The paper is organized into five sections. Following the abstract, in the first section, a review of the results of previous research regarding the vaccination and online media was made, as well as the literature overview in which the motive for this research was found. This section contains an analysis of key aspects of vaccination, arguments pro and against vaccines, vaccines trust, the role of online media, and the importance of social media in strengthening trust in vaccines, as well as the influence of the country development on these questions. This segment also refers to materials and methods and includes a description of research methodology, i.e., data collection and simple, measures and instrument validation. The next part presents the results of research, while the fourth part represents the discussion of the results. Finally, the paper concludes with concluding remarks, a review of the implications, and recommendations for future research studies.

2. Hypotheses Development, Materials, and Methods

Based on the relevant literature and using data obtained from empirical research in three countries: Montenegro, Serbia, and Bosnia and Herzegovina, several hypotheses were developed in order to investigate the relationship between the analyzed variables and parents' attitudes toward vaccination of children, especially from the aspect of online media.

As previously noted, existing research supports the thesis that some of the demographic characteristics may be important in forming parents' attitudes toward vaccination of children. Thus, for example, Brown et al. [53] emphasize the gender and age of parents, while Anderberg et al. [54] point out that decisions about vaccinating children significantly depend on the level of education of parents, because a higher level of education is translated into a higher awareness or the information being perceived differently. Similarly, Walsh et al. [55] relate the age and education of parents. Furthermore, the aim of some research in this area is to determine the extent to which parents' attitudes towards immunization affect coverage (number of vaccinated children) and to assess the level of parents' knowledge about immunization [56]. In addition, a number of these studies highlight the country's level of development as an impact factor, and these studies do not analyze this. In addition, the adequate application of social marketing may influence the change of behavior [57], i.e., it may influence the strengthening of trust, considering the previously mentioned characteristics when creating marketing communication strategies. Thus, the results of previous studies point out that gender, age of parents and their education, as well as knowledge about immunization, may be mentioned as important influencing factors, which the authors wanted to investigate in this research. In accordance with the above, the following hypotheses have been defined:

Hypothesis 1 (H1). *Identified characteristics of respondents have a significant effect on attitudes toward children's vaccination, which reflects on the level of trust in vaccines.*

On the other hand, previous literature suggests that the online media today represent the crucial factor of influence on formation of attitudes in different areas, and that is why their proper use has important role in strengthening trust in vaccines and improvement of public health. Different forms of online marketing may have positive and negative influence [32]. Under the influence of online media, conflicting views on pro-vaccine and anti-vaccine may often be heard [34]. Thus, anti-vaccine articles are more likely to be shared, commented on, and reacted to online than pro-vaccine messages [11]. It is indisputable that media exposure influences the change of parental behavior [21,39]. Hence, the concept of social marketing has more importance and, through various forms and strategies, it plays a significant role in the field of medicine and public health [33]. Thus, in the context of the research topic, online media may be considered as a segment of social marketing, which plays an important role in improving public health. Namely, online media and other forms of marketing communication may have an impact on perceptions and attitudes toward vaccination of children [31], which encourages the importance of social marketing in order to improve public health. In accordance with the above, the following hypotheses have been defined:

Hypothesis 2 (H2). *Online media have a significant impact on parents' attitudes toward children's vaccination, which encourages the importance of adequate implementation of social marketing in the function of improving public health.*

In addition to demographic characteristics and the influence of online media, the authors wanted to analyze other factors that may be relevant, and which, in interaction with other factors, may have a strong influence on the formation of parents' attitudes toward vaccination. According to this, the authors noted that the level of country's development and policy, i.e., the measures that countries take in terms of vaccination may have a significant impact on the formation of attitudes. In this sense, a significant number of countries are trying to develop motivational measures, and we often talk about the obligation to vaccinate and penal policy in case of refusal [58]. For example, despite the implementation of vaccination regulations in Poland, as in other European Union countries, the final decision on vaccination of children is made by their parents or legal guardians [59]. On the other side, experience in the countries of our region shows that developed countries, such as Croatia and Slovenia, have similar policies, while, in countries with lower levels of development, such as Montenegro, Serbia, Bosnia and Herzegovina, there is a stricter vaccination policy, which includes high penalties and provisions in case of refusal of vaccination. In that sense, understanding the attitudes and opinions of parents toward vaccination is essential for planning and undertaking extensive and properly directed educational actions in order to prevent their indecision. Taking these measures, supported by an adequate social marketing strategy, may lead to a strengthening of trust in vaccines, as well as an improvement of public health. Starting from the fact that the countries in which the research was conducted belong to less developed countries, which have relatively similar legislation, people's habits, and that all three countries tend to harmonize public health policies in accordance with European standards, the third hypothesis was formulated:

Hypothesis 3 (H3). *There is no significant difference in parents' attitudes toward children's in the analyzed countries regarding to the impact of online media.*

The conceptual model, based on the defined hypotheses in given in the figure below (Figure 1).

Having in mind motives and goals of the research, the defined hypotheses, results of previously published research, as well as evaluations of theoretical models, the authors developed a form of a questionnaire. The questionnaire was prepared and distributed to 3031 parents in three countries (Montenegro, Serbia, and Bosnia and Herzegovina). Namely, in cooperation with preschool institutions (kindergartens) and parents' associations, the questionnaire was transmitted online (via mailing lists and viber groups) in order to ensure the highest possible representativeness of the sample. The poll lasted for 30 days, and 1593 fully filled in polls were returned, giving the answer rate of 52.55%. This can be considered a high response rate, which is explained by the actuality of the topic itself and the parents' interest to participate in the research. The survey was undertaken in the first quarter of 2020. The questionnaire identified 20 questions, and, for the purpose of analyze of results of the survey, according to identified criteria, 3 variables were defined. The pilot survey, which tended to examine the validity of the content of the questionnaire, was conducted in Montenegro by 15 parents. Based on their suggestions, the final form of the questionnaire was created.

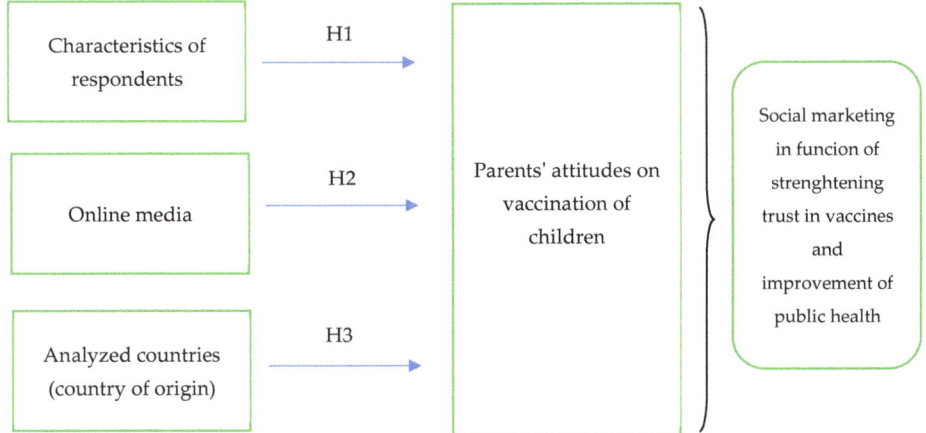

Figure 1. Conceptual model of research. **Source:** Authors.

Cronbach's alpha was used to test the reliability of the study. The calculated values of Cronbach's Alpha are at a satisfactory level and are 0.892 (the Cronbach's alpha values adhered to the suggested minimum value of 0.6), which means that the data are suitable for further analysis [60,61]. We processed the collected data in the SPSS program (Statistics 20) and, during the analysis, we used descriptive statistics, the ANOVA test, the eta coefficient and logistic regression. Analysis of variance (ANOVA) is an analytical model for testing the significance of differences [62,63]. The advantage of this method is that the model considers all the variables, as well as their interaction. Analysis of variance is essentially a special mathematical and statistical procedure that allows testing the significance of the difference between arithmetic means from three or more samples, and within that testing the influence of one or more factors on the variability of a tested numerical feature. Furthermore, in order to further examine the importance of a certain way of using online media to form attitudes, i.e., parents' trust in vaccines, eta-coefficient was used. The Likert scale was treated as an interval scale by placing neither in the place of neutral or moderately [64]. It is obvious that the data itself divide into two categories were the parametric tests is applicable. If the Likert scale data are treated as interval scale data, then the ANOVA test can be used. If the Likert scale data are from 1–5 with equal intervals then the midpoint already exists at 3 [65]. Therefore, the Likert scale is the same as the interval scale, with the difference in the labeling. A Likert scale, finally, label does not create any difference in the data distance since the codes are the same so the usage of parametric tests will get the best results [66].

On the other hand, logistic regression was used in order to obtain a more precise answer to the question of the relationship between the demographic characteristics of the respondents and their attitude towards vaccines based on information from online media. Logistic regression is the most commonly used in order to rank the relative importance of independent variables and to quantify the effect of their interaction [67]. The results of the research are given below.

3. Results

In order to determine the influence of the analyzed factors on parents' attitudes toward children's vaccination and their confidence in vaccines, an analysis of the characteristics of the respondents was performed using the descriptive statistics method, which is presented in Table 1.

Table 1. Characteristics of respondents.

Gender	N	Weighted%	Country	N	Weighted %
Female	1117	70.1	Montenegro	705	44.3
Male	476	29.9	Serbia	520	32.6
			Bosnia and Herzegovina	368	23.1
Age			**Level of education**		
18–24	37	2.3	Primary school	0	0
25–29	163	10.2	Secondary school	610	38.3
30–34	388	24.4	College	174	10.9
35–40	648	40.7	Faculty	638	40.1
41–45	212	13.3	Specialist	102	6.4
More than 45	145	9.1	Master	52	3.3
			PhD	17	1.0
Marital status			**Number of children**		
Married	1429	89.7	1	588	36.9
Extracurricular union	87	5.5	2	719	45.1
Divorced	63	4.0	3	275	17.3
Widower	14	0.9	More than 3	0	0

Based on the descriptive statistics provided in Table 1, it may be concluded that the respondents are predominantly female (as much as 70.1% of the total number of respondents, which may indicate a greater interest of mothers in the mentioned topic), with the largest number between 35 and 40 years (40.7% of respondents). Respondents are married in 89.7% and possess a faculty diploma in 40.1%. The largest number of respondents is from Montenegro (44.3% of respondents, which may be justified by the fact that the research was initiated in this country) and have two children (45.1%). In terms of geographical spread, the demographic of the respondents is as follows: 705 (44.30%) respondents are from Montenegro and 520 (32.60%) from Serbia, while 368 (23.10%) are from Bosnia and Herzegovina.

Furthermore, these characteristics were correlated with the degree of trust that parents have in vaccines, which is shown in Table 2.

Table 2. Table of contingency for attitudes, i.e., trust in vaccines in relation to the characteristics of the respondents.

Rate Your Level of Trust in Vaccines		Gender	Age	Country	Level of Education	Marital Status	Number of Children
I don't trust	Mean	1.08	3.84	1.77	2.81	1.16	1.77
	N	64	64	64	64	64	64
	Std. Deviation	0.270	1.359	0.792	1.006	0.541	0.611
Low level	Mean	1.25	3.87	1.80	3.22	1.26	1.98
	N	244	244	244	244	244	244
	Std. Deviation	0.432	1.068	0.821	1.168	0.777	0.751
Neutral	Mean	1.27	3.43	1.78	3.23	1.11	1.81
	N	444	444	444	444	444	433
	Std. Deviation	0.442	1.243	0.790	1.214	0.381	0.682
High level	Mean	1.36	4.00	1.80	3.60	1.20	1.80
	N	540	540	540	540	540	540
	Std. Deviation	0.481	0.971	0.803	1.271	0.526	0.731
I trust completely	Mean	1.32	3.91	1.78	3.49	1.09	1.66
	N	301	301	301	301	301	301
	Std. Deviation	0.468	1.191	0.762	1.473	0.364	0.678
Total	Mean	1.30	3.80	1.79	3.39	1.16	1.80
	N	1593	1593	1593	1593	1593	1582
	Std. Deviation	0.458	1.148	0.793	1.287	0.516	0.712

The greatest dispersion of data about the average value of the attitude that they do not trust in vaccines was noticed in the question related to the age of the respondents. The standard deviation of this characteristic is 1359. Thus, the age of a randomly selected sample deviates from the average value of all respondents in the amount of 1359 points on the Likert scale, provided that these subjects do not trust vaccines. High data dispersion was also noted for the level of education of respondents in this category of trust in vaccines because the value of the standard deviation is 1006. The two highest values in category I, totally believe, are for education (1473) and age (1191). The analysis of other categories of trust in vaccines also showed that the results are the most dispersed for the level of education and for age because standard deviations have the highest values for these two characteristics of the respondents. The most homogeneous answers refer to the gender and marital status of the respondents.

Based on the contingency table, a graphical presentation (Figure 2) of the participation of individual categories of respondents in terms of characteristics, such as gender, country of origin, age, marital status, and number of children, in combination with their attitude about trust in vaccines was created.

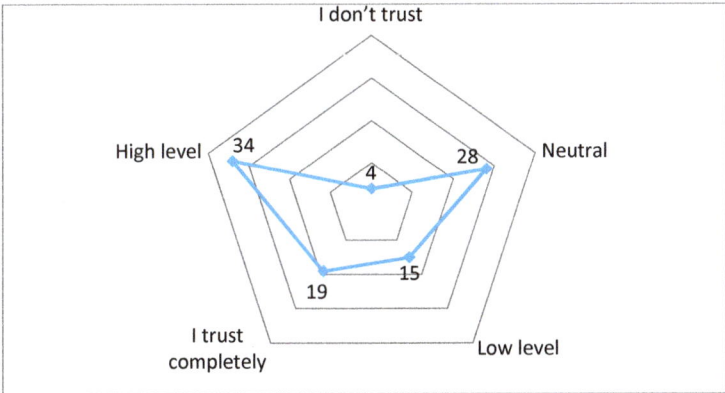

Figure 2. Trust in vaccines.

The analysis of the contingency table showed that the largest number of respondents have high confidence in vaccines (34%), when their characteristics, such as gender, country of origin, age, marital status, and number of children, would be analyzed. However, about one-fifth of respondents do not trust or have a low level of trust in vaccines, which means that certain actions must be taken in order to improve this situation. This was the motive to focus on discovering the reasons why parents do not trust vaccines in one part of the research in order to create set of recommendations which would contribute to the strengthening of trust in vaccines.

Furthermore, characteristics of respondents have been correlated with the attitudes of parents towards vaccines, as shown in Table 3. Since the survey was conducted in three countries, three groups of respondents were available for testing, so it was possible to apply the ANOVA test.

Table 3. ANOVA test of determination of differences based on characteristics of respondents.

Variables			Sum of Squares	DF	Mean Square	F	Sig.
Gender * Attitudes	Between Groups	(Combined)	6.673	4	1.668	8.099	0.000
	Within Groups		327.095	1588	0.206		
	Total		333.768	1592			
Age * Attitudes	Between Groups	(Combined)	87.568	4	21.892	17.279	0.000
	Within Groups		2011.939	1588	1.267		
	Total		2099.508	1592			
Conutry * Attitudes	Between Groups	(Combined)	0.215	4	0.054	0.085	0.987
	Within Groups		1001.492	1588	0.631		
	Total		1001.707	1592			
Level of education * Attitudes	Between Groups	(Combined)	66.847	4	16.712	10.322	0.000
	Within Groups		2570.951	1588	1.619		
	Total		2637.798	1592			
Marital status* Attitudes	Between Groups	(Combined)	5.694	4	1.423	5.401	0.000
	Within Groups		418.487	1588	0.264		
	Total		424.181	1592			
Number of children * Attitudes	Between Groups	(Combined)	14.048	4	3.512	7.037	0.000
	Within Groups		787.024	1577	0.499		
	Total		801.073	1581			

Symbol * represents the combination of two variables.

The starting hypothesis of the ANOVA test indicates the equality of expected values for the characteristics of the respondents, such as gender, age, country of origin, level of education, marital status, and number of children, which the respondents have in relation to their confidence in vaccines. The analysis of the variance of the respondents' data on the above characteristics, given in the previous table, has shown that the expected value for each individual characteristic (except for the state) differs in relation to the attitudes of parents, and that the given characteristics have a significant influence on the formation of attitudes. Based on the obtained results, it is possible to accept hypothesis H1.

Using the conclusion of hypothesis H1, and before testing the justification of the claim of hypothesis H2, it was tried to answer the question of the relationship between the demographic characteristics of respondents (who were the subject of hypothesis H1) and their negative attitude towards vaccines based on information from online media (correlated with hypothesis H2) and for that purpose logistic regression was applied. So, in the continuation of the research, we analyzed the influence of certain characteristics of parents on their attitude not to vaccinate a child, built on the content, which they found by consulting online media. The aim of this part of the analysis was to determine whether there is a certain group of respondents who are more vulnerable to content on online media and, on that basis, refuse to vaccinate a child. In order to determine the relationship between a particular characteristic of respondents and their attitude not to vaccinate a child, under the influence of information found on online media, as mentioned above, we used logistic regression because it is most often used to rank the relative importance of independent variables and to quantify the effect their interactions.

In order to define the variable which represents the negative attitude of parents towards vaccines, formed on the basis of content from online media, we chose the answer to one key question in the survey, which represents this behavior. To define the anti-vaccine attitude, we considered the answer to the question "Texts on online media about the negative effects of the vaccine affect the formation of my attitude to a significant extent." because we believe that other questions about the negative attitude towards vaccines formed on the basis of online media are less focused on forming an attitude and making the final decision not to vaccinate the child. The independent variables in the model are the following key characteristics of the respondents: gender, age, country of origin, level of education, marital status, and number of children in the family. Thus, by assessing logistic regressions, we tried to find an answer to the question of whether men or women, younger or older parents, parents with higher or lower education, etc., are more prone to negative attitudes towards vaccines based on information obtained from online media. The results of the analysis are given below.

Before analyzing the model, we examined its quality by testing the hypothesis that there is no relationship between the dependent and independent variables in logistic regression. The test results are given in the following table (Table 4).

Table 4. Model fitting test for logistic regression of negative attitude of parents towards vaccines formed on the basis of information from online media.

	Model Fitting Information			
Model	Model Fitting Criteria −2 Log Likelihood	Likelihood Ratio Tests		
		Chi-Square	df	Sig.
Intercept Only	2896.054			
Final	2401.083	494.971	72	0.000

In this case, we tested the model by comparing the initial value of the logarithm, i.e., the model without an independent variable, which is 2896.054 with the final model, i.e., the model with an independent variable, which is 2401.083. With 72 degrees of freedom, $\chi 2$ is 494,971, which is significant at the level of 0%. The obtained results show that the model is meaningful and that the null hypothesis about the non-existence of a connection between the independent and dependent variables cannot be accepted.

The results of the evaluation of the logistic regression model are given in the following table (Table 5).

Table 5. Logistic regression of negative attitude of parents towards vaccines formed on the basis of information from online media.

"Texts on Online Media about the Negative Effects of the Vaccine Affect the Formation of My Attitude to a Significant Extent"	B	Std. Error	Wald	DF	Sig.	Exp(B)
Intercept	−17.677	1.467	145.197	1	0	
[Gender = Male]	−1.195	0.295	16.409	1	0.05	0.303
[Gender = Female]	0 a	0		0		
[Age = 18–24]	0.116	0.0056	194.005	1	0	1.122
[Age = 25–29]	0.078	0.0113	294.745	1	0	1.082
[Age = 30–34]	0.194	0.535	16.09	1	0.06	1.214
[Age = 35–40]	−2.145	0.482	7.225	1	0.07	0.117
[Age = 41–45]	−1.296					0.274
[Age = Older than 45]	0 a			0		
[Country = Serbia]	−0.152	0.0134	128.670	1	0.008	0.859
[Country = Montenegro]	−0.189	0.017	123.602	1	0.007	0.828
[Country = Bosnia and Herzegovina]	0 a			0		
[Level of education = High School]	1.291	0.098	173.540	1	0	3.637
[Level of Education = College]	0.043	0.005	73.960	1	0.01	1.043
[Level of Education = Faculty]	0.843	0.096	77.110	1	0	2.323
[Level of Education = Specialist]	0.892	0.129	47.813	1	0.01	2.44
[Level of Education = Master]	0.013	1.559	0.000	1	0	1.013
[Level of Education = PhD]	0 a			0		
[Marital status = Married]	0.17	0.019	80.055	1	0.02	1.185
[Marital status = Common law marriage]	2.458	0.145	287.361	1	0	11.684
[Marital status = Divorced]	0.19	0.017	124.913	1	0	1.209
[Marital status = Widowed]	0 a			0		
[Number of Children = 1]	−1.607	0.39	16.947	1	0	0.2
[Number of Children = 2]	−0.635	0.352	3.255	1	0.071	0.53
[Number of Children = 3]	0 a			0		

a—this variable is et to zero because it is redundant.

At the very beginning, it should be emphasized that all parameters in the regression are statistically significant with a risk of error of 5%. Since we are most interested in commenting on the results of extreme values on the Likert scale, we defined the value 1 as a basis for comparison (I completely disagree), and the value to explain the relationship between demographic characteristics and anti-vaccine attitude based on information from online media was defined with value 5 on the Likert scale (I completely agree). Based on the results of the estimated logistic regression, it is concluded that, if the parent-respondent is a male, i.e., the father, in 69.7% of cases, he will less often form a negative attitude towards vaccines based on information or texts read on online media compared to mothers-respondents. In other words, negative texts about vaccines through online media are not key to forming a negative attitude among fathers-respondents. If the age of the respondents' parents is observed, conclusions on this issue are made on the basis of the reference group of parents, who are older than 45 years. If parents are under the age of 35, they are more likely to form a negative attitude towards vaccines and eventually make the decision not to vaccinate their child by reading texts through online media compared to parents over the age of 45. On the other hand, parents who are between 35 and 45 years old are about 80% less likely to form a negative attitude towards vaccines based on information from online media compared to the parents of the oldest age group of respondents in this survey. Parents from Serbia and Montenegro have between 15 and 18% less chance of forming a negative attitude towards vaccines reading articles on online media compared to parents from Bosnia and Herzegovina. Parents who have any lower level of education than doctors of science, are more likely to form a negative attitude towards vaccines based on information from the online media compared to parents with the title of doctor of science. This conclusion makes sense because parents with the highest level of education are more inclined to check the information and thoroughly process each topic before making such an important decision, such as vaccinating children. Parents who are married, in common law marriage, or divorced are more likely to build a negative attitude towards vaccines by reading content on online media compared to parents who are widowed. And that chance is incomparably higher for parents who are in common law marriage compared to other marital statuses. Finally, if the number of children in a family is observed, parents with less than three children are between 50% and 80% less likely to form a negative attitude towards vaccines based on texts they found on the Internet than parents with three or more children. This conclusion is connected with the fact that parents with a smaller number of children will strive to obtain additional information about vaccines from other sources, so the position on vaccines will not be formed only on the basis of content from the Internet, while parents with more children have a different situation.

Based on this part of the research it may be concluded that the following groups of parents are particularly vulnerable to the influence of online media on attitudes toward vaccines: women, parents of younger age ("millennials"), and parents who are in common law marriage, as well as parents who have more children.

Furthermore, in order to determine the level of influence that online media have on parents' attitudes, an ANOVA test was applied to test the second hypothesis. The results are given in Table 6.

Table 6. ANOVA test of determination of online media on parent's attitudes.

Variables		Sum of Squares	DF	Mean Square	F	Sig.
I regularly read texts on the online media about the negative effects of vaccines * Attitudes	Between Groups (Combined)	51.420	4	12.855	8.610	0.000
	Within Groups	2370.804	1588	1.493		
	Total	2422.223	1592			
Texts on online media about negative effects have more importance than they really should have. * Attitudes	Between Groups (Combined)	194.612	4	48.653	39.038	0.000
	Within Groups	1979.137	1588	1.246		
	Total	2173.749	1592			
The articles on the online media about the negative effects of the vaccine are mostly correct * Attitudes	Between Groups (Combined)	304.422	4	76.106	87.903	0.000
	Within Groups	1374.882	1588	0.866		
	Total	1679.304	1592			
Texts on the online media about the negative effects of the vaccine are mostly based on fears and speculations, not on scientific facts * Attitudes	Between Groups (Combined)	396.950	4	99.238	79.795	0.000
	Within Groups	1974.927	1588	1.244		
	Total	2371.877	1592			
Texts on the online media about the negative effects of the vaccine influence the formation of my attitude to a significant extent * Attitudes	Between Groups (Combined)	564.536	4	141.134	109.449	0.000
	Within Groups	2047.712	1588	1.289		
	Total	2612.249	1592			

Symbol * represents the combination of two variables.

An analysis of the equality of expectancies for the characteristics of research on parents' attitudes toward vaccines in the situation when using online media as a source of information has shown that respondents' attitudes differ significantly depending on which aspect is used as a source of information. The conclusion is that online media has a significant influence on the formation of parents' attitudes toward the vaccination of children, which leads to the acceptance of the hypothesis H2. In addition, the logistic regression itself showed that there is a significant difference in the formation of a negative attitude towards vaccines in different demographic groups of respondents, which is formed on the basis of information from online media.

In order to further examine the importance of a particular way of using online media on formation of attitudes, an eta coefficient was used, in which the squared value represents a relative measure of association. The eta coefficient takes a value between 0 and 1 and represents the proportion of variance in the dependent variable explained by the independent variable. The formula for calculating the eta coefficient is:

$$\eta^2 = \frac{SSeffect}{SStotal}$$

where:

SSeffect = the sum of squares for a given independent variable (factor);
SStotal = the total sum of squares for all factors, interactions, and errors in the ANOVA analysis.

If η^2 is 0.01, then it indicates a small impact, while a moderate impact is indicated for a value of 0.06 and a large influence for a value of 0.14 or greater. The results of the eta coefficient are given in Table 7.

Table 7. Measures of association of online media with attitudes toward vaccines.

Variables	η	η^2
I continuously read texts on the online media about the negative effects of vaccines	0.146	0.021
Texts on online media about negative effects of vaccines have more importance than they should have	0.299	0.090
The articles on the online media about the negative effects of the vaccines are mostly correct	0.426	0.181
Texts on the online media about the negative effects of the vaccines are mostly based on fears and speculations, not scientific facts	0.409	0.167
Texts on the online media about the negative effects of the vaccines influence the formation of my attitude to a significant extent	0.465	0.216

The analysis of the η^2 coefficient has shown that the greatest value in the opinion of parents that the texts on the online media about the negative effects of the vaccine influence the formation of the parents' attitude ($\eta^2 = 0.216$). Then, there is the opinion that these texts are generally correct ($\eta^2 = 0.181$), and thirdly, is the view of parents that these texts have no scientific basis ($\eta^2 = 0.167$), that is, they are based on fears and speculations. On the other hand, when claiming that the texts on the online media about negative effects have more importance than they should have, the value of the η^2 coefficient is significantly 0.090.

In order to examine whether there are differences in the analyzed countries regarding the influence of online media on the formation of attitudes, additional testing has been done and the results are shown in Table 8.

Table 8. ANOVA test examinations of differences by analyzed countries.

Variables		Sum of Squares	DF	Mean Square	F	Sig.
Country * Attitudes toward vaccines/Level of trust in vaccines	Between groups (Combined)	0.215	4	0.054	0.085	0.987
	Within Groups	1001.492	1588	0.631		
	Total	1001.707	1592			

Symbol * represents the combination of two variables.

The analysis of variance showed that the attitudes of the interviewed parents were the same, regardless of whether the respondents were from Montenegro, Serbia, or Bosnia and Herzegovina. Namely, the error made by rejecting the hypothesis that parents' attitude toward trust in vaccines is equal to 98.7%, which is why we cannot reject it. In addition, in the section that follows (Table 9), an analysis of the eta squares for states in relation to attitudes, i.e., trust in vaccines, is presented.

Table 9. Measures of association of countries with attitudes of respondents.

Variables	Eta	Eta Squared
Country * Attitudes toward vaccines	0.015	0.000

Symbol * represents the combination of two variables.

The measure of association, that is, the eta coefficient for the country from which respondents come in relation to respondents' attitudes toward vaccination is 0. In other words, there is no statistically significant difference between the analyzed countries for explaining the influence of online media on parents' attitudes toward vaccines. Based on the results obtained previously, it may be concluded that hypothesis H3 is confirmed. Hence, the ANOVA test and the eta coefficient confirmed that the country of origin of the respondents does not affect their attitude towards the vaccination of children.

4. Discussion

Studies show that immunization, one of the greatest public health achievements, is occasionally hampered by strong biological, social, and cultural reactions of the public [68], which is why the media and communication are extremely important for this issue. In such conditions, online media, which today have become the primary source of information, are of special importance, especially because of the fact that many parents receive information about vaccinations mostly through online sources [10]. However, despite the growing literature on vaccination and the role of online media in modern times, and thus in the field of medicine and public health, we are still trying to explore and understand parents' attitudes about vaccinating children, as well as why and how parents have different levels of trust in vaccines. This is particularly important given the research by Larson et al. [44], who found that socioeconomic status, media information, and attitudes and motivations regarding health care, as well as knowledge and awareness of the need for vaccines, are related to indecision to give the vaccine. This is especially present in less developed countries.

Thence, research on the impact of online media on parents' attitudes towards child vaccination is, according to the authors' knowledge, the first integrated scientific study in three countries of the Western Balkan region—Montenegro, Serbia, and Bosnia and Herzegovina. Therefore, the aim of the research was to investigate the level of influence that online media, as a form of marketing communication, have on the formation of attitudes toward the vaccination of children, in order to direct effectively and efficiently the potentials of this form of communication towards the strengthening and improvement of public health. Discussion of achieved results is presented below.

The obtained results confirmed the hypothesis that the identified characteristics of the respondents (gender, country of origin, age, marital status, and number of children) have a significant influence on attitudes towards vaccination of children, which is correlated with the results of other studies [69] in which demographic characteristics stand out as predictors of vaccines. Furthermore, the contingency analysis showed that the majority of respondents have high confidence in vaccines, when their characteristics, such as gender, country of origin, age, marital status, and number of children would be analyzed. The next largest category are parents who have a neutral attitude, i.e., are indifferent to the vaccination of their children, because this category consists of 27.87% of respondents. In third place are parents who completely trust in vaccines, and they make up 18.9% of all surveyed parents. The penultimate category is that of parents with low confidence in vaccines, and they represent 15.32% of all surveyed parents. In the last place are parents who do not believe in the positive effect of vaccinating their children. They make up only 4.02% of the surveyed parents in this study. Based on the obtained results, we may conclude that more than half of the respondents have a high or complete level of confidence in vaccines. However, about one-fifth of respondents do not trust or have a low level of trust in vaccines, which is correlated with the results of other studies [22–24] which confirm that distrust leads to vaccination rejection. These results suggest that certain actions must be taken in order to improve the existing situation. In that sense, the implementation of social marketing may be of great importance in order to strengthen trust in vaccines. Thus, social marketing in the field of immunization has a general social character, that is, it implies the implementation of marketing strategies in order to achieve specific goals of behavior oriented to the common good. In other words, the adequate implementation of social marketing may influence the change of behavior, that is, it may influence the strengthening of trust in vaccines. Thus, social marketing becomes important factor of improving public health.

Furthermore, the analysis of the variance of the respondents' data on the stated characteristics showed that the expected value for each individual characteristic (except for the country) differs in relation to the attitudes of the parents, i.e., the level of trust in vaccines. These results are in correlation with the results of other studies, in which it is pointed out that important factors of influence are gender, age, level of education, and knowledge about immunization [53–56].

Findings of the research have shown a strong link between online media and parents' attitudes, which is correlated with the results of some studies in other countries [8,32]. Namely, the analysis of equality of expected values for the characteristics of the research on parents 'attitudes towards vaccines in the situation when using online media as a source of information has shown that respondents' attitudes differ significantly depending on which aspect of online media is used as a source of information. In accordance with the above, the results of the descriptive statistics have shown that 37.7% of cases used online health websites, then blogs and forums (33.6%), when collecting online data about vaccines and indicate that the two sources were the most trusted online media outlets. For 11.7% of respondents, Facebook is the primary online source for information about vaccines, while 4.2% prefer other social networks (Twitter, Instagram). The participation of parents who were more informed about the arguments about the pro-vaccine (49.3%) and arguments against the vaccination of children (50.7%) is almost equal, which makes sense, because all those who ask for additional information should want to know both positive and negative arguments on this topic. In collecting information on vaccination through online media, 53.2% of parents stated that their spouse was also involved, while 46.8% of respondents stated that they collected the information for themselves. When asked how they rate their understanding of the material they received through online media, 55.6% of respondents consider their understanding to be average and 16.8% have a complete understanding, while the remaining respondents are not satisfied with their understanding of the information they obtained online. The "pressure" of pro-vaccine campaigns was felt by 13.74% of parents, while 40.55% felt the "pressure" of anti-vaccine campaigns, and the remaining respondents did not feel the pressure of these campaigns. Lastly, it is interesting that only 11.48% of respondents share vaccine information with others online, while 88.52% do not, although they use online sources to inform themselves. These results may be explained by the fact that parents in the analyzed area still use "offline" sources of information to form attitudes about vaccines compared to online media. The most common source of information are doctors, i.e., pediatricians (27.4%), while online media are used in combination with information obtained from doctors or family members and friends. Since this is the way they get information, they still do not have the habit of sharing their views on vaccines to other parents in public, i.e., online. Another reason is that parents in this study stated that they felt "the pressure of the online campaign against vaccines" (39% of respondents), so they did not want to be part of that campaign and impose their views through online media on other parents.

Based on the results obtained through logistic regression, we may conclude that the following demographic groups of parents are especially vulnerable to the formation of attitudes about vaccines: women, because as mothers they are more sensitive and easier to "scare" them with certain texts about harmfulness of vaccines for the health of their children; parents of younger age ("millennials") who are influenced by digital technologies and use them in all spheres of life, including raising children, and it is not surprising that they are the most vulnerable age group of parents, who under the influence of online media form a negative attitude towards vaccines; parents living in common law marriage, as well as parents with more children, one of the key reasons being that more children give little free time to parents to devote to researching and finding additional sources of information to form attitudes about vaccines, so they rely to online sources. Precisely these differences that exist in different demographic groups when forming a negative attitude towards vaccines show the following: parents regularly follow texts about the negative effects of vaccines through online media and, based on this information, form different attitudes towards vaccines (logistic regression, for example, showed that mothers are more likely to form a negative attitude towards fathers, etc.), then that parents look differently at texts from online media about the negative effects of vaccines and thus view differently the importance of this information in forming attitudes towards vaccines ("millennials" will be more often influenced by information from online media compared to parents of older generations, etc.), parents differently estimate the truth of texts from online media about the negative effect of vaccines on children's health (parents with more children are more likely to think these texts are true compared to parents who have one or two children, etc.), and parents react differently to these texts and some of them believe that they are texts that are not based on scientific facts (parents with a doctorate), while there are parents who believe that the texts are quite true (parents with a lower level of education in in relation to doctors of science, etc.), but in the end there are differences in the impact of this information obtained from online media on the final formation of attitudes about vaccines for different demographic categories of parents.

On the other hand, the analysis of the η^2 coefficient has shown that the greatest value in the opinion of parents that the texts on the online media about the negative effects of the vaccine influence the formation of the parents' attitude ($\eta^2 = 0.216$). Namely, the research confirmed that parents were mostly under pressure from the negative campaign about vaccines through the online media (39% of respondents). Then, the research showed that parents trust the information they receive from medical websites the most (51.4% of respondents). Finally, the dominant group in the study consisted of mothers (70.1%), i.e., females, and the results of the logistic regression indicated that mothers were more influenced by the online campaign against vaccines. The combination of these factors has led to the fact that online media really play a significant role in forming the negative attitudes of respondents towards vaccines. Thus, based on the applied methods, we may conclude that online media, as a form of marketing communication, has a significant influence on the formation of parents' position on vaccination of children, that is, trust in vaccines.

On the other hand, the ANOVA test and the eta coefficient confirmed that the country of origin of the respondents does not affect their attitude towards the vaccination of children. However, based on logistical regression, we concluded that, despite the fact that parents who come from these three different countries (Serbia, Montenegro, and Bosnia and Herzegovina) have approximately the same attitudes towards vaccines, the influence of online media on their attitude is different. It turned out that parents from Bosnia and Herzegovina are somewhat more susceptible to forming a negative attitude towards vaccines under the influence of online media than parents from Serbia and Montenegro. One of the potential reasons for this result may be found in the demographic characteristics of the respondents by country. While the demographic structure of the surveyed parents in Serbia and

Montenegro is approximately the same, in Bosnia and Herzegovina, certain deviations have been noticed, which primarily refer to the level of education. Namely, in Bosnia and Herzegovina, there is a smaller number of respondents with the highest education (1.7%) compared to respondents with other lower levels of education. The dominant education is high school (44.2%), which, according to the results of logistic regression, has the greatest chance of forming a negative attitude of parents towards vaccines based on online media.

Finally, the authors tried to investigate whether there was a difference in attitudes of parents coming from different countries, regarding the influence of online media on formation of attitudes. When it comes to potential differences in the analyzed countries, the results of the survey have shown that the attitudes of the parents are the same, regardless of whether the respondents are from Montenegro, Serbia, or Bosnia and Herzegovina ($\eta^2 = 0$). This should not be surprising having in mind the fact that these are developing countries, which have relatively similar legislation in the field of vaccination, and that all of them seek to harmonize public health policies in accordance with European standards. Thus, based on the above analysis, it may be noticed that there is no high value of deviation per state in the relation of the analyzed variable.

Based on all the above, we may conclude that there are a number of factors that affect parents' attitudes toward vaccinating children and that online media are an important factor that determines parental behavior. In addition, research has shown that social marketing may be an important determinant of strengthening trust in vaccines, as well as improving of public health.

5. Conclusions and Implications

Today, information technologies have changed the paradigm of communication between medical professionals and public. The wide availability of information through the penetration of the mass media has played a significant role in encouraging parents [70–72] to form attitudes based on facilitated access to the media, especially when it comes to online media.

Concerns about vaccination have become a global phenomenon and led to the search for answers to the question of who has the greatest influence on the parental attitude toward vaccination: medical professionals, internet, or family and social environment [73]. In this regard, the widespread availability of information through online sources plays a significant role in the formation of attitudes [74]. Accordingly, in recent years, the role of Facebook as a source of pro and antivaccine information has also been analyzed [75,76]. Hence, in this area, social marketing has become especially important, in which activities are aimed at changing or maintaining the behavior of people for the benefit of individuals and society as a whole.

A large number of studies have been published over the years on the degree of exposure to vaccines [18–20]. There is also research on the impact of certain forms of online media (e.g., different forms of social media) on parents' attitudes towards child vaccination. However, although several studies have examined parents' attitudes toward vaccination of children, few of them, according to the authors, have integrated research in the way given in this study. Thus, unlike most previous research on vaccines, in which arguments for or against vaccination were mainly emphasized, the authors wanted to determine if there was a correlation between online media and parents' attitudes towards vaccination through analysis in three countries in the Western Balkans region (Montenegro, Serbia, and Bosnia and Herzegovina), bringing the topic in the context of the application of social marketing in order to strengthen trust in vaccines and improve public health.

The authors developed and empirically tested a model that examined the relationship between influencing factors and parents' attitudes toward vaccination of children. The authors used advanced descriptive statistics, as well as the ANOVA method, which allows to determine the individual influences of the analyzed factors related to the attitudes of parents about the vaccination of children, especially through the prism of online media. Logistic regression was applied to obtain a more precise answer to the question of the relationship between the demographic characteristics of the respondents and their negative attitude towards vaccines based on information from the online media. Furthermore, in order to further examine the importance of a certain way of using online media on the formation of attitudes, i.e., parents' trust in vaccines, the eta-coefficient was used. The analysis of the η^2 coefficient showed that the greatest influence on the formation of attitudes, i.e., parents' trust in vaccines, when we look at the online media, have texts about the negative effects of vaccines that may be found on such sources.

The study has shown that the analyzed variables from the model have a significant influence on parents' attitudes toward vaccination of children, and that they strongly reflect on the level of confidence in vaccines. Further, the study has shown that their impact varied depending on the factor being observed.

These conclusions may create more implications for decision-makers.

Based on the achieved results, the authors suggest that decision-makers should pay more attention to contemporary forms of social marketing, as well as online media, in order to focus their potential more on improvement of public health, as well as to avoid the harmful impact that these forms of communication may have an opinion on vaccines. In a broader sense, the authors conclude that these forms of communication affect not only attitudes about vaccination but the improvement of public health, which opens space for further research on this topic.

Professional support must be present in all forms of application of online media and social marketing in the field of immunization as important segment of public health. In this regard, the provision of information by health professionals and the quality of their information are essential for the decision to vaccinate or otherwise [77,78], which is extremely important for communication through social media, which are very common today.

Decision makers have to be aware that positive attitudes are key to a high level of confidence and that it is necessary to integrate a number of factors in order to maximize the application of social marketing in the field of medicine and public health.

In addition to the practical, the authors believe that this paper has a significant theoretical contribution. Namely, these results, except expanding the base of empirical research on the application of online media and social marketing in order to strengthen the trust in vaccines, offer added value to the existing literature by analyzing this concept in different countries and according to different factors. Additionally, the analysis is brought into the context of improving public health, which makes the work a special value. Finally, this analysis goes beyond the national framework and presents an analysis in a multi-country context, thus contributing to theorizing on the topic of social marketing and online media in the field of medicine and public health in an international context.

Finally, having in mind actual debates on the far-reaching consequences that the world will suffer globally due to external shocks caused by the new Covid-19 corona pandemic, we believe that, in the future, more detailed analyses of the impact of online media on vaccine confidence may be conducted exactly in this area. Not only in less developed countries, but also in developing countries, it is evident that the effects of the pandemic of the new coronavirus Covid-19 will be manifested through direct influences on people's perception and attitudes about vaccination, especially when it comes to vaccination of children. In order to avoid the negative effects that online media may produce, decision-makers need to develop adequate online communication and social marketing strategies, for which the findings offered in this study may be very helpful and useful.

Author Contributions: Conceptualization, B.M., A.J.S., and B.D.; methodology, B.M. and T.B.V.; software, T.B.V.; validation, B.M., A.J.S., and B.D.; formal analysis, B.M., B.D., and E.B.; investigation, B.M. and A.J.S.; resources, B.M., B.D., and E.B.; data curation, B.M., A.J.S., B.D., and T.B.V.; writing—original draft preparation, B.M., A.J.S., and T.B.V.; writing—review and editing, B.M., B.D., and E.B.; visualization, B.D.; supervision, B.M. and B.D. All authors have read and agreed to the published version of the manuscript.

Funding: This research received no external funding.

Conflicts of Interest: The authors declare no conflict of interest.

Appendix A Survey: The Impact of Online Media on Parents' Attitudes toward Vaccination of Children

Respected,

This survey aims to determine the impact of online media on the attitudes of parents about the vaccination of children. The research is conducted for scientific purposes, with the aim of improving the situation in the subject area. The questionnaire contains 20 questions. The research is anonymous, and the results will be observed at the aggregate level.

Thank you for your participation!

1. Gender
   - Male
   - Female

2. Age
   - 18–24
   - 25–29
   - 30–34
   - 35–40
   - 41–45
   - More than 45

3. Country
   - Montenegro
   - Serbia
   - Bosnia and Herzegovina

4. Level of Education
   - Primary school
   - Secondary school
   - College
   - Faculty
   - Specialist
   - Master
   - PhD

5. Marital status
   - Married
   - Extramarital union
   - Divorced
   - Widow

6. Number of Children
   - 1
   - 2
   - 3
   - 4 and more

7. Did you do your own research about vaccines?

- Yes
- No

8. How did you inform yourself about vaccines?

    - Doctors
    - Family/relatives
    - Professional journals
    - Books
    - Flyers/brochures
    - Internet/social networks
    - Mass media (TV, newspapers, etc.)
    - Friends/associates
    - Other (please specify) _____

9. Which internet resources did you use when informing about vaccines?

    - Facebook
    - Other social media (Twitter, Instagram, etc.)
    - Wikipedia
    - Blogs/forums
    - Medical web sites
    - Other web resources (please specify) _____
    - I didn't use internet resources

10. Was your spouse included in collection of data about vaccination through online media?

    - Yes
    - No

11. Please rate your understanding of the materials that you collected through online media:

    - Little or no understanding at all
    - Poor understanding
    - Average understanding
    - Above average understanding
    - Complete understanding

12. During the research on online media, did you inform more about

    - Arguments about pro-vaccine
    - Arguments against vaccine

13. On the basis of information collected through online media, did you ask your child's pediatrician to provide you information about vaccination and/or education?

    - Yes
    - No

14. In which format the pediatrician presented you information?

    - Conversation
    - Brochures/informative sheets
    - Suggested web pages/online sources
    - Referring to media

- Other (please specify)

15. Do you share information about vaccines with other on social media?

    - Yes
    - No

16. Have you ever felt "the pressure" from pro- or anti-vaccine campaigns?

    - Yes, I have felt the "pressure" from pro-vaccines campaigns
    - Yes, I have felt the "pressure" from anti-vaccines campaigns
    - No, I haven't felt the "pressure" from pro-vaccines campaigns
    - No, I haven't felt the "pressure" from anti-vaccines campaigns

17. Rate your level of confidence in vaccines

    - I don't believe at all
    - Low level of trust
    - Neutral
    - High level of trust
    - I really completely believe

18. Please rate your attitude about following statements about vaccination:

    - Vaccination is necessary in order to prevent illnesses
    - I believe my pediatrician
    - Vaccinations should be individual choice of parents
    - Immunity of illness is better than immunity of vaccination
    - Vaccination is ideal: once vaccinated, children may not get the illness against which they were vaccinated
    - It is necessary to have as more vaccinations as possible
    - Without vaccination, a child may become ill and, consequently, cause others to get it.
    - Vaccines are also given for illnesses that children probably will not get.
    - Vaccination is mostly safe for children
    - Vaccines consist of harmful substances
    - Plan of vaccination includes too many vaccines at the same time
    - Children get more vaccines than is useful for them
    - Vaccinations are harmful and they should be avoided
    - I am satisfied with the efforts that the State (relevant institutions) put forth regarding the vaccination

Note: Likert's questions are rated on a scale from 1 to 5, where 1 = I completely disagree, 2 = I disagree, 3 = I cannot judge, 4 = I agree, and 5 = I completely agree.

19. Please rate your attitude about statements about the impact of online media about negative effects of vaccines

    - I regularly read texts in online media about negative effects of vaccines
    - Texts in online media about negative effects of vaccines significantly influence on my attitudes about vaccines
    - Texts in online media about negative effects of vaccines are mostly correct
    - Texts in online media about negative effects of vaccines are mostly based on fears and speculations, not on scientific facts

- Texts in online media about negative effects of vaccines today have more importance than they deserve

Note: Likert's questions are rated on a scale from 1 to 5, where 1 = I completely disagree, 2 = I disagree, 3 = I cannot judge, 4 = I agree, and 5 = I completely agree.

20. Which kind of online informing do you trust most:

- Social networks
- Medical web resources/sites
- Blogs
- Forums
- Online newspapers and magazines
- Other online resources _____

References

1. Camerini, L.; Diviani, N.; Tardini, S. Health virtual communities: Is the self lost in the net? *Soc. Semiot.* **2010**, *20*, 87–102. [CrossRef]
2. Percheski, C.; Hargittai, E. Health information-seeking in the digital age. *J. Am. Coll. Health* **2011**, *59*, 379–386. [CrossRef] [PubMed]
3. Vaterlaus, J.M.; Patten, E.V.; Roche, C.; Young, J.A. #Gettinghealthy: The perceived influence of social media on young adult health behaviors. *Comput. Hum. Behav.* **2015**, *45*, 151–157. [CrossRef]
4. Fox, S.; Duggan, M. Health Online Pew Internet & American Life Project, 2013, 1–4. Available online: http://www.pewinternet.org/~{}/media/Files/Reports/PIP_HealthOnline.pdf%5Cnhttp://www.pewinternet.org/2013/01/15/health-online-2013/# (accessed on 22 February 2020).
5. Eysenbach, G.; Powell, J.; Kuss, O.; Sa, E.R. Empirical studies assessing the quality of health information for consumers on the world wide web. *JAMA* **2002**, *287*, 2691–2700. [CrossRef]
6. Ghenai, A. Health misinformation in search and social media. In *Proceedings of the 2017 International Conference on Information Technology–ICIT December, 2017*; Association for Computing Machinery (ACM): New York, NY, USA, 2017; pp. 235–236.
7. Oyeyemi, S.O.; Gabarron, E.; Wynn, R. Ebola, Twitter, and misinformation: A dangerous combination? *BMJ* **2014**, *349*, g6178. [CrossRef]
8. Piscaglia, L. *Internet and Social Media: Influence on the Parent's Vaccination Decision*; Applied Research Projects; University of Tennessee Health Science Center: Memphis, TN, USA, 2016.
9. Kao, C.M.; Schneyer, R.J.; Bocchini, J.A. Child and adolescent immunizations. *Curr. Opin. Pediatr.* **2014**, *26*, 383–395. [CrossRef]
10. Heikkinen, T.; Tsolia, M.; Finn, A. Vaccination of healthy children against seasonal influenza. *Pediatr. Infect. Dis. J.* **2013**, *32*, 881–888. [CrossRef]
11. Centers for Disease Control and Prevention. Immunization Coverage in the U.S. Centers for Disease Control and Prevention. 2010. Available online: http://www.cdc.gov/vaccines/stats-surv/imz-coverage.htm (accessed on 9 March 2020).
12. Weycker, D.; Edelsberg, J.; Halloran, M.E.; Longini, I.M.; Nizam, A.; Ciuryla, V.; Oster, G. Population-wide benefits of routine vaccination of children against influenza. *Vaccine* **2005**, *23*, 1284–1293. [CrossRef]
13. Jordan, R.; Connock, M.; Albon, E.; Frysmith, A.; Olowokure, B.; Hawker, J.; Burls, A. Universal vaccination of children against influenza: Are there indirect benefits to the community? A systematic review of the evidence. *Vaccine* **2006**, *24*, 1047–1062. [CrossRef]
14. Mirelman, A.J.; Ballard, S.B.; Saito, M.; Kosek, M.; Gilman, R.H. Cost-effectiveness of norovirus vaccination in children in Peru. *Vaccine* **2015**, *33*, 3084–3091. [CrossRef]
15. Shakerian, S.; Lakeh, M.M.; Esteghamati, A.; Zahraei, S.M.; Yaghoubi, M. Cost-effectiveness of rotavirus vaccination for under-five children in Iran. *Iran. J. Pediatr.* **2015**, *25*, 2766. [CrossRef] [PubMed]

16. Feikin, D.R.; Flannery, B.; Hamel, M.J.; Stack, M.; Hansen, P.M. Vaccines for children in low and middle-income countries. In *Reproductive, Maternal, New–Born, and Child Health: Disease Control Priorities*, 3rd ed.; Black, R.E., Walker, N., Laxminarayan, R., Temmerman, M., Eds.; The International Bank for Reconstruction and Development/The World Bank: Washington, DC, USA, 2015; Volume 2, p. 3.
17. Larson, H.J.; De Figueiredo, A.; Xiahong, Z.; Schulz, W.S.; Verger, P.; Johnston, I.G.; Cook, A.R.; Jones, N.S. The state of vaccine confidence 2016: Global insights through a 67-country survey. *EBioMedicine* **2016**, *12*, 295–301. [CrossRef] [PubMed]
18. Smith, J.C.; Appleton, M.; Macdonald, N. Building confidence in vaccines. In *Hot Topics in Infection and Immunity in Children IX*; Springer and LLC: New York, NY, USA, 2013; Volume 764, pp. 81–98.
19. Larson, H.; de Figueiredo, A.; Karafillakis, E.; Rawal, M. *State of Vaccine Confidence in the EU 2018*; European Union: Luxembourg, 2018.
20. Nowak, G.; Cacciatore, M.A. Parents' confidence in recommended childhood vaccinations: Extending the assessment, expanding the context. *Hum. Vaccines Immunother.* **2016**, *13*, 687–700. [CrossRef]
21. Jung, M.; Lin, L.; Viswanath, K. Effect of media use on mothers' vaccination of their children in sub-Saharan Africa. *Vaccine* **2015**, *33*, 2551–2557. [CrossRef] [PubMed]
22. Yaqub, O.; Castle-Clarke, S.; Sevdalis, N.; Chataway, J. Attitudes to vaccination: A critical review. *Soc. Sci. Med.* **2014**, *112*, 1–11. [CrossRef]
23. Larson, II.J.; Jarrett, C.; Eckersberger, E.; Smith, D.M.; Paterson, P. Understanding vaccine hesitancy around vaccines and vaccination from a global perspective: A systematic review of published literature, 2007–2012. *Vaccine* **2014**, *32*, 2150–2159. [CrossRef]
24. Jarrett, C.; Wilson, R.; O'Leary, M.; Eckersberger, E.; Larson, H.J.; SAGE Working Group on Vaccine Hesitancy. Strategies for addressing vaccine hesitancy—A systematic review. *Vaccine* **2015**, *33*, 4180–4190. [CrossRef]
25. Wakefield, A.J. MMR vaccination and autism. *Lancet* **1999**, *354*, 949–950. [CrossRef]
26. Parliament of Montenegro. Law on Protection of the Population from Infectious Diseases. 2018. Available online: http://zakoni.skupstina.me/zakoni/web/dokumenta/zakoni-i-drugi-akti/327/1613-10375-28-2-17-3-4.pdf (accessed on 29 July 2020).
27. Punished 150 Parents Who Did Not Vaccinate Their Children. Available online: https://medicalcg.me/11-februar-kaznjeno-150-roditelja-koji-nisu-vakcinisali-djecu/ (accessed on 29 July 2020).
28. Punished 150 Parents Who Did Not Vaccinate Their Children. Available online: https://www.adriaticnews.eu/2020/02/11/kaznjeno-150-roditelja-bez-vakcine-8-000-djece/ (accessed on 29 July 2020).
29. The World Health Organization (WHO). Ten Threats to Global Health in 2019. Available online: https://www.who.int/news-room/feature-stories/ten-threats-to-global-health-in-2019 (accessed on 30 July 2020).
30. Guillaume, L.R.; Bath, P.A. The impact of health scares on parents' information needs and preferred information sources: A case study of the MMR vaccine scare. *Health Informatics J.* **2004**, *10*, 5–22. [CrossRef]
31. Smith, N.; Graham, T. Mapping the anti-vaccination movement on Facebook. *Inf. Commun. Soc.* **2017**, *22*, 1310–1327. [CrossRef]
32. Betsch, C.; Brewer, N.T.; Brocard, P.; Davies, P.; Gaissmaier, W.; Haase, N.; Leask, J.; Renkewitz, F.; Renner, B.; Reyna, V.F.; et al. Opportunities and challenges of Web 2.0 for vaccination decisions. *Vaccine* **2012**, *30*, 3727–3733. [CrossRef]
33. French, J.; Blair-Stevens, C.; McVey, D.; Merritt, R. *Social Marketing and Public Health: Theory and Practice*, 1st ed.; Oxford University Press: London, UK, 2010; pp. 1059–1082.
34. Flaskerud, J.H. The nanny state, free will, and public health. *Issues Ment. Health Nurs.* **2013**, *35*, 69–72. [CrossRef] [PubMed]
35. Xu, Z.; Guo, H. Using text mining to compare online pro- and anti-vaccine headlines: Word usage, sentiments, and online popularity. *Commun. Stud.* **2017**, *69*, 103–122. [CrossRef]
36. Jones, A.M.; Omer, S.B.; Bednarczyk, R.A.; Halsey, N.A.; Moulton, L.H.; Salmon, D.A. Parents' source of vaccine information and impact on vaccine attitudes, beliefs, and nonmedical exemptions. *Adv. Prev. Med.* **2012**, *2012*, 932741. [CrossRef] [PubMed]
37. Salmon, D.A.; Moulton, L.H.; Omer, S.B.; Dehart, M.P.; Stokley, S.; Halsey, N.A. Factors associated with refusal of childhood vaccines among parents of school-aged children. *Arch. Pediatr. Adolesc. Med.* **2005**, *159*, 470–476. [CrossRef]
38. Tafuri, S.; Gallone, M.; Cappelli, M.; Martinelli, D.; Prato, R.; Germinario, C. Addressing the anti-vaccination movement and the role of HCWs. *Vaccine* **2014**, *32*, 4860–4865. [CrossRef]

39. Wakefield, M.; Loken, B.; Hornik, R.C. Use of mass media campaigns to change health behaviour. *Lancet* **2010**, *376*, 1261–1271. [CrossRef]
40. Dubé, E.; Vivion, M.; MacDonald, N.E. Vaccine hesitancy, vaccine refusal and the anti-vaccine movement: Influence, impact and implications. *Expert Rev. Vaccines* **2014**, *14*, 99–117. [CrossRef]
41. Grant, L.; Hausman, B.; Cashion, M.; Lucchesi, N.; Patel, K.; Roberts, J.; Koerber, A.; Lawrence, H. Vaccination persuasion online: A qualitative study of two provaccine and two vaccine-skeptical websites. *J. Med. Internet Res.* **2015**, *17*, e133. [CrossRef]
42. Kata, A. A postmodern Pandora's box: Anti-vaccination misinformation on the Internet. *Vaccine* **2010**, *28*, 1709–1716. [CrossRef]
43. Cameron, C.D.; Payne, B.K. Escaping affect: How motivated emotion regulation creates insensitivity to mass suffering. *J. Pers. Soc. Psychol.* **2011**, *100*, 1–15. [CrossRef] [PubMed]
44. Larson, H.J.; Cooper, L.Z.; Eskola, J.; Katz, S.L.; Ratzan, S. Addressing the vaccine confidence gap. *Lancet* **2011**, *378*, 526–535. [CrossRef]
45. Bean, S.J. Emerging and continuing trends in vaccine opposition website content*. *Vaccine* **2011**, *29*, 1874–1880. [CrossRef] [PubMed]
46. Quattrociocchi, W. Part 2-Social and Political Challenges: 2.1 Western Democracy in Crisis? World Economic Forum [Internet]. 2017. Available online: http://reports.weforum.org/global-risks-2017/part-2-social-and-political-challenges/2-1-western-democracy-in-crisis/ (accessed on 29 October 2019).
47. Brown, J.; Broderick, A.J.; Lee, N. Word of mouth communication within online communities: Conceptualizing the online social network. *J. Interact. Mark.* **2007**, *21*, 2–20. [CrossRef]
48. Quattrociocchi, W.; Caldarelli, G.; Scala, A. Opinion dynamics on interacting networks: Media competition and social influence. *Sci. Rep.* **2014**, *4*, 4938. [CrossRef] [PubMed]
49. Diekema, D.S. Responding to parental refusals of immunization of children. *Pediatrics* **2005**, *115*, 1428–1431. [CrossRef] [PubMed]
50. Ruiz, J.B.; Bell, R.A. Understanding vaccination resistance: Vaccine search term selection bias and the valence of retrieved information. *Vaccine* **2014**, *32*, 5776–5780. [CrossRef] [PubMed]
51. Davies, P.; Chapman, S.; Leask, J. Antivaccination activists on the world wide web. *Arch. Dis. Child.* **2002**, *87*, 22–25. [CrossRef]
52. Zimmerman, R.; Wolfe, R.E.; Fox, D.; Fox, J.R.; Nowalk, M.P.A.; Troy, J.; Sharp, L.K.; Nasir, L.; Leask, J. Vaccine criticism on the world wide web. *J. Med. Internet Res.* **2005**, *7*, e17. [CrossRef]
53. Brown, K.F.; Fraser, G.; Ramsay, M.M.; Shanley, R.; Cowley, N.; Van Wijgerden, J.; Toff, P.; Falconer, M.; Hudson, M.; Green, J.; et al. Attitudinal and demographic predictors of measles-mumps-rubella vaccine (MMR) uptake during the UK catch-up campaign 2008–09: Cross-sectional survey. *PLoS ONE* **2011**, *6*, e19381. [CrossRef]
54. Anderberg, D.; Chevalier, A.; Wadsworth, J. Anatomy of a health scare: Education, income and the MMR controversy in the UK. *J. Health Econ.* **2011**, *30*, 515–530. [CrossRef] [PubMed]
55. Walsh, S.; Thomas, D.R.; Mason, B.W.; Evans, M.R. The impact of the media on the decision of parents in South Wales to accept measles-mumps-rubella (MMR) immunization. *Epidemiol. Infect.* **2014**, *143*, 550–560. [CrossRef] [PubMed]
56. Ristić, M.; Šeguljev, Z.; Petrović, V.; Vuleković, V.; Dugandžija, T. The influence of sociodemographic characteristics of parents on immunization coverage of children. *Opšta Med.* **2013**, *19*, 1–2.
57. Hoek, J.; Jones, S.C. Regulation, public health and social marketing: A behaviour change trinity. *J. Soc. Mark.* **2011**, *1*, 32–44. [CrossRef]
58. Giubilini, A. *The Ethics of Vaccination*; Palgrave MacMillan: London, UK; LLC: New York, NY, USA, 2019. [CrossRef]
59. Braczkowska, B.; Kowalska, M.; Baranski, K.; Gajda, M.; Kurowski, T.E.; Zejda, J. Parental opinions and attitudes about children's vaccination safety in Silesian Voivodeship, Poland. *Int. J. Environ. Res. Public Health* **2018**, *15*, 756. [CrossRef]
60. Hair, J.F.; Black, W.C.; Babin, B.J.; Anderson, R.E.; Tatham, R.L. *Multivariate Data Analysis*; Prentice Hall Pearson Education: Upper Saddle River, NJ, USA, 2006.
61. Tabachnick, B.G.; Fidell, L.S. *Using Multivariate Statistics*, 5th ed.; Pearson Education: Boston, MA, USA, 2007.
62. Fisher, R.A. Statistical methods for research workers. In *Springer Series in Statistics*; Springer Science and Business Media LLC: New York, NY, USA, 1992; pp. 66–70.

63. Fisher, R.A. *Statistical Methods for Research Workers*; Oliver & Boyd: Edinburgh, UK, 1925; Available online: http://www.haghish.com/resources/materials/Statistical_Methods_for_Research_Workers.pdf (accessed on 29 July 2020).
64. Rinker, T. *On the Treatment of Likert Data*; Department of Learning and Instruction, University of Buffalo: New York, NY, USA, 2016.
65. Carifio, J.; Perla, R. Resolving the 50-year debate around using and misusing Likert scales. *Med. Educ.* **2008**, *42*, 1150–1152. [CrossRef]
66. Norman, G. Likert scales, levels of measurement and the "laws" of statistics. *Adv. Health Sci. Educ.* **2010**, *15*, 625–632. [CrossRef]
67. Hosmer, D.W.; Lemeshow, S. *Applied Logistic Regression*; John Wiley & Sons: New York, NY, USA, 2000.
68. Wade, G.H. Nurses as primary advocates for immunization adherence. *MCN, Am. J. Matern. Nurs.* **2014**, *39*, 351–356. [CrossRef]
69. Lee, S.; Riley-Behringer, M.; Rose, J.C.; Meropol, S.B.; Lazebnik, R. Parental vaccine acceptance: A logistic regression model using previsit decisions. *Clin. Pediatr.* **2016**, *56*, 716–722. [CrossRef]
70. Tones, K.; Green, J. *Health Promotion: Planning and Strategies*; Sage: London, UK, 2004.
71. Kar, S.B.; Pascual, C.A.; Chickering, K.L. Empowerment of women for health promotion: A meta-analysis. *Soc. Sci. Med.* **1999**, *49*, 1431–1460. [CrossRef]
72. Ehrhardt, A.A.; Sawires, S.; McGovern, T.; Peacock, D.; Weston, M. Gender, empowerment, and health: What is it? how does it work? *J. Acquir. Immune Defic. Syndr.* **2009**, *51*, S96–S105. [CrossRef] [PubMed]
73. Charron, J.; Gautier, A.; Jestin, C. Influence of information sources on vaccine hesitancy and practices. *Med. Mal. Infect.* **2020**, 1–7. [CrossRef] [PubMed]
74. Lane, S.; Macdonald, N.E.; Marti, M.; Dumolard, L. Vaccine hesitancy around the globe: Analysis of three years of WHO/UNICEF joint reporting form data-2015-2017. *Vaccine* **2018**, *36*, 3861–3867. [CrossRef]
75. Gandhi, C.K.; Patel, J.; Zhan, X. Trend of influenza vaccine Facebook posts in last 4 years: A content analysis. *Am. J. Infect. Control.* **2020**, *48*, 361–367. [CrossRef] [PubMed]
76. Owłasiuk, A.; Bielska, D.; Gryko, A.; Marcinowicz, L.; Czajkowski, M.; Kleosin, K.N.P.H.C.I. Child vaccination programme in family doctor practices in 1997–2015: A cross-sectional study in Białystok, Poland. *Pediatr. Med. Rodz.* **2018**, *14*, 189–200. [CrossRef]
77. Czajka, H.; Czajka, S.; Biłas, P.; Pałka, P.; Jędrusik, S.; Czapkiewicz, A. Who or what influences the individuals' decision-making process regarding vaccinations? *Int. J. Environ. Res. Public Health* **2020**, *17*, 4461. [CrossRef]
78. Lewandowska, A.; Lewandowski, T.; Rudzki, G.; Rudzki, S.; Laskowska, B. Opinions and knowledge of parents regarding preventive vaccinations of children and causes of reluctance toward preventive vaccinations. *Int. J. Environ. Res. Public Health* **2020**, *17*, 3694. [CrossRef]

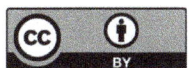

© 2020 by the authors. Licensee MDPI, Basel, Switzerland. This article is an open access article distributed under the terms and conditions of the Creative Commons Attribution (CC BY) license (http://creativecommons.org/licenses/by/4.0/).

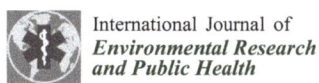

Article

Topic Modeling and User Network Analysis on Twitter during World Lupus Awareness Day

Salvatore Pirri [1,*], Valentina Lorenzoni [1], Gianni Andreozzi [1], Marta Mosca [2] and Giuseppe Turchetti [1]

[1] Institute of Management, Scuola Superiore Sant'Anna, 56127 Pisa, Italy; v.lorenzoni@santannapisa.it (V.L.); g.andreozzi@santannapisa.it (G.A.); giuseppe.turchetti@santannapisa.it (G.T.)
[2] Rheumatology Unit, Department of Clinical and Experimental Medicine, Università di Pisa, 56126 Pisa, Italy; marta.mosca@med.unipi.it
* Correspondence: s.pirri@santannapisa.it; Tel.: +39-328-032-2201

Received: 20 June 2020; Accepted: 24 July 2020; Published: 28 July 2020

Abstract: Twitter is increasingly used by individuals and organizations to broadcast their feelings and practices, providing access to samples of spontaneously expressed opinions on all sorts of themes. Social media offers an additional source of data to unlock information supporting new insights disclosures, particularly for public health purposes. Systemic lupus erythematosus (SLE) is a complex, systemic autoimmune disease that remains a major challenge in therapeutic diagnostic and treatment management. When supporting patients with such a complex disease, sharing information through social media can play an important role in creating better healthcare services. This study explores the nature of topics posted by users and organizations on Twitter during world Lupus day to extract latent topics that occur in tweet texts and to identify what information is most commonly discussed among users. We identified online influencers and opinion leaders who discussed different topics. During this analysis, we found two different types of influencers that employed different narratives about the communities they belong to. Therefore, this study identifies hidden information for healthcare decision-makers and provides a detailed model of the implications for healthcare organizations to detect, understand, and define hidden content behind large collections of text.

Keywords: social media; Twitter; systemic lupus erythematosus (SLE); network analysis; topic modeling; text analysis

1. Introduction

In recent years, the way in which researchers' results, discoveries, and knowledge have been disseminated has changed significantly. The advancement of Internet technology has enabled the rise of social media platforms such as Facebook, Twitter, Reddit, and others to serve as channels where people interact, share opinions, and debate. These forums create communities where people establish relationships and interactions among themselves.

These online communities can influence and can be influenced by other online communities. This spread of influence plays a major role in the spreading of information, some of which may affect people's offline behavior [1].

Content produced on social media can spread quickly throughout these communities, triggering rumors and cascading effects that can deeply influence political decisions, economic choices, social well-being, perceptions, and beliefs [2].

The use of social media text analysis and social network detection is not new in the public health field. Many studies have investigated the areas of forecasting clinical surveillance [3,4] and misinformation within and across health communities [5]. These studies contain considerable evidence suggesting that technology has been useful in the health domain, generating considerable awareness on social media, and helping people who live in remote areas [6] or who have little access to treatment [7].

Most of these studies have focused on epidemic and infectious diseases, while in the field of chronic diseases efforts have been mainly devoted to well-known diseases like diabetes or cardiovascular disease [8]. To our knowledge, little effort has been made to investigate the online communities' dynamics around rare and complex rheumatic diseases, such as systemic lupus erythematosus (SLE), which is a chronic autoimmune disease whose management is still challenging due to the variety and complexity of the symptoms. These challenges greatly impact SLE patients' quality of life and social activities [9]. Additionally, SLE also faces significant and complex unmet needs that must be dealt with [10], such as diagnostic delay and high burden of therapy [11], which puts pressure on healthcare costs.

Despite this lack of deep investigation of the social media interaction phenomenon for this complex rheumatic disease, patient associations, healthcare communities, blog pages, and patients are active on social media in order to seek information and increase awareness among the general public. In most cases, patients use these channels for emotional and peer health support [12,13], often searching for new treatments or healthcare decision suggestions [14].

Literature Review

Literature on social media analysis has been previously analyzed in different applications that explore the pivotal role played by people's perspective and community interactions to obtain worthwhile information for healthcare decision-making [15]. Applications of social media analysis for collecting information on behavioral patterns have previously been proposed under different conditions and with different purposes. In cancer, for instance, content analysis of discussions related to medication use and side effects [16] showed how the internet can be a valuable way for individuals to report side effects, and how healthcare professionals can support an effective medication adherence plan by monitoring the social media discussion. Another example can be found in tweets about diabetes and diets [17], emphasizing how some users acting as diabetes advocates can spread information and serve as opinion leaders, thus influencing others' attitudes and behavior [18].

Other studies have reported the beneficial effects of higher patient satisfaction and patient engagement when hospitals create valuable social media interaction and strategy, providing better value for the hospitals adopting such a policies [19].

A recent literature review [20] that explored the effects of social media interaction on patient and healthcare professional relationships pointed out how patients mainly use social media for social support, which is represented through information support, emotional support, esteem support, and network support.

One of the main advantages of Twitter is the fact that users can express themselves freely, reducing the bias effect that often affects other types of investigation methods, such as online surveys or interviews [21]. On the other hand, it is important to consider the risks of using Twitter in social and healthcare research given the unrepresentativeness of the user community, the spread of misinformation, and difficulties in verifying the credibility of sources.

However, we believe that perspectives and views held by community members and expressed on social media platforms represent a good proxy of feelings and attitudes that might influence decision-making of other communities or users. Identifying as precisely as possible the content of these feelings and attitudes would improve the development of a tailored strategy for public health issues.

Analyzing the network dynamics and the role played by key users in the network community (such as influencers and opinion leaders) offers a gatekeeping tool to understand how information enters, flows, and spreads throughout the communities, and who drives it.

2. Methods

The objectives of this study were (1) to investigate and identify the common themes that spread on Twitter during World Lupus Day and to (2) detect the communities' network dynamics, identifying "influencers" and their communities' features.

2.1. Proposed Methodology

Using Twitter public streaming API, tweets released on the 10th of May 2019 containing at least one of the following words or hashtags were collected and analyzed: #WorldLupusDay, #lupus, #SystemicLupusErythematosus, or #SLE. A total number of 4434 (including retweets) tweets took into account information (i.e., time, location, sources, retweets, retweet count, follower count, and friend count) were collected. Tweets came from 2813 unique users. R software was used for the analyses.

A comprehensive analysis flow is presented in Figure 1. Following the scheme of social media analytics [22], it is possible to extract patterns, discover hidden information, and outline network interactions among online communities by mining the health discussions.

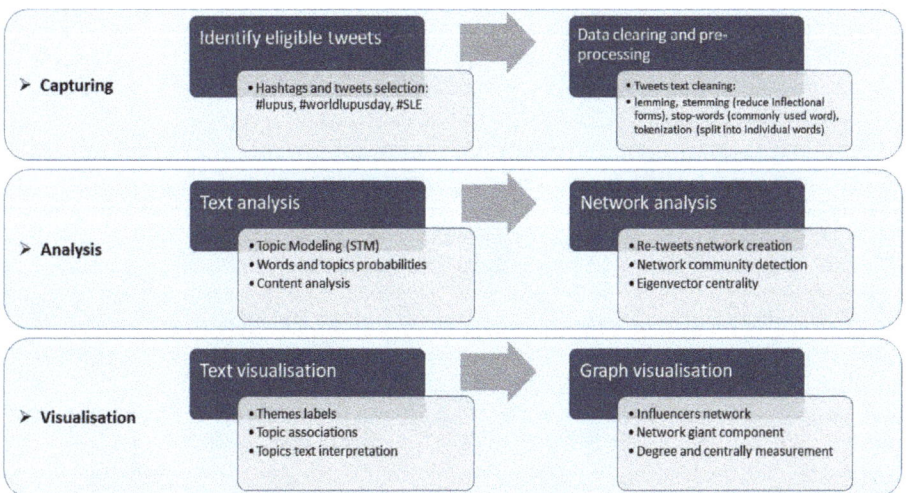

Figure 1. Framework workflow of social media Twitter analysis.

In stage one (capturing), we collected tweet texts and information containing keywords or hashtags released on Lupus Day through the Twitter API. Next, data-cleaning and pre-processing were applied to the entire dataset obtained. In stage two, we performed data analysis using two main techniques: (a) text analysis/natural processing languages through word frequencies, n-gram, and topic modeling, and (b) network analysis and measurements (statistics and scores of the network under investigation). Stage three focused on results visualization. Visualization techniques, such as bar-charts, histograms, network graphs, and other visualization types, assumed a key role in interpreting and presenting results.

2.2. Data Cleaning and Pre-Processing

Data were gathered to employ retweet [23] packages belonging in the R software. On the basis of data collected, the influencer score and network influence score were calculated. The influencer score represents a proxy to identify the small percentage of users who have a large connection (followers) to a large audience who follow them and have established a sort of trust in which their posted content creates perceived influence [24]. On the other hand, the network influence score, which is based on the number of retweets received by other users, represents a sort of endorsement of a specific content or message shared. The further a tweet spreads, the more influence the user has.

We can summarize the two scores by saying that the first score is more oriented toward the enormous attraction of followers one is able to obtain based on shared lifestyles, opinions, and textual content [25]. The second score is more based on the attention and endorsement that a tweet content (or a set of tweets) is able to achieve, being shared throughout a user network in a certain span of time [26].

Despite the efforts and increasing interest in properly measuring and assessing an influencer's score, when detecting a user's ability to maximize and spread content and thus shape followers' perceptions and behavior there is still a clear lack of widely recognized measures that are able to do so [27]. Nevertheless, some studies, especially from marketing literature [28,29], have developed robust measures to gain solid proxies of the social media influencers' effect. In our study, we obtained the influencers score, aggregating the performance of Twitter indicators addressed by Anger Isabel and Kittl Christian [30]. The score index was calculated as the average of the sum of three different ratios: the ratio between the number of followers over the number of following (R_f); the retweets and mention ratio (R_{rt}), which is calculated as total retweet count over the total number of tweets created; and the interaction ratio (R_i) obtained dividing total retweets count by the number of followers. The aggregation of three independent ratios reduced the possibility of misinterpretation based on the mass-followers effect. Nevertheless, it is important to keep in mind that other measures exist, which could integrate even more sophisticated scores [29].

2.3. Network Analysis

The scoring index for the network influence score (ii) takes into account typical approaches from social network analysis, which considers independent indexes from graph theory [31], i.e., betweenness centrality, out-degree, PageRank, and others. To detect influencer users in the network dynamics, we considered retweets as a proxy to represent an endorsement to the tweet content shared by the user. The modularity [32] detection algorithm was employed to identify communities (clusters) that compose retweet network. Basically, the modularity algorithm divides a network into a set of clusters where each node (user) belongs to only one cluster. It measures the strength of the identified clusters in the network where modularity group nodes exhibit high density with each other. The Force Atlas 2 [33] algorithm was employed to visualize the network layout. It is a force-based algorithm that draws linked nodes closer while pushing unrelated nodes farther, addressing hubs in clusters. This visualization provides a readable representation of the entire graph.

As a score index, the eigenvector centrality [34] was employed to determine the influencer nodes. Eigenvector centrality is a measure of the node's importance in the entire network weighed on the nodes' connection. For our purposes, this was the most suitable index to identify influencer nodes [35]. To calculate and compute the network analysis, score, and visualizations, we used Gephi software [36].

2.4. Text Analysis and Topic Modeling

Topic modeling is a branch of unsupervised methodology for the natural processing language applied to analyze and extract topics from a corpus of documents. This approach fit the text analysis for Twitter content quite well. Considering, the unsupervised nature of the topic modelling method, it was possible to identify the thematic structure (topics) within the set of tweet texts without any prior data manipulation, like text-labeling or training dataset. Topic modeling application allowed the discovery of the thematic structure in a large corpus of text, making it possible to organize, summarize, and visualize the latent themes and patterns present in any kind of text corpus [37].

The most common topic modeling approach used was the latent Dirichlet allocation (LDA) [38], which is a generative probabilistic model assuming that a document is composed of a set of (latent) topics, where each topic is composed of a set of words. This approach can be thought of as a classification method instead of a numerical feature or collection of words one could group together in a meaningful way. See Figure A1 in the Appendix A for more details.

A recent application that can expand the ability of the LDA framework to gain valuable results from a large corpus of text is structured topic modeling (STM) [39]. STM provides the possibility of considering metadata associated with the text, such as the author of the tweet, the associated numerical score, and other characteristics of the overall dataset using document-level covariates. After identification of the latent topic, using the stm R package [40], we estimated the effect influencer score and network influencer score as covariates had on topic prevalence, exploring whether and which topics had a higher probability of appearing in tweet texts, aiming to investigate whether different topics were used in different ways. See Figure A2 in the Appendix A.

3. Results

From the dataset composed of 4434 tweets, a network to analyze the network influencer score was created involving 2813 unique users and employing a direct graph. Each node represented a user and the edge between two nodes was established when a user's tweet was retweeted. We considered the giant component network and the smaller disconnected components were dropped out (18.3%). More details on the network analysis are provided in the Appendix A. See Figures A6 and A7.

The size of the nodes was proportional to the number of social connections based on the number of retweets a specific user received. Nodes and edges had the same color if they were linked to each other, making the detection of communities possible. The node position in the network was determined by a heuristic that attempted to locate nodes connected closer together, which thus revealed the communities' structure. See Figure 2.

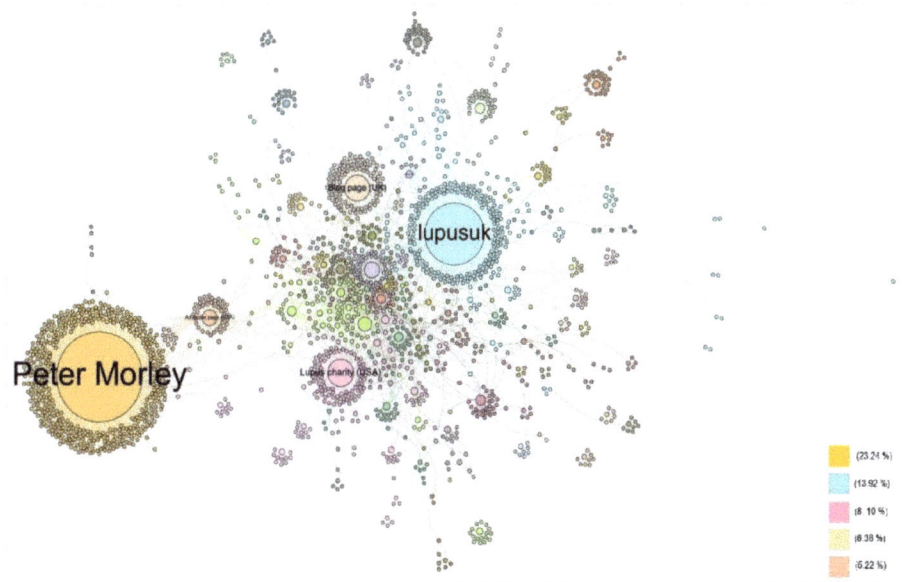

Figure 2. Retweet network analysis.

The community detection algorithm found 25 communities (clusters). The top five communities accounted for more than 55% of all network connections. Applying the eigenvector centrality algorithm to detect the most influential users, five nodes emerged as the most influential. These five users received more attention, intended as the number of retweets, allowing them to catalyze a vast amount of attention based on their tweet text content shared. We asked the top influencers identified for their permission to display their account name. Four of them consented to display their names; for the others, we used anonymized acronyms to identify the account type.

As reported in Table 1, only one account appeared in both influencer scores. This was due to the fact that the two scores were intended to measure different dynamics. Nevertheless, considering the specificity of the dataset collected, in this case it was also true that two different types of influencers played a different role and showed different features in attracting attention based on their posted content. Interestingly, the highest scored user was Peter Morley, whose network is weakly connected with the rest of the main users' connections. He is easily visible in Figure 2 with his peripheral position in the network structure.

Table 1. Top scored influencers.

Title	Screen Name	Influencer Score	Screen Name	Network Influencer Score
1	Integrated clinical Hospital; USA	35.182	Peter Morley	0.99
2	information boards Blog; UK	26.257	lupusuk	0.66
3	Physiopedia	21.259	Information boards Blog; UK	0.37
4	Newspaper; South Africa	20.830	Advocate page; USA	0.28
5	Radio; Nigeria	12.814	Lupus charity; USA	0.24
6	HibbsLupusTrust	12.271	Charity; UK	0.18

After the influencer score analysis and the network relationship measurement, tweet text analysis was employed. We adopted STM on the entire tweet text dataset.

When performing STM, several steps need to be addressed before reaching the final evaluation, including the identification of the proper number of topics (k) that better represents the number of themes in the text corpus. Different approaches exist; no one is more correct than the others. In our analysis, we based the optimal number of latent topic on "Griffiths" [41] and "CaoJuan" [42], which are metric scores implemented in the ldatuning package [43] that use the log-likelihood method via Gibbs sampling. Griffiths metrics maximize likelihood, while CaoJuan metrics minimize divergence between topics. As a result, the optimal number of topics (k) for our dataset was 12 topics. In the Appendix A, Figure A3, the optimal number of topic plots is provided.

Another step in the STM that needs to be addressed before reaching the final evaluation is the choice of the model that best estimates the possible outcome. There are different initialization parameters that need to be evaluated, discarding models with low likelihood values [40]. Even in this case, there is no ground truth approach. However, assessing the quality of the models by considering the trade-off between semantic coherence [44] and exclusivity [39] for each topic within the model is one of the most suitable approaches. The semantic coherence metric is related to pointwise mutual information that measures the most probable words in a specific topic that occur together. The exclusivity measure includes information on word frequency employed in the FREX metric [45]. These measures provide the distinctness of the topics, making possible a comparison of the highest scores, ensuring the quality of the model selected. Plots and results of the selected model are provided in the Appendix A Figures A4 and A5.

The results of the topic model are shown in Figure 3. Specific words were linked to specific topics accordingly with their (beta) β probabilities of belonging to the topic. Topic labels were not automatically generated. Label selection was the moment when researchers analyzed the results after the parameter setting to check what emerged from the model's execution, and to decide whether the emerged allocation was coherent, or if more model executions were needed. In our case, for each topic a specific label was identified using the authors' judgment obtained through an open discussion until a consensus was reached. Indeed, topics were interpreted and labelled on the basis of the probability of each word belonging to each specific topic.

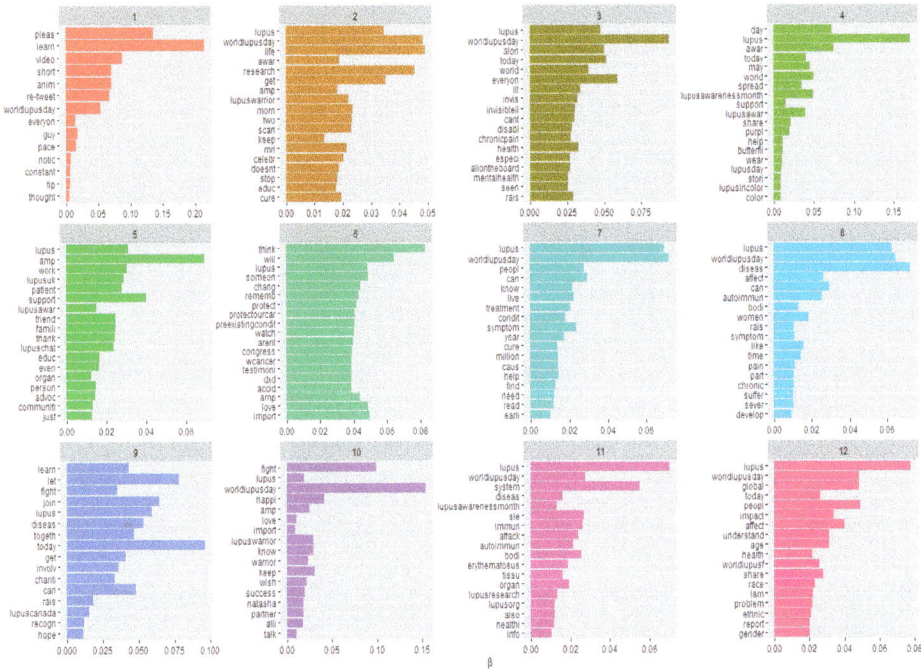

Figure 3. Topics and themes identified in the tweet text corpus.

In doing so, we also checked the most representative tweets related to the topics, to better understand the meaning of the topics by inspecting highly correlated tweet texts. A sample of the topics and the associated tweets are reported in Table 2.

Table 2. Most representative tweet texts and topic label selection.

Learning and sharing (topic 1):
"To anyone with Lupus, it does get better. With time you learn your triggers, you learn to pace yourself and most importantly you learn to listen to your own body."; "Help us spread awareness for #lupus on #WorldLupusDay!" "Learn more about #lupus brain fog and get tips for coping with it in our article at."
Information and advice (topic 2):
"Do eat a healthy, balanced diet try to stay active when you're having a flare-up try walking or swimming get lots of rest try relaxation techniques to manage stress"; "stress can make symptoms worse." "For information about available support, please take a look at our article here."
Feeling loneliness (topic 3):
"Invisible. For everyone with a disability or an illness that can't be seen. YOU are not alone, WE are not alone. Today is #WorldLupusDay and we are especially thinking of everyone in the world who has #Lupus #invisibleillness #chronicpain #health #mentalhealth."
"In conjunction of special day for this invisible illness I would like to encourage everybody to appreciate your health and for all Lupus fighter in the world."

Table 2. *Cont.*

Spread awareness (topic 4):
"MAY 10 is WORLD LUPUS DAY! Spread Lupus Awareness share the Lupus In Color Butterfly Woman. Spread Lupus Awareness Today!"; "Today is World Lupus Day! Show me your purple! #LupusAwarenessMonth,"; "I chose purple, and you?"

Social support (topic 5):
"Today around the world #Lupus advocates, patients, and amp; supporters are working hard to spread #LupusAwareness. For #WorldLupusDay we'll highlight our #LupusChat community members, advocates, caregivers, doctors, and friends who work tirelessly daily to educate others about Lupus."
"Just because something doesn't directly affect you doesn't make it irrelevant. Sending out strength and encouragement to everyone battling lupus, extra love to my queen."

Advocating (topic 6):
"Government would prefer narcotics or sleep medication, which isn't natural and addictive but that's ok they get their money from the big old pharma companies #kickbacks #opioidcrisis but they're getting paid right?!?"; "#WorldLupusDay; Sen Resolution presented (…) We encourage ALL our legislators to join them."; "If you think #PreExistingConditions protections aren't important, remember someone you love could have an accident, that will change how you think about this."

Patient stories (topic 7):
"My scars are my war wounds, my proof that I survived. They show me that I am..."
"Lupus is a long-term condition causing inflammation to the joints, skin and other organs. There's no cure, but symptoms can improve if treatment starts early. Read about the symptoms here … "

Disease description (topic 8):
"#Lupus is a severe + life-changing autoimmune disease that can affect any organ in the body. Yet it is also an illness where "but you don't look sick" is truly apt as the pain, suffering + heavy duty meds aren't always visible."; "Symptoms can flare up and settle down, often the disease flares up (relapses) and symptoms become worse for a few weeks, sometimes longer."
"How lupus is diagnosed? As lupus symptoms can be similar to lots of other conditions, it can take some time to diagnose."

Involvement (topic 9):
"Learn more about the disease and how you can get involved with the charity at"; "Let's Join Together to Fight Lupus! #WorldLupusDay"; "Did you know that over 1:1000 Canadian men, women and children are living with lupus? Let's join together in the fight against #lupus!"

Encouraging (topic 10):
"Keep fighting and know we are fighting with YOU!"; "to all the Lupus Warriors still fighting every day. You're amazing and you're strong. Keep the faith."; "To all those living with Lupus around the world, keep fighting and may your efforts to awareness be successful."

Body symptoms (topic 11):
"As well as the 3 main symptoms, you might also have: weight loss, swollen glands, sensitivity to light (causing rashes on uncovered skin), poor circulation in fingers and toes (Raynaud's)"; "#Lupus is a long-term autoimmune disease in which the body's immune system becomes hyperactive and attacks normal, healthy tissue."; "The immune system protects the body against infections and diseases. However, in Lupus, the immune system starts attacking the body's healthy tissue, leading to organ damage and chronic inflammation."

Communities effect (topic 12):
"lupus affects approx. 5 million people globally yet there is still a lack of awareness amongst general public and healthcare professionals? On #WorldLupusDay join us in encouraging greater understanding of this condition."; "Today is #WorldLupusDay. Lupus is a global health problem that affects people of all nationalities, races, ethnicities, genders and ages! There are about 200,000 cases diagnosed in Kenya.";
"Lupus is a global health problem that affects people of all nationalities, races, ethnicities, genders and ages."

From the topic model results, clearly latent themes behind the tweet texts discussion emerged, underlining a hidden structure that aimed to share something more than just awareness messages or informative content. Some topics that emerged appeared to be similar yet still covered different issues and tackled different narratives, which attracted the attention of different users. To capture the effects that different topics may have on different types of users, we employed a measurement of the covariate impact. As previously mentioned, the main difference between the LDA and STM is the possibility of incorporating metadata and estimating the relationship between the selected covariates and the topics [40].

Figures 4 and 5 show the estimated proportion of topics more likely to be used and discussed according to the value of influencer score and network influencer score in the contents of their tweets. Topics whose estimates lie on the right side (corresponding to positive values of the *x*-axis) were more likely to be discussed/used by influencer, and conversely for the left side.

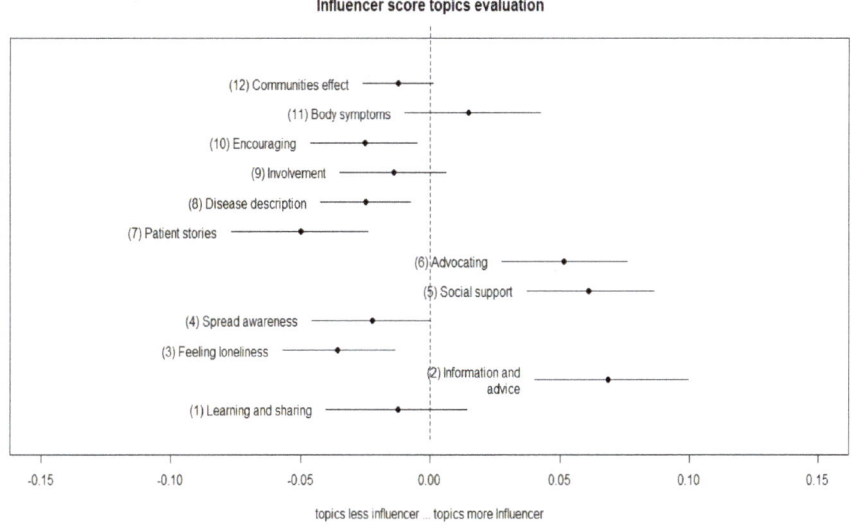

Figure 4. Estimated topic proportion to be discussed by influencer score.

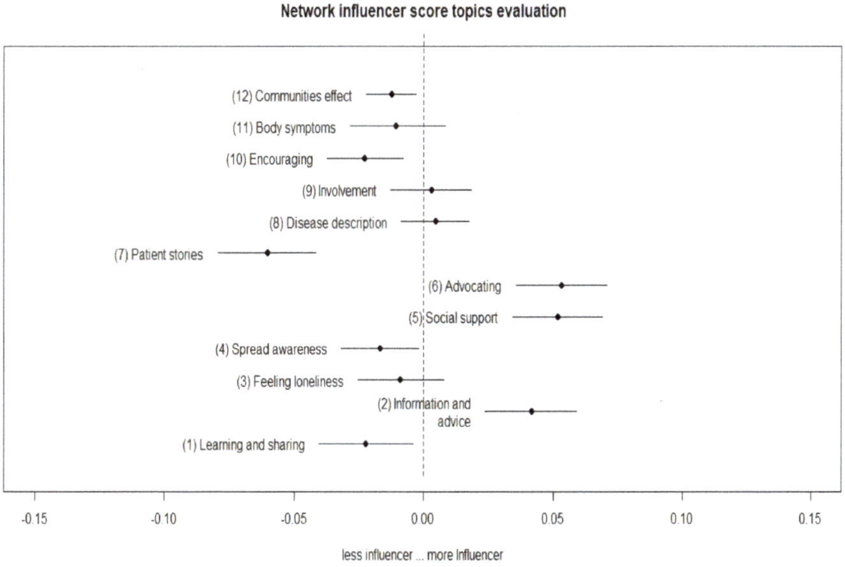

Figure 5. Estimated topic proportion to be discussed by network influencer.

Such an approach made it possible to evaluate the uncertainty surrounding the coefficient, performing a regression where the topic-proportions were the outcome variable, based on the covariance matrix. The results allowed the estimation of topic proportion as a function of covariate data, which further produces confidence intervals around the estimated topic [39].

Interestingly, the results of the estimated topic prevalence showed that some topics and their prevalence were different between the two types of influencer. In particular, topic number 6, the advocacy theme, was largely associated with the network influencer tweet content. We assumed that this kind of topic and the related discussion attracted an enormous amount of attention from a specific type of user related to network influencers. In other words, it was more probable that the topic was related with advocates' content, i.e., in favor of new policy law, health policy attention, or in support of specific collective actions. This can attract specific attention and spread the narrative under discussion faster and more deeply in specific communities.

Topics 8 (disease description) and 9 (involvement) received less attention from the general public and were more likely to occur in the influencers' network communities, which may be more attracted to news or information about possible new treatments or sustaining program involvement.

Instead, topic 11 (body symptoms description) was more likely to receive attention from general influencers. Thus, the public was more interested in understanding the illness and its manifestations.

The STM also allowed an exploration of the correlations between topics to evaluate topics more likely to be discussed in the same tweet. Figure 6 shows pairwise correlation coefficients between identified topics. Positive correlations (in blue) indicate that both topics were more likely to be discussed in a tweet, and vice versa for the negative correlation coefficient (in red). A positive correlation appeared between topics 1 and topic 8, addressing discussions about the disease description and the way in which it was possible to learn and share information on SLE.

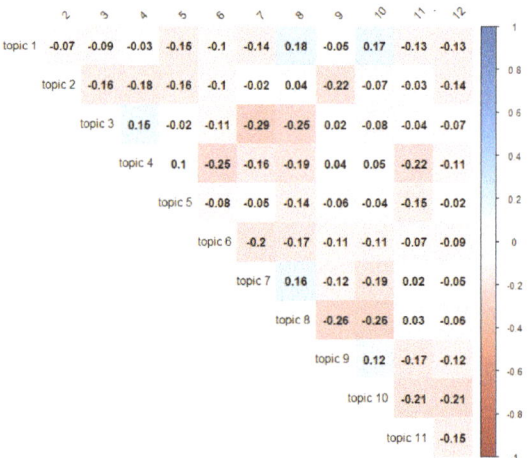

Figure 6. Correlation topics matrix.

A fairly negative correlation appeared between topics 3 and topic 7, which referred to patient stories and loneliness. It is our opinion that these two topics were less likely to be discussed in a tweet together because patient stories tended to describe the illness' physical symptoms, while tweets about loneliness were more a consequence of the disease and tended to be oriented as messages in order to feel less alone. However, as previously mentioned, there was no positive or negative correlation in our results, so we did not have enough information to make more assumptions. Further research could explore more deeply how topics are related and discussed with each other and evolve over time.

4. Discussion

Twitter enables millions of users to share information worldwide in real time. This phenomenon allows policymakers, healthcare stakeholders, and other people to influence and be influenced by opinions and discussions that flow across online social communities, making it possible to share valuable information and practices more quickly and easily than ever before. Such a possibility has become a rich source of value for information-gathering and practical dissemination, in particular for complex and low-intensity diseases like Lupus [46].

Interactivity among online communities makes it possible to renovate not only the healthcare organizations' online approach but the manner in which people's attitudes and intentions regarding health behavior might be influenced [47]. However, valuable information is complex to detect and depict, considering how vast and fast social media platforms work, too often spreading rumors or misinformation [48].

For these reasons, investigating the dynamics played by online communities during specific events like the World Lupus Day can offer a powerful tool to stakeholders for identifying and setting up policy strategies for gathering valuable information and sharing good practices. This ability can offer a concrete tool for decision-makers in dealing with information asymmetry [49], obtain valuable new elements for the decision-making process, promote trust across the identified communities, and promote health-seeking behavior [50].

In our study, we sought to analyze latent themes spread on Twitter during World Lupus Day and detect online user communities' behavior by measuring the users' retweet network.

We measured and found two different types of influencers in our analysis, who behaved and acted differently. There was one type of influencer who was more generally public-oriented, measured on the ratio between the number of followers and the ability to amplify the content they posted, and a second type of influencer, more based on the retweets and network attention count, as an endorsement of their tweet content.

Network influencer users, mostly led by patient organizations, have many followers who tend to have intense connections among themselves, and show more interest in specific topic discussions about the role of social support and policy advocacy. General influencers show less network connection and appear to attract more followers with content related to general disease advice.

Many topics discussed by the two types of influencer were in common. However, the attention posed in some topics were different. This is well represented by the discussion order of topics 2 (Information and advice), 5 (social support), and 6 (advocating), which are swapped in the likelihood order.

Another difference between the topics was posed by the fact that general influencers discussed body symptoms (topic 11), whereas the network influencer discussed topics related to patient involvement (topic 9) and diseases description (topic 8).

To the best of our knowledge, this study is the first to employ a combination of methods to explore deeply latent topic discussions and online communities' interactions regarding a low-prevalence disease like Lupus. Unlike other kinds of diseases such as diabetes, HIV, or stroke, where the vast population offers more opportunities for investigation, low-prevalence or rare diseases can benefit greatly from the application of such methodologies to identify unmet needs or improve the network of care and treatment for patient communities. Therefore, it is critical for public health institutions to systematically explore how to effectively use interactive features on social media to attract public attention and maintain communication with the public.

Further research should also evaluate a qualitative analysis of the selected topics, offering insights that can help improve the judgement in understanding the topic relationships [51].

5. Limitations

For all its strengths, this study has limitations. We based our analysis on just one specific day that may not describe all the dimensions and themes about Lupus Awareness Month. Data collection relied on a public Twitter API was able to detect 4434 tweets in English, which may have led to a loss of some tweets.

In the dataset, most accounts were based in the UK or USA due to the language choice. Only a tiny percentage of accounts reported the geographical location, making it impossible to properly explore specific geographic characteristics at the country level. Therefore, future studies could take into account and explore a longer period, consider other languages, and evaluate geographic and ethnic effects that play a role in Lupus.

We used structural topic modeling to analyze tweet texts, while other methods may offer other types of classification based on natural processing language or deep learning suitable for tweet texts [52]. However, despite these limitations, this study provides an extensive and detailed methodological approach offering useful insights into social media platform dynamics regarding Lupus, which is still little investigated.

6. Conclusions

Applying the combination of topic modeling and user network analysis, we were able to detect two main types of user communities with specific types of concerns and topic discussions and define different narratives employed by influencers.

The findings of this study provided a detailed example of the implications for healthcare organizations when detecting, understanding, and defining topic discussions and communicative functions available on Twitter. We thus provided an overview of the valuable opportunity to identify appropriate user audiences and share what might be suitable content to engage and interact them, going beyond word frequency, hashtag counts, and online community detection. The importance of considering public health issues involves the complexity embedded in any kind of low-prevalence/rare disease where the low number of patients makes it hard to obtain valuable information, increasing public awareness, and impact on health behavior.

Future research should consider the geographical location and related characteristics of health communication strategies to provide insights able to implement health information dissemination for health practitioners and policymakers.

This type of research can fill the knowledge gap between clinical epistemological uncertainty and patient experiential knowledge when dealing with lupus. We believe that the proposed approach may have a significant role in public health, applying such research indicators and methodologies to aid decision-makers in designing interventions and effective communication strategies.

Author Contributions: Conceptualization, S.P.; methodology, S.P. and V.L.; software, S.P. and G.A.; formal analysis, S.P., V.L., G.A., and G.T.; writing—original draft preparation, S.P., V.L., M.M., and G.T.; writing—review and editing, S.P., V.L., G.A., M.M., and G.T.; supervision, M.M. and G.T.; All authors have read and agreed to the published version of the manuscript.

Funding: This research received no external funding.

Acknowledgments: We would like to acknowledge Peter Morley, Paul Howard at LUPUS UK, Rachael Lowe at Physiopedia, and John Hibbs at the Hibbs Lupus Trust for their support and consent in sharing their Twitter account name. Their efforts add tangible value to increasing the awareness for Lupus. We would like to thank the Data Protection Officer and legal-ethical advisor of Scuola Superiore Sant'Anna for providing advice on how to collect and manage data in compliance with current privacy legislation. Furthermore, we would like to extend our gratitude to Simone Ticciati for helping us draft the manuscript.

Conflicts of Interest: The authors declare no conflict of interest.

Appendix A

1. Topic Modeling

The heuristic of the probabilistic topic modeling can be seen in Figure A1.

LDA and other topic models are part of the larger field of probabilistic modeling [1]. Generative probabilistic modeling consider data as arising from a generative process that includes hidden variables. This generative process defines a joint probability distribution over both observed and hidden random variables.

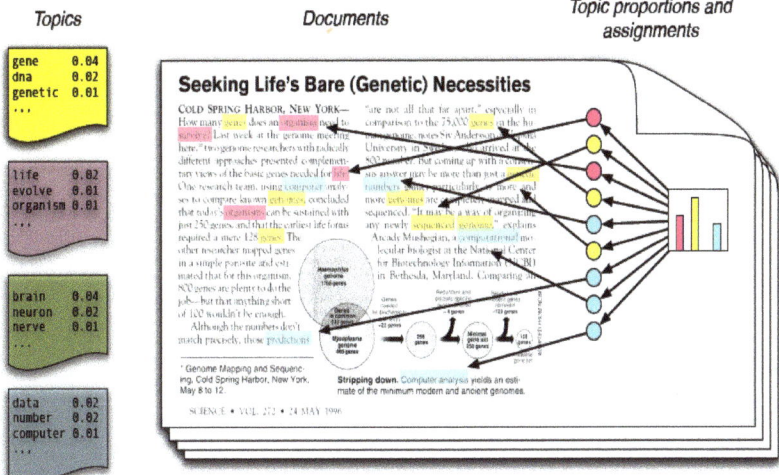

Figure A1. Source: David M. Blei. "Probabilistic topic models". Communications of the ACM (Association for Computing Machinery); 2012, Vol. 55 No. 4, Pages 77–84. 10.1145/2133806.2133826.

The joint distribution to compute the conditional distribution of the hidden variables is given to the observed variables. This conditional distribution is also called the posterior distribution.

Structural topic modeling extends to the LDA framework. STM allows for correlations among topics. Covariate data including document metadata influences topic prevalence within documents. STM also uses (document-specific) covariate data to define distributions for word use within a topic [2].

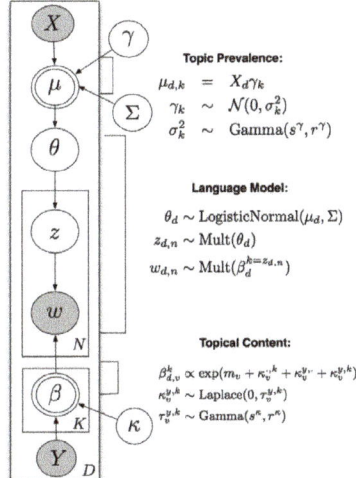

Figure A2. Structural topic modeling, in plate notation, in: (Roberts ME, Stewart BM, Tingley D, Airoldi EM. The structural topic model and Applied Social Science 2013).

We employed the ldatuning package [3] using the log-likelihood method via Gibbs sampling. Specifically, we used the "Griffiths" [4] and "CaoJuan" [5] metrics scores.

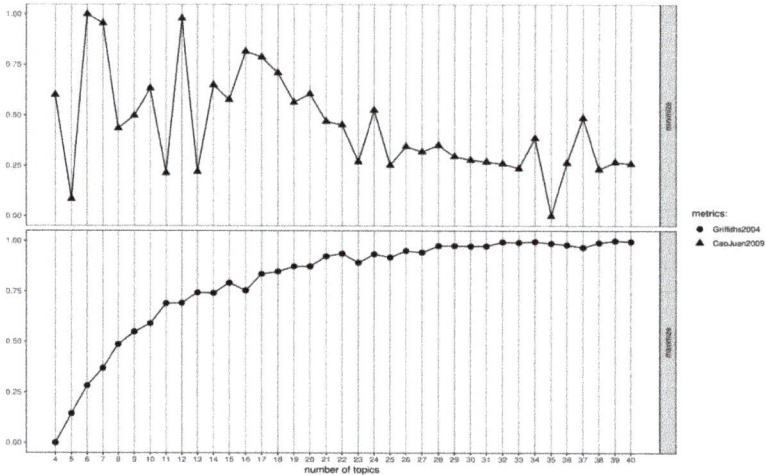

Figure A3. Find optimal number of topics.

2. STM Evaluation

The semantic coherence and exclusivity values were associated with each topic. Numerals represent the average for each model and dots represent topic specific scores.

Each model has semantic coherence and exclusivity values associated with each topic. Figure A4 plots these values and labels each with its topic number.

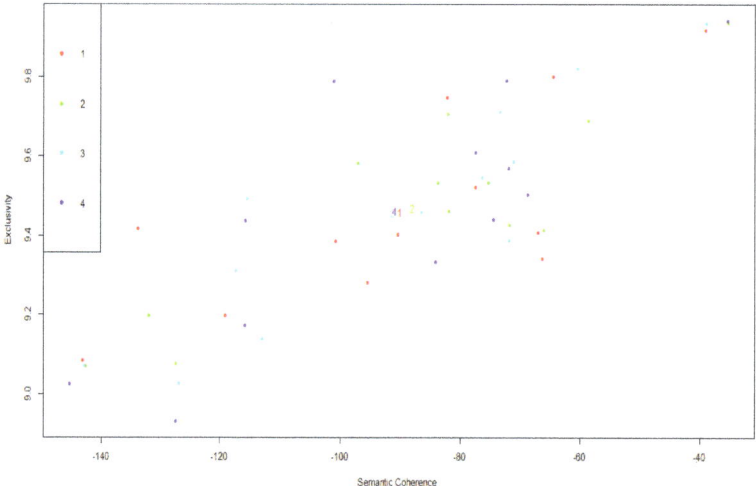

Figure A4. Topic models selection in STM packages.

3. Network Construction

We used a directed graph network G to represent social connections and information flows for Twitter users. In $G = (V, E)$, V denotes the set of nodes (Twitter users) and E denotes the set of edges (social connections) in G. An edge $e_{ij} \in E$ corresponds to a set of node pairs (v_i, v_j) that connects node v_i and v_j in G. To define an edge in the network, we include the lists of users they retweeted. Retweet networks consist of directed links indicating that one user has retransmitted a tweet from another user.

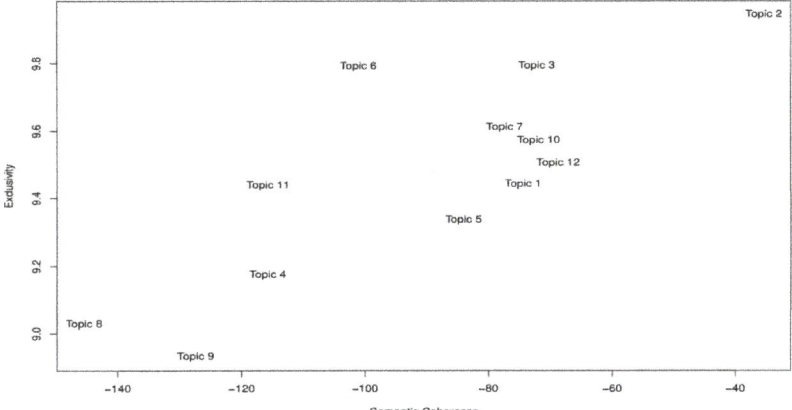

Figure A5. Plots result pf the selected model semantic coherence and exclusivity for each 12 topics.

Eigenvector centrality (EC) is a method of computing the approximate importance of each node in a network [6]. The rationale behind this centrality measure is that a node is thought to be more important if it is directly connected to important nodes. This relationship to other highly connected nodes indicates a high level of influence.

The modularity algorithm measures [7] the strength of division of a network into clusters or communities and was applied to detect the number of clusters (communities) in the retweets network.

$$Q = \frac{1}{2m} \sum_{i,j} \left[A_{ij} - \frac{K_i K_j}{2m} \right] \delta(c_i\ c_j) \qquad (A1)$$

where A_{ij} represents the weight of the edge between i and j, $k_i = \sum A_{ij}$ is the sum of the weights of the edges attached to vertex i, C_i is the community to which vertex i is assigned, the δ function $\delta(u, v)$ is 1 if $u = v$ and 0 otherwise, and $m = \frac{1}{2} \sum_{ij} A_{ij}$.

4. Gephi Network Parameter Results

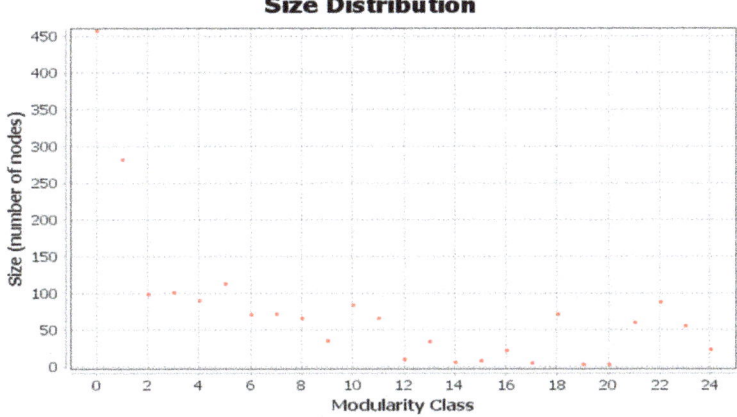

Figure A6. Community size distribution.

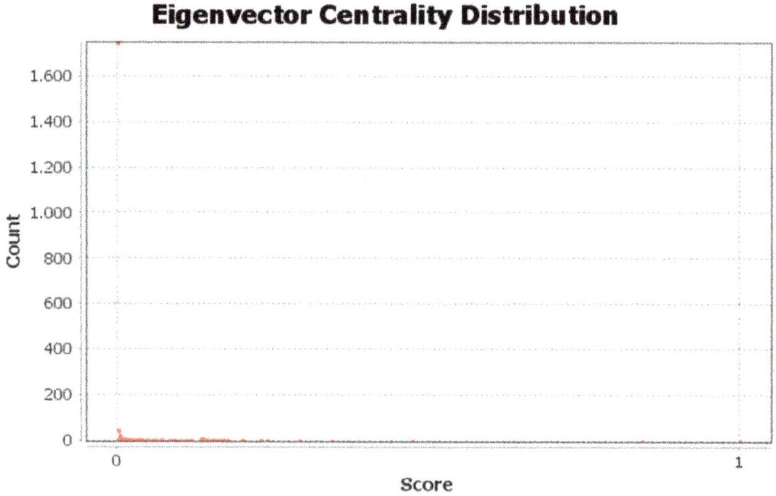

Figure A7. Eigenvector distribution of retweet network data.

References

1. Weng, L.; Menczer, F.; Ahn, Y.-Y. Virality prediction and community structure in social networks. *Sci. Rep.* **2013**, *3*, 2522. [CrossRef] [PubMed]
2. Vosoughi, S.; Roy, D.; Aral, S. The spread of true and false news online. *Science* **2018**, *359*, 1146–1151. [CrossRef]
3. Paul, M.J.; Dredze, M.; Broniatowski, D. Twitter Improves Influenza Forecasting. *PLoS Curr.* **2014**, *6*. [CrossRef] [PubMed]
4. Smolinski, M.S.; Crawley, A.W.; Baltrusaitis, K.; Chunara, R.; Olsen, J.M.; Wójcik, O.; Santillana, M.; Nguyen, A.; Brownstein, J.S. Flu Near You: Crowdsourced Symptom Reporting Spanning 2 Influenza Seasons. *Am. J. Public Health* **2015**, *105*, 2124–2130. [CrossRef] [PubMed]
5. Oliver, J.E.; Wood, T. Medical Conspiracy Theories and Health Behaviors in the United States. *JAMA Intern. Med.* **2014**, *174*, 817–818. [CrossRef]
6. Miah, S.J.; Hasan, N.; Hasan, R.; Gammack, J. Healthcare support for underserved communities using a mobile social media platform. *Inf. Syst.* **2017**, *66*, 1–12. [CrossRef]
7. Thomas, M.; Narayan, P. The Role of Participatory Communication in Tracking Unreported Reproductive Tract Issues in Marginalized Communities. *Inf. Technol. Dev.* **2016**, *22*, 117–133. [CrossRef]
8. Young, S.D.; Rivers, C.; Lewis, B. Methods of using real-time social media technologies for detection and remote monitoring of HIV outcomes. *Prev. Med. (Baltim)* **2014**, *63*, 112–115. [CrossRef]
9. Golder, V.; Morand, E.F.; Hoi, A.Y. Quality of Care for Systemic Lupus Erythematosus: Mind the Knowledge Gap. *J. Rheumatol.* **2017**, *44*, 271–278. [CrossRef] [PubMed]
10. Stockl, A. Complex syndromes, ambivalent diagnosis, and existential uncertainty: The case of Systemic Lupus Erythematosus (SLE). *Soc. Sci. Med.* **2007**, *65*, 1549–1559. [CrossRef] [PubMed]
11. Gergianaki, I.; Bertsias, G. Systemic Lupus Erythematosus in Primary Care: An Update and Practical Messages for the General Practitioner. *Front. Med.* **2018**, *5*, 161. [CrossRef] [PubMed]
12. Reuter, K.; Danve, A.; Deodhar, A. Harnessing the power of social media: How can it help in axial spondyloarthritis research? *Curr. Opin. Rheumatol.* **2019**, *31*, 321–328. [CrossRef]
13. Crowe, A.L.; McKnight, A.J.; McAneney, H. Communication Needs for Individuals with Rare Diseases Within and Around the Healthcare System of Northern Ireland. *Front. Public Health* **2019**, *7*, 236. [CrossRef] [PubMed]
14. Tenderich, A.; Tenderich, B.; Barton, T.; Richards, S.E. What Are PWDs (People With Diabetes) Doing Online? A Netnographic Analysis. *J. Diabetes Sci. Technol.* **2019**, *13*, 187–197. [CrossRef] [PubMed]

15. Rathore, A.K.; Kar, A.K.; Ilavarasan, P.V. Social Media Analytics: Literature Review and Directions for Future Research. *Decis. Anal.* **2017**, *14*, 229–249. [CrossRef]
16. Mao, J.J.; Chung, A.; Benton, A.; Hill, S.; Ungar, L.; Leonard, C.E.; Hennessy, S.; Holmes, J.H. Online discussion of drug side effects and discontinuation among breast cancer survivors. *Pharmacoepidemiol. Drug Saf.* **2013**, *22*, 256–262. [CrossRef] [PubMed]
17. Backa, K.E.; Holmberg, K.; Ek, S. Communicating diabetes and diets on Twitter—A semantic content analysis. *Int. J. Netw. Virtual. Organ.* **2016**, *16*, 8–24. [CrossRef]
18. Xu, W.W.; Chiu, I.-H.; Chen, Y.; Mukherjee, T. Twitter hashtags for health: Applying network and content analyses to understand the health knowledge sharing in a Twitter-based community of practice. *Qual. Quant.* **2015**, *49*, 1361–1380. [CrossRef]
19. Smith, K.T. Hospital Marketing and Communications Via Social Media. *Serv. Mark. Q.* **2017**, *38*, 187–201. [CrossRef]
20. Smailhodzic, E.; Hooijsma, W.; Boonstra, A.; Langley, D.J. Social media use in healthcare: A systematic review of effects on patients and on their relationship with healthcare professionals. *BMC Health Serv. Res.* **2016**, *16*, 442. [CrossRef]
21. Althubaiti, A. Information bias in health research: Definition, pitfalls, and adjustment methods. *J. Multidiscip. Healthc.* **2016**, *9*, 211–217. [CrossRef] [PubMed]
22. Fan, W.; Gordon, M.D. The power of social media analytics. *Commun. ACM* **2014**, *57*, 74–81. [CrossRef]
23. Kearney, M.W. Packagrtweet: Collecting Twitter Data. R Package Version 0.6.9e 'Rtweet' Title Collecting Twitter Data. 2019. Available online: https://cran.r-project.org/package=rtweet (accessed on 17 August 2019).
24. Lou, C.; Yuan, S. Influencer Marketing: How Message Value and Credibility Affect Consumer Trust of Branded Content on Social Media. *J. Interact. Advert.* **2019**, *19*, 58–73. [CrossRef]
25. Abidin, C. Communicative intimacies: Influencers and Perceived Interconnectedness. *Ada J. Gender New Media Technol.* **2015**, *8*, 1–16. [CrossRef]
26. Kefi, H.; Indra, S.; Abdessalem, T. Social media marketing analytics: A multicultural approach applied to the beauty & cosmetics sector. In Proceedings of the Pacific Asia Conference on Information Systems PACIS, Chiayi, Taiwan, 27 June–1 July 2016; Available online: https://www.semanticscholar.org/paper/Social-media-marketing-analytics-%3A-a-multicultural-Kefi-Indra/98a22035e89e2d2573f1115d3e0b1dfc7ee82300 (accessed on 17 December 2019).
27. Ananda, A.S.; Hernández-García, Á.; Lamberti, L. N-REL: A comprehensive framework of social media marketing strategic actions for marketing organizations. *J. Innov. Knowl.* **2016**, *1*, 170–180. [CrossRef]
28. Jiménez-Castillo, D.; Sánchez-Fernández, R. The role of digital influencers in brand recommendation: Examining their impact on engagement, expected value and purchase intention. *Int. J. Inf. Manag.* **2019**, *49*, 366–376. [CrossRef]
29. Arora, A.; Bansal, S.; Kandpal, C.; Aswani, R.; Dwivedi, Y. Measuring social media influencer index- insights from facebook, Twitter and Instagram. *J. Retail. Consum. Serv.* **2019**, *49*, 86–101. [CrossRef]
30. Anger, I.; Kittl, C. Measuring influence on Twitter. In *ACM International Conference Proceeding Series*; ACM Press: New York, NY, USA, 2011; p. 1.
31. Pavlopoulos, G.A.; Secrier, M.; Moschopoulos, C.N.; Soldatos, T.G.; Kossida, S.; Aerts, J.; Schneider, R.; Bagos, P.G. Using graph theory to analyze biological networks. *BioData Min.* **2011**, *4*, 10. [CrossRef]
32. Blondel, V.D.; Guillaume, J.-L.; Lambiotte, R.; Lefebvre, E. Fast unfolding of communities in large networks. *J. Stat. Mech. Theory Exp.* **2008**, P10008. [CrossRef]
33. Jacomy, M.; Venturini, T.; Heymann, S.; Bastian, M. ForceAtlas2, a continuous graph layout algorithm for handy network visualization designed for the Gephi software. *PLoS ONE* **2014**, *9*, e98679. [CrossRef]
34. Bonacich, P.; Lloyd, P. Eigenvector centrality and structural zeroes and ones: When is a neighbor not a neighbor? *Soc. Netw.* **2015**, *43*, 86–90. [CrossRef]
35. Meera Gandhi, G. Identification of Potential Influencers in Facebook Using Network Graph Metrics. 2014. Available online: http://www.digitalxplore.org/up_proc/pdf/88-140479998117-21.pdf (accessed on 18 December 2019).
36. Leonard, M.; Graham, S.; Bonacum, D. The human factor: The critical importance of effective teamwork and communication in providing safe care. *Qual. Saf. Health Care* **2004**, *13*, 361–362. [CrossRef]
37. Blei, D.M. Probabilistic topic models. *Commun. ACM* **2012**, *55*, 77–84. [CrossRef]
38. Blei, D.M.; Ng, A.Y.; Jordan, M.I. Latent Dirichlet allocation. *J. Mach. Learn. Res.* **2003**, *3*, 993–1022.

39. Roberts, M.E.; Stewart, B.M.; Tingley, D.; Lucas, C.; Leder-Luis, J.; Gadarian, S.K.; Albertson, B.; Rand, D.G. Structural topic models for open-ended survey responses. *Am. J. Pol. Sci.* **2014**, *58*, 1064–1082. [CrossRef]
40. Roberts, M.E.; Stewart, B.M.; Tingley, D. Stm: An R package for structural topic models. *J. Stat. Softw.* **2019**, *91*. [CrossRef]
41. Griffiths, T.L.; Steyvers, M. Finding scientific topics. *Proc. Natl. Acad. Sci. USA* **2004**, *101*, 5228–5235. [CrossRef] [PubMed]
42. Cao, J.; Xia, T.; Li, J.; Zhang, Y.; Tang, S. A density-based method for adaptive LDA model selection. *Neurocomputing* **2009**, *72*, 1775–1781. [CrossRef]
43. Murzintcev, N. Package 'Ldatuning' Title Tuning of the Latent Dirichlet Allocation Models Parameters Description Estimates the Best Fitting Number of Topics. 2019. Available online: https://cran.r-project.org/web/packages/ldatuning/ldatuning.pdf (accessed on 21 December 2019).
44. Mimno, D.; Wallach, H.M.; Talley, E.; Leenders, M.; McCallum, A. Optimizing semantic coherence in topic models. In Proceedings of the EMNLP 2011—Conference on Empirical Methods in Natural Language Processing, Edinburgh, Scotland, UK, 27–31 July 2011; Association for Computational Linguistics: Stroudsburg, PA, USA, 2011; pp. 262–272.
45. Airoldi, E.M.; Bischof, J.M. Improving and Evaluating Topic Models and Other Models of Text. *J. Am. Stat. Assoc.* **2016**, *111*, 1381–1403. [CrossRef]
46. Wheeler, L.M.; Pakozdi, A.; Rajakariar, R.; Lewis, M.; Cove-Smith, A.; Pyne, D. 139 Moving with the Times: Social Media Use Amongst Lupus Patients. *Rheumatology* **2018**, *57*, key075-363. [CrossRef]
47. Jiang, S. Functional interactivity in social media: An examination of Chinese health care organizations' microblog profiles. *Health Promot. Int.* **2019**, *34*, 38–46. [CrossRef]
48. Wang, Y.; McKee, M.; Torbica, A.; Stuckler, D. Systematic Literature Review on the Spread of Health-related Misinformation on Social Media. *Soc. Sci. Med.* **2019**, *240*, 112552. [CrossRef] [PubMed]
49. Haas-Wilson, D. Arrow and the Information Market Failure in Health Care: The Changing Content and Sources of Health Care Information. *J. Health Polit. Policy Law* **2001**, *26*, 1031–1044. [CrossRef]
50. Fletcher-Brown, J.; Pereira, V.; Nyadzayo, M.W. Health marketing in an emerging market: The critical role of signaling theory in breast cancer awareness. *J. Bus. Res.* **2018**, *86*, 416–434. [CrossRef]
51. Nikolenko, S.I.; Koltcov, S.; Koltsova, O. Topic modelling for qualitative studies. *J. Inf. Sci.* **2017**, *43*, 88–102. [CrossRef]
52. Al Moubayed, N.; McGough, S.; Awwad Shiekh Hasan, B. Beyond the topics: How deep learning can improve the discriminability of probabilistic topic modelling. *PeerJ Comput. Sci.* **2020**, *6*, e252. [CrossRef]

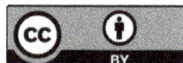 © 2020 by the authors. Licensee MDPI, Basel, Switzerland. This article is an open access article distributed under the terms and conditions of the Creative Commons Attribution (CC BY) license (http://creativecommons.org/licenses/by/4.0/).

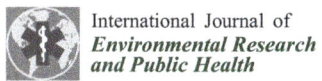 International Journal of
Environmental Research and Public Health

Article

Exploring the Social Media on the Communication Professionals in Public Health. Spanish Official Medical Colleges Case Study

Carlos de las Heras-Pedrosa [1],*, Dolores Rando-Cueto [1], Carmen Jambrino-Maldonado [2] and Francisco J. Paniagua-Rojano [1]

[1] Department of Advertising and Public Relations, Universidad de Málaga 29071 Málaga, Spain; lrandocueto@uma.es (D.R.-C.); fjpaniagua@uma.es (F.J.P.-R.)
[2] Department of Economics and Business Administration, Universidad de Málaga, 29071 Málaga, Spain; mcjambrino@uma.es
* Correspondence: cheras@uma.es

Received: 2 June 2020; Accepted: 1 July 2020; Published: 6 July 2020

Abstract: The purpose of the study is to analyze the role that social media have on the practice of health professionals working in information and communication department of Spanish official medical college. Social media in health fields have experienced growing participation of users and are increasingly considered a credible form of communication. This paper examines the use of social media as communication tool by the Official Medical Colleges (OMC) of Spain. According to the National Institute of Statistics, in 2019 there were 267,995 registered medical professionals in the 52 OMC in Spain. This research is based on a qualitative methodological technique through semi-structured interviews, with the aim of identifying the profiles of the people who lead the information in the professional organizations of the OMC. Of the colleges, 73.07% participated. The findings show that information is essential for the OMC and most of them have at least one experienced communication professional. Social media are essential tool in their work and Twitter (87.5%) and Facebook (81.3%) are considered the most relevant social media according to their interests. These tools are believed to be very useful for informing, establishing relationships and listening to users.

Keywords: health communication; social media; public health; Spanish official medical colleges; stakeholders

---

1. Introduction

Nowadays, health communication plays an important role for citizens [1] and, therefore, contributes to social sustainability. Society is increasingly using the Internet in a bid to obtain health information, share experiences related to pathologic processes or find people with similar physical or psychological conditions [1,2]. Since information and communication technologies are being used in the field of health, terms such as e-patient or e-health are widely used, which is evidence of the increasing role citizens play in making decisions about their well-being [3,4].

Terrón [5] offers his perception from an anthropological point of view. In his opinion, the interest in health communication in a country like Spain has increased significantly due to the growing need for lifestyles that entail greater social well-being. This idea is reinforced in the feedback required by the supply and demand of information. Thus, interest in what is communicated grows as more information is offered [5,6].

The Internet has become the most important "loudspeaker" for patients' expectations and demands. This fosters the emergence of associations that support patients' rights to make their voices heard [5].

As a result, this makes patients feel stronger as they are members of a collectively supported platform on which they can express their needs and the needs of their environment.

Social media play a relevant role in this sense, with a progressive increase observed in terms of their use in the health field [3,7]. Factors such as the accessibility, immediacy or their potential to communicate bidirectionally with different audiences allow active communication [8]. Health centers are aware of the potential of social media and use them to promote interaction and collaboration between patients, relatives and professionals [9].

However, the democratization of information through social media [10] in the field of health means that social networks, blogs or mobile social media have developed peer communication with an increasingly participative audience, but above all, it has also made it more credible. Therefore, it confers greater communicational power to citizens and professionals in the sector when their messages reach a greater number of people [11,12].

These channels have become the preferred communication instruments for health corporations, by facilitating participation and collaboration with their stakeholders and allowing, thanks to a two-way communication, the control of the quality and efficiency of the institution [6,13], but also for the education of citizens with new healthy lifestyle habits [14,15]. It is also a key tool for communicating health alerts, the creation of networks of groups of patients with the same pathologies, or professionals for research purposes [12,16].

These real-time interactive information platforms provide a free online resource [17]. Therefore, another advantage of social media for the health sector is its low cost [7,18,19]. They are, therefore, a very effective two-way communicative tool for communication with stakeholders, such as sector professionals and patients [20].

The most popular health-related social media are those specifically intended for patients [1,21]. Nevertheless, other sectors of the population could also play a central role and benefit from the knowledge circulating on these networks if they became stakeholders of such information channels. Swan [1] suggests that agents in the health field who are meant to take care of patients, researchers and other agents involved in this area could take part more actively [21]. In the patient's view, social media are the best instrument for real-time interaction, enabling the exchange of information and participation not only simply as patients or users, but also as groups or associations [22]. In the case of professionals, social media are used primarily for the dissemination of results, research, networking or teaching, among others [23].

However, this issue has disadvantages, the democratization of communication via social media entails, in some cases, a lack of veracity and information control [19]. Anyone may stir-up anxiety within society with their opinions or unconfirmed facts [6], as well as harmful criticisms or falsehoods directed at health professionals or health institutions [24]. It would not be ignored both the legal problems and lack of privacy, such as damage to professional image, violation of patient privacy, etc. [7,19,23]. In order to solve this problem, health institutions and professional organizations, such as Official Medical Colleges (OMC), have developed prevention guidelines and guides to good practices [7] aimed at protecting institutions in this area on a legal, clinical and organizational level [25–28]. OMC, together with health institutions, play a crucial role in developing recommendations for the use of social media. For this reason, the work of professionals with an expert profile in information and health is essential.

The choice of the official medical associations for this research is determined by the obligation that doctors must be registered to be able to practice the medical profession representing all the doctors in the country.

In detail, this work attempts to answer the following research questions:

RQ_1: Are the official medical colleges in Spain valid interlocutors with their stakeholders?

RQ_2: Do the communication professionals of the Spanish official medical colleges mainly use social media for their work as a source of information and verification?

RQ_3: Do social media have any involvement in the agenda setting of the official medical colleges?

This study is structured as follows. It begins with a review of the existing literature focused on the importance of communication professionals and the use of social media in the health sector. Next, an analysis of the official medical colleges is carried out within the health field in Spain and analyzing the stakeholders with which it is related. Second, the methodology used is presented. This research work is carried out with a qualitative technique through semi-structured interviews with the communication experts of official medical colleges with the support of the Atlas.ti. Third, the most important research results are shown. The main contribution is a framework with strategic communication keys and the use of social media as an essential element of information. Finally, conclusion, managerial implications in health sector and limitations of the study are discussed.

2. Theoretical Background

2.1. Communication in Health and Social Media

Scientific literature regarding health communication highlights the necessity of the professionals practicing it to adapt to the changes brought about by the rapid invasion and evolution of social media.

With social media, access to information has changed, currently people do not rely exclusively on traditional or government media but trust the social media for essential information from the health sector [29]. Nowadays, social media such as blogs, websites or social networks such as Twitter, Facebook, Instagram, etc. are increasingly used by the population to acquire health knowledge [30].

It is necessary to design new strategies and challenges to cope with the apparition of a new style of network communication in real time [31]. Health professionals can make use of the new communication scenarios and their position as authoritative and credible sources in order to promote and defend health [32].

The professional practice of those who develop informative content for the media has been recognized for over a decade. As Arkin points out [33], in a study focusing on the American population, social media, as a leading source of health information, could potentially save lives in the event of a health crisis [29]. Nevertheless, those who develop informative content can also be alarmist and spread false information in the news or the coverage they offer.

Therefore, while the media selects the version of reality that it transmits and offers its own views on matters, it has the power to give this information the importance it considers appropriate [5]. It could be added that citizens search for increasing health communication, not only in what could be considered reliable sources, such as health professionals, but also in the media, so it seems necessary for the media to proceed responsibly [6]. Due to this fact, the media must offer true, transparent and coherent information [34].

Social media provide such health communication specialists with valuable information about patients' experiences with which they can monitor public reaction to health problems. They also highlight the potential of such information for the development of health policies [35]. An example are medical blogs, which are frequently visited by the most important media outlets [36].

However, Leask, Hooker and King [32] also highlight how the role of specialists in charge of communication is losing relevance. This incurs a disappearance of the basic technical knowledge that is necessary to transmit health communication correctly. One of the new challenges is developing tools to verify contents, given the risk of spreading inaccurate or false information generated by the ever-increasing speed with which information emerges [31].

Rumors, conflicting news and speculation are characteristics of the messages circulating within social media. According to Hermida [37], it is the responsibility of media professionals to select, contextualize and verify the enormous amount of information. In this sense, it is not conceivable that the health communicator is dependent on sources, funders, or other informants with certain interests to reliably inform society and not be detrimental to the well-being or the quality of life of society [38]. Therefore, ethics and responsibility at work, as well as a commitment to society, are key elements of the communicator. This is how better care is offered to the population [39]. This work is reflected when organizational interests are transferred in order to reinforce the welfare or quality of life of citizens.

However, the veracity of the information lies with the communication professional, the determination of correct information now becomes complicated due to, among other aspects, the vast amount of information generated by social media. Knowing how to use them for professional purposes is no easy task and a new type of reasoning is required. In spite of this, the authors both defend this new scenario, saying that the communicative potential of social media is "far from being negligible" [40] (p. 67).

As well as verification and credibility of the information spread through social media, other aspects of social media that the studies under analysis expose are the effects that these produce in professional practice [41]; the use that professionals make of them [42] and their importance for communicators or the weight they bear regarding information [43].

Since McCombs and Shaw proposed the theory of agenda-setting in 1972 [44,45] to explain how the media influence the shaping of public opinion, its application to research has been intense and fruitful. In the process of establishing the news that attracts the attention of the audience, each media has tried to play a differentiated role [46]

The change of the hierarchical structures regarding the organization of the information by the spaces of conversation, connectivity and the creation of a community that have provoked social media is one of the changes highlighted by Hermida, Lewis and Zamith [41] in the exercise of communication professionals who work on social media. There is no longer a single paradigm for the structure of news as proposed by Almaguer [46], but there are many different ways of developing content. Even if corporations seem particularly interested in social media as a vehicle to market news content, increase traffic to their websites, and strengthen relations with the customers, communication professionals, on the other hand, mainly use social media to talk about what they are working on or share opinions or ideas. This implies that the content provided by corporations does not enrich the media agenda. On the contrary, according to these authors, news that refers to social media as the source of information is rare or infrequent [42].

Lariscy et al. [43] not only put the emphasis on the attention that corporations should expend in terms of the content that is disseminated through social media, in addition, they point out that the task of communication or public relations professionals are to closely monitor the information issued from the entities for which they work and possibly involve those who are the originators of the content [47], considering that social media contribute to the construction of the agenda setting [48–50].

Different studies highlight the potential of hospital social media and how society can profit from them. In this way, Shepherd et al. [51] place these in a favorable and expanding environment, which favors personal relationships. De la Peña and Quintanilla [52] (p. 495), describe the role they play for citizens as "a virtual community where they can find stimulation, get answers to specific questions related to health and a place to share success stories" and Koteyko et al. [53] add that this tool has great potential to promote initiatives.

To the field of hospital information, the content producers would be health professionals and management and service professionals, together with users of the health system, patients and family members, among others.

Influencing the importance of information supervision, social media is considered as an effective instrument to promote communication between public administrations and different stakeholders [48,54]. Specifically, in the sector in charge of communication through social media within the field of specialized health care, scientific publications that focus on the practice of communication professionals specialized in health are scarce [49,50,55].

However, as well as these publications that underline the benefits of health communication by means of social media, there are others that focus on their harmful effects or potential dangers. Among these dangers are the loss of privacy or security regarding shared information [50,56] and the lack of specialized training, both in health and in the management of social media among communication professionals [57,58].

2.2. Official Medical Colleges (OMC) in Spain

In many countries, registration in the medical association is legally mandatory for all doctors who practice medicine temporarily or permanently. Thus, in Europe, as examples, there are the *Conseils de l'Ordre des Médecins* in France, the *Fédération des Médecins Suisses*, the general medical council in the United Kingdom, the *Ordre des Médecins* in Belgium or the *Colegio Oficial de Médicos* in the case of Spain. The first regulations in Spain of the official medical colleges date from April 12, 1898, but it is not until the Royal Decree of May 28, 1917 where the compulsory registration in the college to practice the medical profession is definitively approved.

Professional colleges play an essential role. This relevance of professional services lies in the protection of the rights and interests of citizens who receive them.

Throughout diverse regulations on professional associations in Spain, the sector has undergone different transformations, but maintains the same structure that it originally had. The law defines professional associations as legal public corporations, protected by the law and recognized by the State, with their own legal personality and full capacity for the fulfilment of their purposes, which empowers them as entities that represent and defend the profession that each college has and points out the obligatory registration for the professional exercise which is regulated by law.

In the present case, the Spanish official medical college promotes the scientific work of doctors and connects this collective with patients and society. Most importantly, its ethical code committees ensure that health institutions adhere to the norms.

There are currently 52 official medical colleges in Spain with a territorial structure. The number of doctors registered at the official medical colleges have been increasing year-by-year to reach a total of 267,995 in 2019, as represented by Table 1.

Table 1. Number of doctors registered at the Spanish official medical colleges. Series 2015–2019.

	2015	2016	2017	2018	2019
Doctors	242,840	247,958	253,796	260,588	267,995

Source: Instituto Nacional de Estadística. 2019 [59].

The number of registered medical professionals per 1000 inhabitants is 5.66 on average. By autonomous communities, the representation is as follows (Figure 1).

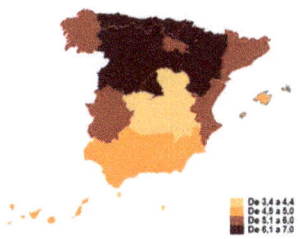

Figure 1. Registered medical professionals in 2019. Quota per 1000 habitants. Source: Instituto Nacional de Estadística. 2019 [59].

Official Medical Colleges and the Relationships with Stakeholders

The situational theory of Grunig's audiences [60] identifies stakeholders as groups formed by people who unite them with a problem or end of a similar nature and of which they are aware and so they group together to adopt a proactive attitude focused on action, in its attempt of resolution.

The professional management of communication according to Grunig and Hunt [61] identifies three weaknesses and three strengths. The weaknesses are: (a) the saturation of the communicative channels due to the lack of well-documented and orderly information that ends up becoming irrelevant to the public, (b) frequently this information overshadows the true relevant facts of interest and (c) it ends up generating distrust in interest groups because of the sense of deception. The strengths are: (a) it approaches and sensitizes the entities with their stakeholders, by establishing a more dynamic and bidirectional communication, (b) it acts as a clear and concise spokesperson for issues of public interest and (c) it promotes the knowledge of the various stakeholders through information in formal and informal communication media.

For Ruiz de Azua [62], health communication management requires an open and empathetic communication style that generates public trust. It is most effective when health professionals try to stimulate the population to take positive action or abstain from a harmful act. However, trust is essential, public mistrust of other stakeholders such as health experts and representatives of health institutions can increase for a variety of reasons, one of the priorities being access to conflicting information collected in the social media.

Mainardes, Raposo and Alves [63] emphasize the importance of identifying and aligning stakeholders with the strategic objectives of their institutions, given that they themselves play a vital role in the development of management strategies. Therefore, any serious and reputable entity needs to develop and implement its strategy through specific expert structures created with the objective of directing relations with its audiences. Due to the powerful position and performance they entail [64], proactive care of these can become a huge advantage for the reputation of the official medical colleges.

Therefore, an express knowledge of the stakeholders and the relationship that must exist between them is essential [65]. Next, the following Figure 2 establishes the public map that relates to the official medical colleges. Beginning with the main audience to which they are directed as their own members are, guiding them in good ethical practices, in technological advances and in health research. Continuing with healthcare professionals such as nurses, psychologists, therapists, physiotherapists, etc., including the providers where pharmacists and health engineers will be highlighted and ending with patients, their families, health institutions, hospitals, government or the media and society itself in general. In short, once the map of the stakeholders is represented, the prioritized objectives will be established in order to design the communication strategies and policies appropriate to each one of said audiences.

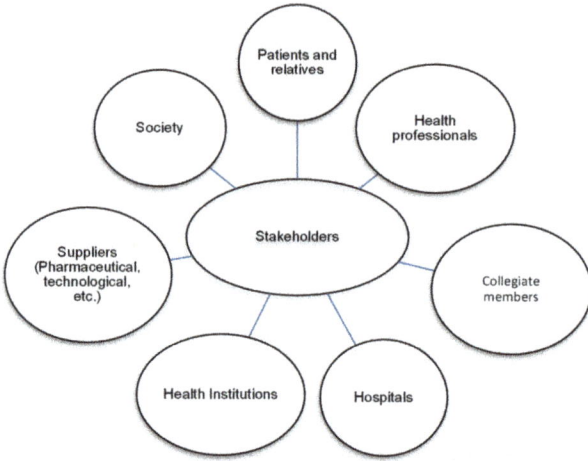

Figure 2. Stakeholders of Spanish official medical colleges. Source: Adapted from Freeman [66].

For this reason, this study focuses on the degree of knowledge that such professional college have regarding current communication tools, among which social media plays an influential role that affects the information that reaches its stakeholders. The Spanish official medical colleges must continue transmitting reliable information using language that is appropriate for the whole population. Therefore, the existence of specialized communication professionals who are at the vanguard of communication languages, mechanisms and strategies is so important.

3. Methods

A qualitative method through semi-structured interviews has been applied with the aim of delving deeper into the use of social media by communication professionals specializing in health. The choice is relevant as the main contribution of this qualitative study is to explore and understand some features of the communication of these colleges.

Qualitative research (QR) is useful for analyzing and understanding interpersonal relationships, behavioral experiences and variables such as opinions, perceptions, motivations and attitudes [67,68]. These variables are of interest in the field of communication. Moreover, the flexible and eminently inductive nature of QR is particularly suitable for seeking explanations for communication phenomena. Atlas.ti is the tool used to systemize the data and provide the desirable insights.

However, given the novelty of the issues being discussed and the need to ensure that the views of the most important actors were obtained, the flexibility of semi-structured interviews greatly outweighed the limitations on statistical analysis that would result [69–72]. In fact, flexibility both in designing and refining the interview guides and in actually conducting the interviews is probably the most important key to success in using this technique. This kind of interviewing also allowed the research to explore some of the underlying motives more directly [73]. Hence, semi-structured interviews using a deductive approach [74] were chosen in order to allow the participants a degree of freedom to explain their thoughts and to highlight areas of particular interest and expertise that they felt they had [75], as well as to enable certain responses to be questioned in greater depth, and in particular to bring out and resolve apparent contradictions.

The research team developed a protocol for semi-structured guides, that included five phases: (1) identifying the prerequisites for using semi-structured interviews; (2) retrieving and using previous knowledge; (3) formulating the preliminary semi-structured interview guide; (4) pilot testing the guide; and (5) presenting the complete semi-structured interview guide.

The interviews were carried out by the authors.

All 52 of the OMC in Spain were contacted, addressing the person in charge of communication or, whenever this information was not publicly available, addressing the Dean as the head representative. Of the OMCs, 38 showed interest in participation; they represented 73.07% of the total. The high participation of the OMC allowed to obtain information from a highly representative group. For this reason, it was considered interesting to include some statistical data, which are reflected in tables.

The guide included three predefined categories. At first in order to know the profile the professional who lead the communication in the official medical colleges, they were asked some data about their functions and tasks, as well as the labor seniority, based on a validated tool by European Monitor Communication studies [76]. It was also considered important to know first of all aspects related to gender and age and especially those related to their work situation and whether there were communication cabinets in the OMC and whether the professionals responsible for them were experts with communication training.

The first category was regarding the involvement of the official medical colleges' stakeholders. The role of health institutions, health professional, hospital groups, patients and family members or society were discussed. This debate helped us to have enough knowledge to map the stakeholders with whom they were dealing.

Second, we were interested in knowing the importance of communication professionals in the OMC and their use of social media for their work. The main reasons why they use social media in their professional routine (as a source of information, to interact with its stakeholders, as a communication channel, to establish professional relationships, to search for stories or to contrast information) were discussed in the interviews.

Finally, the third category was related OMC as producers of heath information. Social media has brought opportunities and challenges in health field, so we were interested about how social media contribute to the construction of agenda-setting in the health sector.

4. Results

Going into detail concerning with the qualitative technique, it is shown a descriptive analysis of the participant in order to present a general view of its make-up and highlight the main relationships between variables and their significance for the population (Table 2).

Table 2. Demographic factors.

		Frequency	Percent
Gender	Male	12	32.70
	Female	26	67.30
Age	26–29	0	0
	30–39	22	57.90
	40–49	8	21.05
	50–65	8	21.05
Employment situation	Communication Cabinet OMC	35	92.10
	Freelance	3	7.90
Job experience	Less to 5 years	0	0
	5 to 10 years	17	42.10
	More than 10 years	21	57.90

Both their years of work experience in the health communication sector and their activity in social media validate their extensive knowledge in the field.

Over half of the interviewees, is between 30 and 39 years old, whereas the rest is over 40. All of them were part of the working-age population when social media appeared, according to the mapping of birth with the evolution of social media that Boyd and Ellison made in 2008 [77,78].

The number of years of professional experience is also worthy of attention. Over half of the professionals have worked for over ten years and the rest have worked for between five and ten years. This is significant if it is considered that specializing in the health sector, which since the 90 s has been affected by a "superabundance of information" [79], implies years of professional experience in order to provide quality information.

As it was indicated before three categories were predefined. Table 3 summarily describes the themes obtained of participants.

Regarding RQ_1, the experts highlighted that the most important stakeholders for the OMC are their own collegiate members that corresponds to all medical professionals enrolled in their district, with which they maintain regular bidirectional communication. When considering that they should be informed of all the concerns and investigations that are carried out by all health professionals. Followed by public and private hospitals. Patients and their families showed scarce representativity. Finally, society in general and health institutions were the groups with the lowest score (Figure 3). Comparing Figure 3 with the theory of Freeman's stakeholders seen in Figure 2, the only groups that are not represented are the suppliers (pharmaceutical, technological, etc.) and other health's professional (nurses, physiotherapists, etc.).

Table 3. Main Themes.

Theme	Description
The role of OMC as interlocutor with stakeholders.	References that coincide in the same stakeholders, focusing mainly on the collegiate members, then in the hospitals and health institutions and finally in the patients and society. All OMC communicators confirm that there is bilateral communication with them.
Social media as a work tool for this professional.	References indicate that they use social media to learn about advances in the health field, connection with other health institutions, professionals and verification of fake news.
The importance of social media in the communication strategies of the OMC and the implementation of its agenda setting.	References to social media as a useful tool for bidirectional communication in the preparation of agenda setting. Social media is changing communication pattern, although it is recognized social media is not the only source used for the realization of the agenda setting There is no total agreement among those interviewed that social media is the best channel of information in the context of health crises.

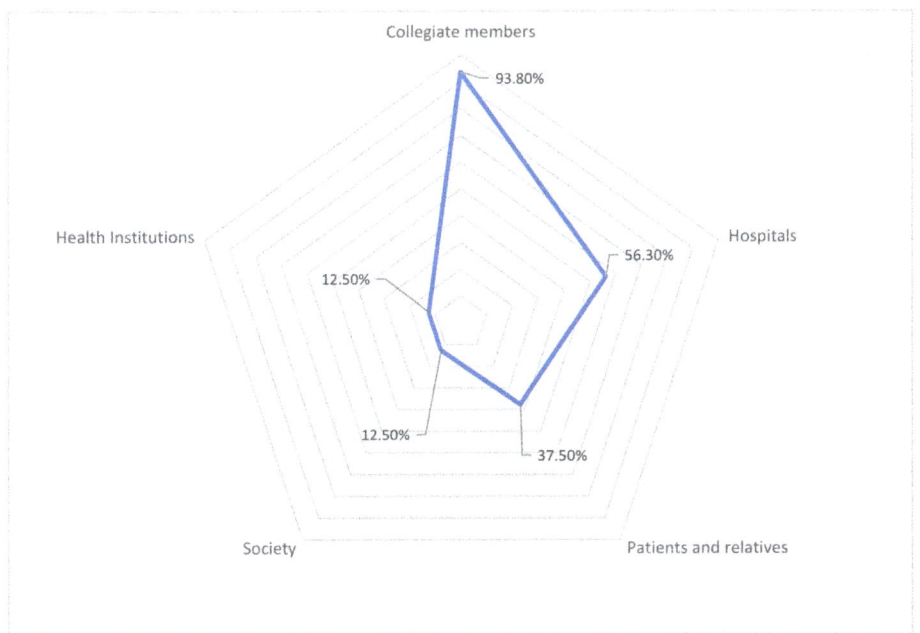

Figure 3. Official medical colleges (OMC) relations with their primary stakeholders. The percentage indicates the relationship with each stakeholder. Source: In-house elaboration.

Regarding question RQ_2, all official medical colleges participants in this investigation have an organized communication department, in which one to three people work—either specialists in the field and graduates in Journalism and/or Public Relations. In addition, these are organized in a communication network of professional medical colleges, to exchange experiences, and even organize an annual congress to present and share their initiatives. Recently, they have dedicated these conferences to social media strategies, and they have also worked in the fight against the dissemination of fake health news or crisis communication.

In terms of usability, the recurrent use of social media as an instrument of work exposed in the scientific literature referred to is corroborated in the results obtained in the interviews. The fact that all respondents use social media in their work may reflect the challenge of incorporating social media. Most indicated that their usage times are growing annually. The following table reflects the number of hours/days of social media use to collect or disseminate information (Table 4).

Table 4. Use of social media per day (%).

Communication Experts	Use of Social Media per Day (%)
Less than 1 h	23.80
Between 1 and 2 h	51.20
Between 2 and 5 h	13.50
More than 5 h	11.50

It is important to highlight that, despite the fact that 18.8% of those interviewed consider that social media hinders their work because excessive information published results in intoxication of the content, most of the respondents think that social media make their job easier and lead them to other sources of information (Table 5).

Table 5. Usefulness of social media for daily work.

Usefulness of Social Media for Daily Work	Utility (%)
Make work easier and increase the possibilities for information sources.	75.00
Hinder their work because there is too much information and sometimes intoxication.	18.80
Increase the workload and time spent	6.20

Nevertheless, social media have become a source of information that is relevant or very important for most professionals (Table 6).

Table 6. Social media as an information source in your work.

Social Media as an Information Source	(%)
Very important	62.50
Important	25.00
Low importance	12.50

It was highlighted by respondents that content generated by unofficial sources or by users was not sufficiently rigorous.

With regard to health-related accounts. All of them visit the corporate social media of hospitals and/or health institutions and evaluate their content as relevant (Table 7). None of the respondents considers the content found on hospital or health institutions social media to be "not important at all".

Table 7. Importance of the social media related to the health sector.

Importance of the Social Media Related to the Health Sector	(%)
Very important	12.50
Important	56.20
Not so important	12.50
Neutral	18.80
Not important at all	0

The participants use social media as a "source of information", which is one of the main aims for using them. In addition, the respondents highlight that this motivation is followed by keeping up with what is happening in their professional field. The aims that follow in the ranking of importance emerging from the interview are "as a source of information for the organization they work for", "as the main content focus", "establishing professional connections", "monitoring competition", "as a source of information as specialized journalist", "verifying information" and "finding stories" (Figure 4).

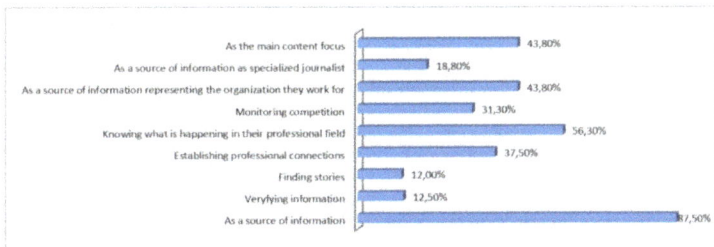

Figure 4. Main aims in the use of social media. Source: In-house elaboration.

In the case of social media as a source of information, the difference between the percentage of Twitter and Facebook users increases, so that Twitter emerges as the top social media chosen by specialized professionals. All of them point out social media as the main channel in the future.

In particular, out of the social media that they use, specialized health professionals in Spain resort most often to Twitter and Facebook (Table 8).

Table 8. Social media used most frequently.

Social Media	Use (%) The Percentage Indicates the Level of Use with Each Social Media.
Facebook	81.30
Twitter	87.50
LinkedIn	12.50
Pinterest	0
Google +	18.80
Specialized scientific and health networks	18.80
Instagram	6.30

All of the interviewers visit social media that are managed by health institutions, follow by health professionals accounts and researchers. Almost a third of the participants mention patient collectives that also communicate by social media.

In terms of credibility, the most credible accounts are those of health institutions, to which 87.5% refer. They are followed by the accounts of health professionals and researchers in the health sector. If the public and private hospitals are considered separately, the public hospitals accounts enjoy greater credibility than those in the private hospitals. The patient collectives accounts are the least credible. The accounts of citizens expressing themselves on the topic of health and who do not belong to any association do not enjoy any credibility (Table 9).

The argument that the respondents give for their answers is scientific rigor, which is considered to be greater in the case of health institutions. The communication on these social media is contemplated dependable because it is supported by the institution they represent and the professionalism of is specialists.

Table 9. Health-related social media.

Accounts Social Media	Consult (%)	Credibility (%)
	The Percentage Indicates the Relationship with Each Account Social Media.	
Health institutions	100.00	87.50
Health professionals and researchers	56.30	31.30
Public hospitals	56.30	18.80
Private hospitals	50.00	12.50
Patient collectives	31.30	12.50
Citizens	0	0

It is necessary to point the low level of credibility in public and private hospitals. The professional proposes changes in hospital social media, such as contents that are not biased according to institutional interests, more information about health in general and about health promotion in particular that can be communicated to the citizenship. Another suggestion has been to give a relevant role to the hospital professionals as co-creators of contents.

In their responses, communication professionals of OMC do not coincide in their opinions about how institutions avoid managing communication through social media in the event of a health crisis. It is widely recognized in the literature that social media offer immediate circulation of messages and this makes them valuable for such professional communication.

The speed with which information can be spread through social media in emergency situations, catastrophes and socially critical events which are dangerous for public health makes them essential for professionals specializing in health.

With respect to RQ_3, the participants think that social media is a useful tool for establishing bidirectional communication with their registered doctors, health institutions, hospitals and patient associations. Likewise, the contents generated in their social media accounts have scientific rigor that is very useful for society.

The professional of OMC defend that unlike the beginning of the decade, when the participation of the official medical colleges in Spain in social media was insignificant, today its activity is remarkable. This can be noticed in the significant increase both in the number of followers of their social media and in the volume of information they generate. The voice of the professionals of these entities in social media acquires special relevance in order to promote accurate information that preserves the quality of life and well-being of citizens.

The interviewees consider that official medical colleges have the capacity and the authority to become the voice for health institutions in their role as official sources in matters of health, using its own social media accounts at times when citizens claim a continuous supply of information.

5. Conclusions

However, organizations and professional associations in the health field are increasingly examining the potential of social media to allow members to share knowledge and engage their publics [54], these activities in official medical colleges were under researched [5,24].

Spanish official medical colleges, with a total of 52 locations distributed in each of the Spanish provinces and with 267,995 registered doctors, are considered one of the most important health institutions in the country.

Unlike other health institutions, communication is essential for the official medical colleges in Spain. Therefore, they have communication cabinets with professionals specialized in communication with extensive knowledge in the work they develop as part of their staff with more than five years' experience. Their professionals have degrees in journalism and/or public relations and are mostly women.

They have shown a strong relationship with stakeholders such as health professionals, health institutions, hospitals, patients and their families and society in general. Consequently, it can be stated that RQ$_1$ can be answered in the affirmative, the official medical colleges represented by their communication experts are valid interlocutors with their stakeholders.

OMC' professionals analyzed and verified the social media information of their stakeholders. Social media are a valid source of information for aspects related to new developments in the field of health.

All the communication professionals consulted use social media for their work. Twitter and Facebook are the most widely used; Twitter being the most popular (87.5%), followed by Facebook (81.3%). It coincides with Ahmed [80], that points out the most important social media for health conversations is Twitter, where it is also possible to extract tweets for academic research purposes. Through social media there can be the possibility of key debates and relationships with other stakeholders related to health topics.

The credibility of the corporate social media of health institutions and hospitals, based on the veracity of the information they publish, is well appreciated by communication professionals at the official medical colleges of Spain. However, it is significant that a percentage of the participants considered that these hospital contents are not sufficiently complete to serve their interests, and therefore are unsatisfactory.

The value afforded by the communication established by hospitals through their corporate social media has been useful in analyzing the influence of these contents on the daily practice of professionals specialized in health working in the communication departments of the Spanish official medical colleges. The contribution of these professionals, as intermediaries between the health institutions and the society in the construction of reality, has revealed strengths and weaknesses of hospital social media.

With the purpose of bringing the professionals on both sides closer together and making their relationship more successful those in charge of hospital communication, would must rise to the challenge of active listening to the communication specialists of the Spanish official medical colleges.

This finding coincides with Castilla [24]. Those in charge of setting the health agenda have expressed that in such circumstances, they would become more permeable to information coming from hospital social media, which would play a more significant role as relevant sources of information. This fact would reverse the percentages of credibility obtained in this respect.

These professionals find social media relevant, they know their potential and value the volume of information that they can access through them, even if their contents make up only portion of their agenda-setting. In this sense, most professionals consider that social media are one more tool that they can use in their work, but few of them include them how only as a source of content. Fulfilling research question three.

There is no total consensus among those interviewed that social media is the best channel of information in the context of health crises. For them there is much noise on social media with unconfirmed or fake news.

Most of the experts suggest social media as the main communication channel with stakeholders in the future.

Limitations and Future Research Lines

First, since this is an exploratory study of the behavior of official medical colleges, it is not possible to measure development in the medium term, and a lengthier study is needed in order to advance. Other qualitative research techniques such as content analysis on social media could be integrated in order to perform more in-depth analysis. Second, research has only focused on Spain, so further empirical research should be conducted in different regions, which would be of interest to make comparisons with other countries. The limitations identified are the basis for the design of future lines of research.

Author Contributions: All authors contributed equally to this study. All authors have read and agreed to the published version of the manuscript.

Funding: This research has received funds from a Plan Propio of University of Malaga.

Acknowledgments: Our special gratitude to the Official Medical colleges participants.

Conflicts of Interest: The authors declare no conflicts of interest.

References

1. Swan, M. Emerging Patient-Driven Health Care Models: An Examination of Health Social Networks, Consumer Personalized Medicine and Quantified Self-Tracking. *Int. J. Environ. Res. Public Health* **2009**, *6*, 492–525. [CrossRef] [PubMed]
2. Van de Belt, T.H.; Engelen, L.J.; Berben, S.A.; Teerenstra, S.; Samsom, M.; Schoonhoven, L. Internet and social media for health-related information and communication in health care: Preferences of the Dutch general population. *J. Med. Internet Res.* **2013**, *15*, e220. [CrossRef] [PubMed]
3. Tonia, T. Social media in public health: Is it used and is it useful? *Int. J. Public Health* **2014**, *59*, 889–891. [CrossRef] [PubMed]
4. Prasad, B. Social media, health care, and social networking. *Gastrointest. Endosc.* **2013**, *77*, 492–495. [CrossRef] [PubMed]
5. Terrón Blanco, J.L. La comunicación para la salud en España, algunos apuntes. *Rev. Española de Comun. y Salud* **2007**, *10*, 23–24.
6. Vance, K.; Howe, W.; Dellavalle, R.P. Social internet sites as a source of public health information. *Dermatol. Clin.* **2009**, *27*, 133–136. [CrossRef] [PubMed]
7. Ventola, C.L. Social media and health care professionals: Benefits, risks, and best practices. *Pharm. Ther.* **2014**, *39*, 491–520. Available online: https://www.ncbi.nlm.nih.gov/pmc/articles/PMC4103576/ (accessed on 27 August 2019).
8. Mangold, W.G.; Faulds, D.J. Social media: The new hybrid element of the promotion mix. *Bus. Horiz.* **2009**, *52*, 357–365. [CrossRef]
9. Sánchez, M.T.; Armayones, M.; Fernández-Luque, L.; Gómez-Zúñigay, B.; Pousada, M. Análisis del uso del video sanitario online en una muestra de redes sociales en España: Implicaciones para la promoción de la salud. *RevistaeSalud. Com* **2012**, *8*, 1–13. Available online: https://dialnet.unirioja.es/servlet/articulo?codigo=4205991 (accessed on 27 August 2019).
10. De las Heras Pedrosa, C.; Jambrino-Maldonado, C.; Iglesias-Sánchez, P.P.; Lugo-Ocando, J. Importancia de las relaciones con los públicos en la reputación en un destino turístico inteligente. Propuesta de un modelo sostenible. *Rev. Int. Relat. Public.* **2019**, *9*, 117–138. [CrossRef]
11. Andersen, K.N.; Medaglia, R.; Enriksen, H.Z. Social media in public health care: Impact domain propositions. *Gov. Inf. Q.* **2012**, *29*, 462–469. [CrossRef]
12. Bjerglund-Andersen, N.; Söderqvist, T. *Social Media and Public Health Research*; University of Copenhagen, Faculty of Science: Copenhagen, Denmark, 2012. Available online: http://www.bjerglund.files.wordpress.com/2012/11/final-social-media-and-public-health-research1.pdf (accessed on 28 August 2019).
13. Griffis, H.M.; Kilaru, A.S.; Werner, R.M.; Asch, D.A.; Hershey, J.C.; Hill, S.; Ha, Y.P.; Sellers, A.; Mahoney, K.; Merchant, R.M. Use of Social Media across US Hospitals: Descriptive Analysis of Adoption and Utilization. *J. Med. Internet Res.* **2014**, *16*, e264. [CrossRef] [PubMed]
14. Merchant, R.M.; Elmer, S.; Lurie, N. Integrating Social Media into Emergency-Preparedness Efforts. *N. Engl. J. Med.* **2011**, *365*, 289–291. [CrossRef] [PubMed]
15. Kass-Hout, T.; Alhinnami, H. Social media in public health. *Br. Med. Bull.* **2013**, *108*, 5–24. [CrossRef]
16. Roman, L.A. Using Social Media to Enhance Career Development Opportunities for Health Promotion Professionals. *Health Promot. Pract.* **2014**, *15*, 471–475. [CrossRef]
17. Zhao, J.; Wang, J. Health Advertising on Short-Video Social Media: A Study on User Attitudes Based on the Extended Technology Acceptance Model. *Int. J. Environ. Res. Public Health* **2020**, *17*, 1501. [CrossRef]
18. Gomes, C.; Coustasse, A. Tweeting and Treating: How Hospitals Use Twitter to Improve Care. *Health Care Manag.* **2015**, *34*, 203–214. [CrossRef]
19. Bernhardt, J.M.; Alber, J.; Gold, R.S. A social media primer for professionals: Digital do's and don'ts. *Health Promot. Pract.* **2014**, *15*, 168–172. [CrossRef]

20. Blázquez Fernández, C.; Cantarero Prieto, D.; Pascual Sáez, M. Promoting the use of health information and communication technologies in Spain: A new approach based on the ICT-H. *Rev. ICONO14 Rev. Científica de Comun. y Tecnol. Emerg.* **2015**, *13*, 238–259. [CrossRef]
21. Chou, W.S.; Hunt, Y.M.; Beckjord, E.B.; Moser, R.P.; Hesse, B.W. Social media use in the United States: Implications for health communication. *J. Med. Internet Res.* **2009**, *11*, e48. [CrossRef]
22. Krowchuk, H.V.; Lane, S.H.; Twaddell, J.W. Should Social Media be Used to Communicate With Patients? *MCN Am. J. Matern. Chil. Nurs.* **2010**, *35*, 6–7. [CrossRef] [PubMed]
23. Chretien, K.C.; Kind, T. Social Media and Clinical Care. *Circulation* **2013**, *127*, 1413–1421. [CrossRef] [PubMed]
24. Castilla, G. La Comunicación en salud desde el punto de vista de una sociedad médica. *Rev. Española de Comun. y Salud* **2016**, *7*, 129–132. [CrossRef]
25. Lambert, K.M.; Barry, P.; Stokes, G. Risk management and legal issues with the use of social media in the healthcare setting. *J. Healthc. Risk Manag.* **2012**, *31*, 41–47. [CrossRef]
26. Househ, M. The use of social media in healthcare: Organizational, clinical, and patient perspectives. *Stud. Health Technol. Inform.* **2013**, *183*, 244–248. [CrossRef]
27. Dizon, D.S.; Graham, D.; Thompson, M.A.; Johnson, L.J.; Johnston, C.; Fisch, M.J.; Miller, R. Practical guidance: The use of social media in oncology practice. *J. Oncol. Pract.* **2012**, *8*, e114–e124. [CrossRef]
28. Childs, L.M.; Martin, C.Y. Social media profiles: Striking the right balance. *Am. J. Health Syst. Ph.* **2012**, *69*, 2044–2050. [CrossRef]
29. Nazir, M.; Hussain, I.; Tian, J.; Akram, S.; Mangenda Tshiaba, S.; Mushtaq, S.; Shad, M.A.A. Multidimensional Model of Public Health Approaches Against COVID-19. *Int. J. Environ. Res. Public Health* **2020**, *17*, 3780. [CrossRef]
30. Mhasawade, V.; Elghafari, A.; Duncan, D.T.; Chunara, R. Role of the Built and Online Social Environments on Expression of Dining on Instagram. *Int. J. Environ. Res. Public Health* **2020**, *17*, 735. [CrossRef]
31. Brandtzaeg, P.B.; Lüders, M.; Spangenberg, J.; Rath-Wiggins, L.; Følstad, A. Emerging Journalistic Verification Practices Concerning Social Media. *Journal. Pract.* **2015**, *10*, 323–342. [CrossRef]
32. Leask, J.; Hooker, C.; King, C. Media coverage of health issues and how to work more effectively with journalists: A qualitative study. *BMC Public Health* **2010**, *10*, 535. [CrossRef]
33. Arkin, E.B. Opportunities for Improving the Nation's Health through Collaboration with the Mass Media. *Public Health. Rep.* **1990**, *105*, 219–223. [PubMed]
34. Medina Aguerrebere, P. La gestión de la reputación online de las marcas hospitalarias: Una propuesta de modelo. *ZER* **2017**, *22*, 53–68. [CrossRef]
35. Moorhead, S.A.; Hazlett, D.E.; Harrison, L.; Carroll, J.K.; Irwin, A.; Hoving, C. A New Dimension of Health Care: Systematic Review of the Uses, Benefits, and Limitations of Social Media for Health Communication. *J. Med. Internet Res.* **2013**, *15*, e85. [CrossRef] [PubMed]
36. Kovic, I.; Lulic, I.; Brumini, G. Examining the Medical Blogosphere: An Online Survey of Medical Bloggers. *J. Med. Internet Res.* **2008**, *10*, e28. [CrossRef] [PubMed]
37. Hermida, A. Tweets and truth. *Journal. Pract.* **2012**, *6*, 659–668. [CrossRef]
38. Gavilán, E.; Iriberri, A. Medios de Comunicación como agentes que facilitan la medicalización de la vida: El ejemplo de la andropausia. *Rev. de Comun. y Salud* **2014**, *4*, 49–67. [CrossRef]
39. Barrero, A.E.; Palacios, J.A. Reflexiones sobre el papel del comunicador social y competencias del comunicador en las organizaciones. *Poliantea* **2015**, *11*, 197–221. [CrossRef]
40. Kaplan, A.M.; Haenlein, M. Users of the world, unite! The challenges and opportunities of Social Media. *Bus. Horiz.* **2010**, *53*, 59–68. [CrossRef]
41. Hermida, A.; Lewis, S.C.; Zamith, R. Sourcing the Arab spring: A case study of Andy Carvin's sources on twitter during the Tunisian and Egyptian revolutions. *J. Comput. Mediat. Commun.* **2014**, *19*, 479–499. [CrossRef]
42. Paulussen, S.; Harder, R.A. Social Media References in Newspapers. *Journal. Pract.* **2014**, *8*, 542–551. [CrossRef]
43. Lariscy, R.W.; Avery, E.J.; Sweetser, K.D.; Howes, P. An examination of the role of online social media in journalists' source mix. *Public Relat. Rev.* **2009**, *35*, 314–316. [CrossRef]
44. McCombs, M.; Shaw, D. The agenda-setting function of mass media. *Public Opin. Q.* **1972**, *36*, 176–187. [CrossRef]

45. McCombs, M.; Shaw, D. The agenda-setting function of mass media. *Agenda Setting J.* **2017**, *1*, 105–116. [CrossRef]
46. Almaguer, R. Prensa diaria y elecciones: ¿contribución o seguimiento de la agenda? In *Sociedad, Desarrollo y Movilidad en Comunicación*; Nieto, J., Ed.; Universidad Autónoma de Tamaulipas: Tamaulipas, México, 2010; pp. 201–216.
47. Russell, K.M.; Lamme, M.O. Theorizing public relations history: The roles of strategic intent and human agency. *Public Relat. Rev.* **2016**, *42*, 741–747. [CrossRef]
48. Păun, M. Perceptions on the Effectiveness of Communication between Public Institutions and Journalists through Social Media. *Styles Commun.* **2009**, *1*, 121–140. Available online: http://journals.univ-danubius.ro/index.php/communication/article/viewFile/145/138 (accessed on 28 August 2019).
49. Rando-Cueto, D.; Paniagua-Rojano, F.J.; de las Heras-Pedrosa, C. Factores influyentes en el éxito de la comunicación hospitalaria vía redes sociales. *Rev. Lat. de Comun. Soc.* **2016**, *71*, 1170–1186. [CrossRef]
50. Antheunis, M.L.; Tates, K.; Nieboer, T.E. Patients' and health professionals' use of social media in health care: Motives, barriers and expectations. *Patient Educ. Couns.* **2013**, *92*, 426–431. [CrossRef]
51. Shepherd, A.; Sanders, C.; Doyle, M.; Shaw, J. Using social media for support and feedback by mental health service users: Thematic analysis of a twitter conversation. *BMC Psychiatry* **2015**, *15*, 2–9. [CrossRef]
52. De la Peña, A.; Quintanilla, C. Share, like and achieve: The power of Facebook to reach health-related goals. *Int. J. Consum. Stud.* **2015**, *39*, 495–505. [CrossRef]
53. Koteyko, N.; Hunt, D.; Gunter, B. Expectations in the field of the Internet and health: An analysis of claims about social networking sites in clinical literature. *Sociol. Health Illn.* **2015**, *37*, 468–484. [CrossRef] [PubMed]
54. Hara, N.; Foon Hew, K. Knowledge-sharing in an online community of health-care professionals. *Inf. Technol. People* **2007**, *20*, 235–261. [CrossRef]
55. Antonacci, G.; Fronzetti Colladon, A.; Stefanini, A.; Gloor, P. It is rotating leaders who build the swarm: Social network determinants of growth for healthcare virtual communities of practice. *J. Knowl. Manag.* **2017**, *21*, 1218–1239. [CrossRef]
56. Joseph Mattingly, T. Innovative patient care practices using social media. *J. Am. Pharm. Assoc.* **2015**, *55*, 288–293. [CrossRef] [PubMed]
57. Rando-Cueto, D.; de las Heras-Pedrosa, C. Presencia y estrategias de comunicación de hospitales andaluces en las redes sociales. *Cuad. Artes. de Comun.* **2014**, *92*, 155–173. [CrossRef]
58. Rando-Cueto, D.; de las Heras-Pedrosa, C. Análisis de la comunicación corporativa de los hospitales andaluces vía twitter. *Rev. Opción* **2016**, *32*, 557–576. [CrossRef]
59. Instituto Nacional de Estadística. Profesionales Sanitarios Colegiados. 2019. Available online: https://www.ine.es/prensa/epsc_2019.pdf (accessed on 1 April 2020).
60. Grunig, J.E. Theory and practice of interactive media relations. *Public Relat. Q.* **1990**, *35*, 18–23.
61. Grunig, J.E.; Hunt, T. *Managing Public Relations*; Holt, Rinehart and Wilson: Fort Worth, TX, USA, 1984.
62. Ruiz de Azua, S.; Ozamiz-Etxebarria, N.; Ortiz-Jauregui, M.A.; Gonzalez-Pinto, A. Communicative and Social Skills among Medical Students in Spain: A Descriptive Analysis. *Int. J. Environ. Res. Public Health* **2020**, *17*, 1408. [CrossRef]
63. Mainardes, E.W.; Raposo, M.; Alves, H. Universities Need a Market Orientation to Attract Non-Traditional Stakeholders as New Financing Sources. *Public Organ. Rev.* **2014**, *14*, 159–171. [CrossRef]
64. Jambrino-Maldonado, C.; De las Heras-Pedrosa, C. Building a model of corporate reputation observatory for a tourist destination. *Tour. Manag. Stud.* **2013**, *1*, 66–76. [CrossRef]
65. Wenger, E. Communities of Practice and Social Learning Systems. *Organization* **2000**, *7*, 225–246. [CrossRef]
66. Freeman, R.E. Formulating Strategies for Stakeholders. In *Strategic Management*; Cambridge University Press: Cambridge, UK, 2010; pp. 126–153. [CrossRef]
67. Imms, M.; Ereaut, G. *An Introduction to Qualitative Market Research*; SAGE Publications Ltd.: London, UK, 2013. [CrossRef]
68. Belk, R.W. *Handbook of Qualitative Research Methods in Marketing*; Edward Elgar Publishing Limited: Cheltenham, UK, 2006. [CrossRef]
69. Gummesson, E. *Qualitative Methods in Management Research*, 2nd ed.; Sage: Thousand Oaks, CA, USA, 2000.
70. Chrzanowska, J. *Interviewing Groups and Individuals in Qualitative Market Research*; Sage: London, UK, 2002.
71. Ruiz-Olabuénaga, J.I. *Teoría y Práctica de la Investigación Cualitativa*; Deusto Digital: Bilbao, Spain, 2012.

72. Malhotra, N.K. Questionnaire Design and Scale Development. In *The Handbook of Marketing Research: Uses, Misuses, and Future Advances*; Grover, R., Vriens, M., Eds.; Sage Publications Ltd: London, UK, 2006; pp. 115–168. [CrossRef]
73. Horton, J.; Macve, R.; Struyven, G. Qualitative Research: Experiences in Using Semi-Structured Interviews. In *The Real Life Guide to Accounting Research*; Elsevier Ltd.: London, UK, 2004; pp. 339–357. [CrossRef]
74. Azungah, T. Qualitative research: Deductive and inductive approaches to data analysis. *Qual. Res. J.* **2018**, *18*, 383–400. [CrossRef]
75. Walker, R. *Applied Qualitative Research*; Gower: Aldershot, UK, 1985.
76. Zerfass, A.; Tench, R.; Verhoeven, P.; Verçid, D.; Moreno, A. *European Communication Monitor 2018. Excellence in Strategic Communication-Key Issues, Leadership, Gender and Mobile Media. Results of a Survey in 42 Countries*; EACD/EUPRERA: Brussels, Belgium; Quadriga Media Berlin: Berlin, Germany, 2018. Available online: http://www.zerfass.de/ECM-WEBSITE/ECM-2016.html (accessed on 27 August 2019).
77. Boyd, D.; Ellison, N. Social Network Sites: Definition, History, and Scholarship. *J. Comput. Mediat. Commun.* **2007**, *13*, 210–230. [CrossRef]
78. Colás-Bravo, P.; González-Ramírez, T.; De-Pablos-Pons, J. Young People and Social Networks: Motivations and Preferred Uses. *Comunicar* **2013**, *20*, 15–23. [CrossRef]
79. Mercado, M.T. La especialización periodística como salida a la crisis de los medios. In *Prospectivas y Tendencias Para la Comunicación en el Siglo XXI*; Salas, M.I., Mira., E., Eds.; CEU Ediciones: Madrid, Spain, 2013; pp. 59–78.
80. Ahmed, W.; Marin-Gomez, X.; Vidal-Aloball, J. Contextualising the 2019 E-Cigarette Health Scare: Insights from Twitter. *Int. J. Environ. Res. Public Health* **2020**, *17*, 2236. [CrossRef] [PubMed]

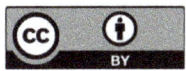

© 2020 by the authors. Licensee MDPI, Basel, Switzerland. This article is an open access article distributed under the terms and conditions of the Creative Commons Attribution (CC BY) license (http://creativecommons.org/licenses/by/4.0/).

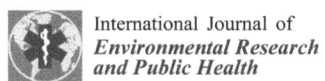
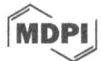

Article

Primary Care Professionals' Acceptance of Medical Record-Based, Store and Forward Provider-to-Provider Telemedicine in Catalonia: Results of a Web-Based Survey

Josep Vidal-Alaball [1,2,3,*], Francesc López Seguí [4,5], Josep Lluís Garcia Domingo [3], Gemma Flores Mateo [6], Gloria Sauch Valmaña [1,2], Anna Ruiz-Comellas [2,7], Francesc X Marín-Gomez [1,2] and Francesc García Cuyàs [8]

1. Unitat de Suport a la Recerca de la Catalunya Central, Fundació Institut Universitari per a la recerca a l'Atenció Primària de Salut Jordi Gol i Gurina, 08272 Sant Fruitós de Bages, Spain; gsauch.cc.ics@gencat.cat (G.S.V.); xmarin.cc.ics@gencat.cat (F.X.M.-G.)
2. Health Promotion in Rural Areas Research Group, Gerència Territorial de la Catalunya Central, Institut Català de la Salut, 08272 Sant Fruitós de Bages, Spain; aruiz.cc.ics@gencat.cat
3. Department of Economics and Business, University of Vic-Central University of Catalonia, 08500 Vic, Spain; jlgarcia@uvic.cat
4. TIC Salut Social-Generalitat de Catalunya, 08005 Barcelona, Spain; flopez@ticsalutsocial.cat
5. CRES&CEXS-Pompeu Fabra University, 08003 Barcelona, Spain
6. Unitat d'anàlisi i qualitat. Xarxa Sanitària i Social de Santa Tecla, 43003 Tarragona, Spain; gfloresm@xarxatecla.cat
7. Centre d'Atenció Primària Sant Joan de Vilatorrada, Gerència Territorial de la Catalunya Central, Institut Català de la Salut, 08250 Sant Joan de Vilatorrada, Spain
8. Sant Joan de Déu Hospital, Catalan Ministry of Health, 08950 Esplugues de Llobregat, Spain; francesc.garcia@umedicina.cat
* Correspondence: jvidal.cc.ics@gencat.cat; Tel.: +34-936930040

Received: 11 May 2020; Accepted: 2 June 2020; Published: 8 June 2020

Abstract: While telemedicine services enjoy a high acceptance among the public, evidence regarding clinician's acceptance, a key factor for sustainable telemedicine services, is mixed. However, telemedicine is generally better accepted by both patients and professionals who live in rural areas, as it can save them significant time. The objective of this study is to assess the acceptance of medical record-based, store and forward provider-to-provider telemedicine among primary care professionals and to describe the factors which may determine their future use. This is an observational cross-sectional study using the Catalan version of the Health Optimum questionnaire; a technology acceptance model-based validated survey comprised of eight short questions. The online, voluntary response poll was sent to all 661 primary care professionals in 17 primary care teams that had potentially used the telemedicine services of the main primary care provider in Catalonia, in the Central Catalan Region. The majority of respondents rated the quality of telemedicine consultations as "Excellent" or "Good" (83%). However, nearly 60% stated that they sometimes had technical, organizational or other difficulties, which might affect the quality of care delivered. These negatively predicted their declared future use ($p = 0.001$). The quality of telemedicine services is perceived as good overall for all the parameters studied, especially among nurses. It is important that policymakers examine and provide solutions for the technical and organizational difficulties detected (e.g., by providing training), in order to ensure the use of these services in the future.

Keywords: telemedicine; primary health care; acceptability of health care; surveys and questionnaires

1. Introduction

Aside from emerging evidence on the clinical impact of telemedicine, which has shown that it can provide effective health services at a lower cost [1–3], telemedicine services enjoy a high degree of acceptance among the public, as studies show that it saves them significant time [4–7]. In addition, it has been shown that avoiding travel to health centers can reduce air pollution in the context of the current climate crisis [8,9]. While clinician acceptance is a key factor for sustainable telemedicine services [10–12], evidence is mixed. A comprehensive systematic review reported that clinicians were highly satisfied with both store-and-forward and real time telemedicine [13]. However, other evidence suggested a subtle/nuanced effect: although services are generally well accepted by professionals, they express concerns regarding the increased workload that this might entail [14,15]. Such concerns appear to be more prevalent among primary care physicians than among nursing staff, who also express a fear that telemedicine could potentially undermine their professional autonomy [16]. While some studies suggest that telemedicine is better accepted by patients who live in rural areas [17], professionals in these fields are also more satisfied with the service as it facilitates contact with hospital specialists, improving their professional development [18,19]. Other studies also show the benefits of telemedicine for professionals in terms of professional development [20,21], as well as suggesting that it enabled them to approach their patients with greater knowledge [22].

The Catalan Health Care System dispenses services for 7.6 inhabitants, providing universal coverage through a tax-based system. Administratively, it is composed by a single public payer and multiple service providers publicly or privately owned, with an integrated system. Some of its peculiarities are the role of community and primary health care and the increasing use of information technologies and digital health [23]. In Catalonia, telemedicine is used in numerous areas, such as screening, diagnosis and the treatment of disease, asynchronously in particular. The most widely used are interconsultations between primary and hospital care professionals and teleconsultations between primary care professionals and patients [24]. With regard to the former, evidence suggests that they are cost-effective, serve to reduce face-to-face visits and that the economic benefit is mainly enjoyed by the patient [2]. Regarding the latter, recent studies show that they can also be useful in reducing face-to-face visits mainly for administrative reasons [25,26]. If, as these experiences suggest, telemedicine is shown to be socially desirable, it is important that healthcare professionals (who are the ones who make the decision to use it) are satisfied with it, even though it may not be of any particular benefit to them, meaning that they are active promoters of such services.

Numerous questionnaires attempt to study the acceptance of healthcare professionals regarding telemedicine [27–29]. Among them is the validated Catalan version of the "Health Optimum Questionnaire" [30], inspired by the areas and simplicity of the technology acceptance model [31]. In this context, the objective of this study was to assess the acceptance of telemedicine services among primary care professionals in the Catalan central region using the aforementioned questionnaire, and to describe the factors which may determine the use of telemedicine services in the future.

2. Methods

2.1. Study Questionnaire

This is an observational cross-sectional study using the Catalan version of the Health Optimum questionnaire, a Technology Acceptance Model-based validated survey which aims to measure the degree of satisfaction with telemedicine services and describing the factors that can determine its future use [30]. The questionnaire, consisting of 8 short questions with 3 or 5 response options using a Likert scale, is based on the two main concepts of ease of use and comprises three dimensions of perceived usefulness: individual context, technological context and implementation or organizational context [31]. An internet polling tool was used to anonymously send the questionnaire to all primary health care professionals who potentially had contact with the four medical record-based, store and forward provider-to-provider telemedicine specialties (teledermatology, teleulcers, teleophthalmology and teleaudiometry) of the 17 primary health care teams in the counties of Bages, Moianès and Berguedà of the Catalan Central Region of the Catalan Health Institute (the main primary care provider in Catalonia). The poll was sent by the Institute's Central Catalonia Research Unit to 661 healthcare professionals' email addresses on 18 May 2018. A reminder was sent on 30 May and the questionnaire was definitively closed on 8 June 2018.

The first question asked whether the health professional had used a telemedicine service at any time. If the response was "Yes", they continued with the questionnaire, while if the response was "No", the questionnaire ended. The survey received a total of 163 responses (response rate: 24.7%). Those who stated that they had never used a telemedicine service (40) or did not complete the survey (15) were excluded from the analysis. Thus, the sample under analysis is comprised of 108 participants (Figure 1).

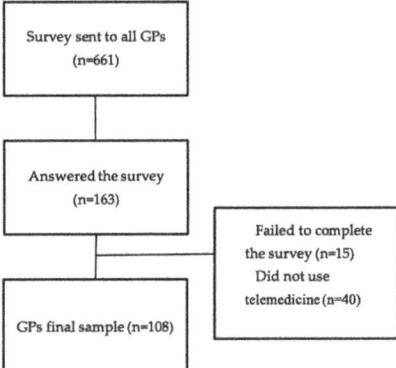

Figure 1. Participant Flow.

When numbers are small, Chi-square tests can give inaccurate results. This problem can be solved by grouping some of the answers. In questions 1 and 2, we grouped together the positive variables "excellent" and "good" on one hand and the negative variables "regular" and "bad" on the other. In question 3, "much better" was grouped with "better", and "worse" with "much worse". In question 4, "very comfortable" was grouped with "somewhat conformable", and "somewhat uncomfortable" with "very uncomfortable". The Chi-square was recalculated after grouping the variables and no differences were found in the results.

Linear correlations between questions were calculated, in order to better describe possible relations and to try to summarize information for future studies on the quality of telemedicine. For this purpose, the 112 participants who replied to some of the questions were included. Only Pearson correlation coefficients (PCC) higher than 0.5 were considered. A multivariate linear regression model was used to assess which variables could predict the future use of telemedicine services.

The programs Epi InfoTM v7.2.2.1 (Centers for Disease Control and Prevention, Atlanta, GA, USA) and SPSS v23 (SPSS IBM Inc., Chicago, NY, USA) were used for statistical analyses. Results were considered significant with $p < 0.05$. The study protocol was approved by the University Institute for Primary Care Research (IDIAP) Jordi Gol Health Care Ethics Committee (Code P16/046).

2.2. Sample Characteristics

Besides the questionnaire, the poll collected additional information to supplement the data with background characteristics of the respondents (Table 1). The typical profile was a 48-year-old woman, a General Practitioner, who mostly used the teledermatology service. The respondents declared having used one or more telemedicine service a total of 1515 times during the previous year, an average of 14.02 (with a median of 5 and a mode of 3) per respondent.

Table 1. Sample Characteristics.

Demographics		N
Women n (%)		83 (76.85)
Age (Mean, SD, min–max)		48.4 (9.1) (26–64)
Times used (Mean, SD, min–max)		14.02 (20.82) (1–100)
Professional role n (%)	Physicians	54 (50)
	Nurses	52 (48.15)
	Other	2 (1.85)
Telemedicine services used n (%) (respondents could choose more than one option)	Teledermatology	85 (52.15)
	Teleulcers	64 (39.26)
	Teleaudiometry	46 (28.22)
	Other	14 (8.59)

3. Results

3.1. Survey Results

The main results of the questionnaire are shown above (Figure 2).

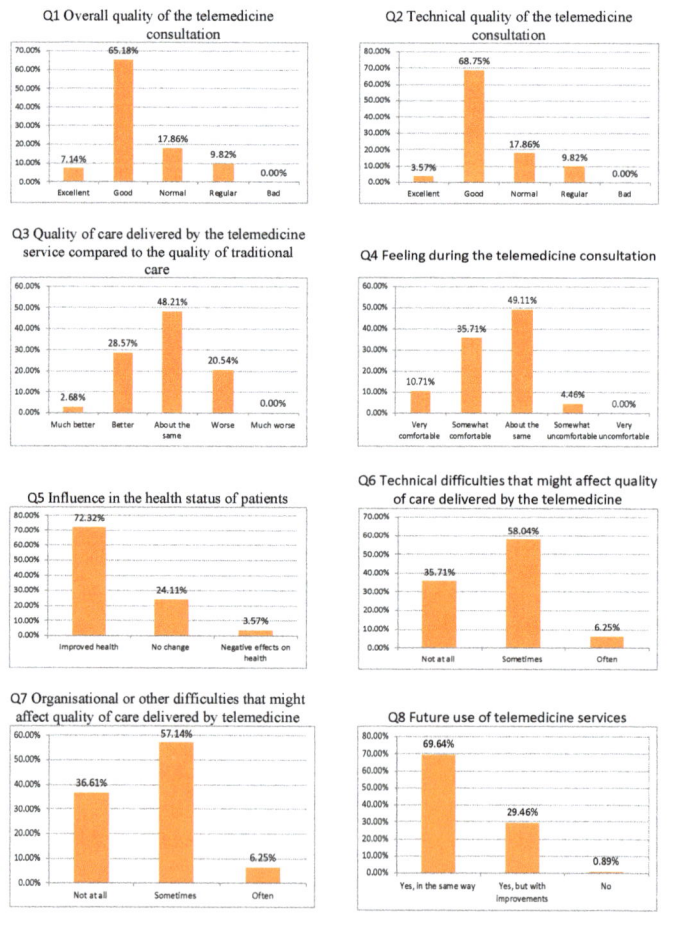

Figure 2. Survey Results.

The majority of participants rated the quality of telemedicine consultations as excellent (65.18%) or good (17.86%). They also mostly rated the technical quality of telemedicine consultations as good (68.75%). When comparing the quality of care delivered by the telemedicine service with the quality of traditional care, nearly half of the respondents stated that the quality was about the same; around 30% considered the quality of care to be better or much better, and just 20% considered the quality of care to be worse.

Half of the participants responded that they feel as comfortable during the telemedicine consultation as in a face-to-face consultation, while the rest felt somewhat comfortable or very comfortable. More than 70% of respondents considered that telemedicine services could improve patients' health status. However, nearly 60% of respondents stated that they sometimes had technical, organizational or other difficulties which might affect the quality of care delivered by telemedicine services.

Finally, when asked about future use of telemedicine services, nearly 70% of respondents wanted to continue to use the services in the same way, whilst the rest wanted to use the service but with some improvements. The mean and standard deviation of the responses are shown in Table 2.

Table 2. Main Survey Results.

Question	Mean	SD
Q1 How would do you rate the overall quality of the telemedicine consultation? *	3.70	0.74
Q2 How would you rate the technical quality of the telemedicine consultation? *	3.66	0.70
Q3 How would do you rate the quality of care delivered by the telemedicine service when compared to the quality of traditional care? *	3.13	0.76
Q4 Did you feel comfortable during the telemedicine consultation? *	3.53	0.74
Q5 Do you feel that the telemedicine consultation service may influence your patients' health status? **	2.69	0.54
Q6 Did you experience technical difficulties that might affect the quality of care delivered by the telemedicine service? **	2.29	0.58
Q7 Did you experience organisational or other difficulties that might affect the quality of care delivered by the telemedicine service? **	2.30	0.58
Q8 Would you continue to use the telemedicine service? **	2.69	0.48

* Q1 to Q4 are 5-point Likert whilst ** Q5 to Q8 are 1–3.

3.2. Sensitivity Analysis.

We looked at differences in responses to the eight questions in the questionnaire according to professional categories, identifying significant statistical differences in three cases. First, with respect to question 3, nursing staff rated the quality of care delivered by the telemedicine services as significantly better compared with medical staff ($p < 0.001$). Second, regarding question 6, medical staff reported having experienced more technical difficulties than nursing staff ($p < 0.05$). Finally, with regard to question 7, medical staff stated having experienced more organizational and other difficulties that might have affected the quality of care delivered by the telemedicine services than nursing staff ($p < 0.001$) (Table 3). The differences in responses by gender and age have no statistical differences between groups.

Looking at differences in responses to the eight survey questions, in relation to the number of times respondents have used any of the various telemedicine services in the previous year, significant statistical differences were found in three questions. Respondents who used telemedicine services more often rated the quality of care of these services as significantly worse, compared with respondents who use them less often (Figure 3) ($p < 0.05$). They also stated having experienced more technical difficulties and more organizational and other difficulties compared with respondents that used telemedicine services less often ($p < 0.001$).

Table 3. Differences in Responses by Professional Categories.

Rating the Quality of Care Delivered by the Telemedicine						
Professional category	About the same	Better	Much better	Worse	Much Worse	Total
Medical staff	26	7	2	19	0	54
Nursing staff	24	24	1	3	0	52
TOTAL	50	31	3	22	0	106
Technical difficulties that might affect the quality of care						
Professional category	Often	Sometimes	Not at all	Total		
Medical staff	5	39	10	54		
Nursing staff	2	24	26	52		
TOTAL	7	63	36	106		
Organizational or other difficulties that might affect the quality of care						
Professional category	Often	Sometimes	Not at all	Total		
Medical staff	5	39	10	54		
Nursing staff	2	22	28	52		
TOTAL	7	61	38	106		

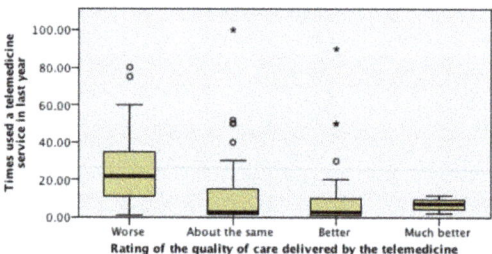

Figure 3. Quality of Care of the Telemedicine Consultation, by Number of Times Used.

3.3. Multivariate Linear Regression Model

A positive correlation (PCC = 0.728) was found between the overall quality of the telemedicine consultation and the rating of the technical quality of said consultation, between the overall quality of the telemedicine consultation and the future use of telemedicine (PCC = 0.583), and between the technical quality of the telemedicine consultation and the future use of telemedicine (PCC = 0.505). A negative correlation (PCC = 0.531) was found between organizational and other difficulties that might affect the quality of care delivered by the telemedicine service and the future use of telemedicine. We found no correlation between the perceived quality of telemedicine rendered and the perceived barriers of use (Table 4).

The multivariate linear regression showed two variables to be good predictors for the future use of telemedicine services: the overall quality of the telemedicine consultation ($p < 0.005$) which positively affects the future use, and organizational (or other) difficulties that might affect the quality of care delivered by the telemedicine service ($p < 0.001$), which negatively impacts the future use (Table 5).

Table 4. Linear Correlations between Q1–Q8.

		Rating of The Overall Quality of the Telemedicine Consultation	Rating of the Technical Quality of the Telemedicine Consultation	Rating of the Quality of Care Delivered by the Telemedicine	Feeling during the Telemedicine Consultation	Influence in the Health Status of the Patients	Technical Difficulties That Might Affect the Quality of Care Delivered by the Telemedicine Service	Organisational or Other Difficulties That Might Affect the Quality of Care Delivered by the Telemedicine Service	Future Use of Telemedicine Services
Rating of the overall quality of the telemedicine consultation	Pearson Correlation Sig. (2-tailed) N	1 112	0.728 ** 0 112	0.388 ** 0 112	0.468 ** 0 112	0.346 ** 0 112	−0.271 ** 0.004 112	−0.422 ** 0 112	0.583 ** 0 112
Rating of the technical quality of the telemedicine consultation	Pearson Correlation Sig. (2-tailed) N	0.728 ** 0 112	1 112	0.419 ** 0 112	0.480 ** 0 112	0.384 ** 0 112	−0.379 ** 0 112	−0.363 ** 0 112	0.505 ** 0 112
Rating of the quality of care delivered by the telemedicine	Pearson Correlation Sig. (2-tailed) N	0.388 ** 0 112	0.419 ** 0 112	1 112	0.301 ** 0.001 112	0.322 ** 0.001 112	0.256 ** 0.007 112	−0.353 ** 0 112	0.308 ** 0.001 112
Feeling during the telemedicine consultation	Pearson Correlation Sig. (2-tailed) N	0.468 ** 0 112	0.480 ** 0 112	0.301 ** 0.001 112	1 112	0.324 ** 0 112	−0.054 0.569 112	−0.312 ** 0.001 112	0.384 ** 0 112
Influence in the health status of the patients	Pearson Correlation Sig. (2-tailed) N	0.346 ** 0 112	0.384 ** 0 112	0.322 ** 0.001 112	0.324 ** 0 112	1 112	−0.183 0.054 112	−0.162 0.088 112	0.348 ** 0 112
Technical difficulties that might affect the quality of care delivered by the telemedicine service	Pearson Correlation Sig. (2-tailed) N	−0.271 ** 0.004 112	−0.379 ** 0 112	−0.256 ** 0.007 112	−0.054 0.569 112	−0.183 0.054 112	1 112	0.506 ** 0 112	−0.331 ** 0 112
Organisational or other difficulties that might affect the quality of care delivered by the telemedicine service	Pearson Correlation Sig. (2-tailed) N	−0.422 ** 0 112	−0.363 ** 0 112	−0.353 ** 0 112	−0.312 ** 0.001 112	−0.162 0.088 112	0.506 ** 0 112	1 112	−0.531 ** 0 112
Future use of telemedicine services	Pearson Correlation Sig. (2-tailed) N	0.583 ** 0 112	0.505 ** 0 112	0.308** 0.001 112	0.384** 0 112	0.348* 0 112	−0.331 ** 0 112	−0.531 ** 0 112	1 112

** Correlation is significant at the 0.01 level (2-tailed); For correlations, we used the 112 participants who answered this part of the questionnaire.

Table 5. Multivariate Linear Regression.

Model	Unstandardized Coefficients B	Std. Error	Standardized Coefficients Beta	t	Sig.
(Constant)	1.817	0.336		5.404	0.000
Rating of the overall quality of the telemedicine consultation	0.209	0.072	0.322	2.918	0.004
Organizational and other difficulties that might affect the quality of care delivered by the telemedicine service	−0.268	0.077	−0.322	−3.495	0.001

Dependent variable: Q8 Would you continue to use the telemedicine service?

4. Discussion

In a public health system such as the one found in Catalonia, in which health professionals can choose between telemedicine and usual care (you cannot force them to use telemedicine), understanding the "drivers" of acceptance is essential, so that its use is widespread. The short questionnaire used in this study has allowed an easy, massive and real-time measurement of professional acceptance. If telemedicine is shown to be socially desirable, it is important that health professionals (who are the ones who make the decision to use it) are satisfied, although it may not be of particular benefit to them, so that they become active promoters. This study shows that, in general, the professionals in central Catalonia who responded to the survey are pleased with the telemedicine services available to them and that they will continue to use them as they are currently designed. They state that these services have an overall perceived quality similar to usual care; they do not show any anxiety when using them and believe that they can improve the health of their patients.

However, the Catalan public health system needs to improve in terms of the technical and organizational difficulties which the professionals claim to have suffered while using the services; key elements for their acceptance: since those who had difficulties would be more reluctant to use the services in the future. It is worth noting that none of the healthcare professionals received any training prior to the utilization of the telemedicine services, and nor did new health professionals who joined the primary care teams. If the healthcare professionals had received some form of training, they would probably have had fewer of the difficulties which negatively affect the use of the services. Furthermore, the results show that we can expect a high degree of acceptance by nurses in managing a systemic change towards models with more telemedicine services, unlike that which was shown in other studies [16].

Respondents who used the telemedicine services more often rated the quality of care of these services significantly lower than respondents who use them less often and reported having experienced more technical difficulties and more organizational and other difficulties, compared with respondents who used telemedicine less often. The fact that those who use the tools more are more critical is a wake-up call to technical managers of telemedicine services, suggesting that their experiences should be incorporated into the development of the technology.

Limitations

In relation to the sample universe, there was an overall response rate of just 24.7% among all physicians, nurses and dentists from the counties of Bages, Moianès and Berguedà, regardless of whether they used a telemedicine service or not. However, the 108 participants can be seen as a representative sample of the professionals who use telemedicine in this area, since it is not expected that many more professionals use it, although the exact number has not been recorded. Considering that nurses make up almost half of the sample, the socio-demographic profile of the participants is quite similar to that shown by analyses of primary care professionals in Catalonia [32].

Using a web-based survey implies a possible bias in obtaining answers from those with better technology management. It is also possible, for example, that more people in favor of telemedicine services responded to the survey. Professionals who had negative experiences may have not responded to the questionnaire. Moreover, because the data are based on self-reported measurements, they are potentially highly correlated. It should also be borne in mind that this survey was conducted in a semi-rural context, where previous studies have shown that, in general, there is a greater acceptance of telemedicine [18,19]. In the future, it would be interesting to see if the same results are reproduced in an urban context.

We are aware that the simplicity of the eight questions questionnaire might imply that the tool loses some capacity to capture specific insights. However, the questionnaire was specifically designed to be simple to use and was validated in a previously published study, showing a high reliability index [30].

We performed correlations using ordinal qualitative variables, as we thought that it could help us to understand relations among the factors we were dealing with, such as satisfaction, difficulties and future use. We also used a multivariate linear regression model as a qualitative exercise to propose possible relations between variables, and also in order to propose the key questions to measure the success of teledermatology. These results should not be interpreted as a basis on which to draw firm conclusions or certainties, or to quantify relations, but rather to observe possible relations and to find possible indicators of success. Finally, it should be mentioned that, in future studies, these results should be compared with other perspectives, such as users/patients or healthcare administrators.

5. Conclusions

We assessed the acceptance of telemedicine services amongst health professionals in the Catalan central region, using a short validated questionnaire. Results show that the quality of the services are overall perceived as good for all the parameters studied. Although no great enthusiasm was shown, the results are good, especially among nursing professionals. The healthcare professionals also reported that the technical quality is good, although they often experience technical and organizational problems. It is noteworthy that less than 1% intend to stop using telemedicine in the future. It is necessary that policymakers address the technical and organizational difficulties which professionals have encountered (e.g., by providing training), if they are to ensure the use of these services in the future.

Author Contributions: Conceptualization, J.V.-A., G.F.M., J.L.G.D. and G.S.V.; Data curation, J.V.-A.; Formal analysis, J.V.-A., J.L.G.D and F.L.S.; Investigation, J.V.-A. and J.L.G.D.; Methodology, J.V.-A. and J.L.G.D.; Project administration, J.V.-A. and F.G.C.; Resources, F.X.M.-G.; Supervision, J.V.-A. and J.L.G.D.; Validation, F.L.S.; Visualization, A.R.-C. and F.X.M.-G.; Writing—original draft, J.L.G.D., G.S.V. and F.G.C.; Writing—review and editing, J.V.-A., G.F.M., F.X.M.-G., A.R.-C. and F.L.S. All authors have read and agreed to the published version of the manuscript.

Funding: This research received no external funding.

Acknowledgments: This study was conducted with the support of the Secretary of Universities and Research of the Department of Business and Knowledge at the Generalitat de Catalunya. We are also grateful to the staff at the Technical and Support Area of Gerència Territorial de la Catalunya Central for their help during data collection. This is part of Josep Vidal-Alaball's PhD thesis, publicly available at the University of Vic, doctoral thesis repository: http://dspace.uvic.cat/xmlui/handle/10854/5626.

Conflicts of Interest: The authors declare no conflict of interest.

Abbreviations

PCC: Pearson Correlation Coefficient

References

1. Vidal-Alaball, J.; Domingo, J.L.G.; Cuyàs, F.G.; Peña, J.M.; Mateo, G.F.; Rosanas, J.D.; Valmaña, G.S. A cost savings analysis of asynchronous teledermatology compared to face-to-face dermatology in Catalonia. *BMC Health Serv. Res.* **2018**, *18*, 650. [CrossRef] [PubMed]
2. López Seguí, F.; Franch Parella, J.; Gironès García, X.; Mendioroz Peña, J.; García Cuyàs, F.; Adroher Mas, C.; García-Altés, A.; Vidal-Alaball, J. A Cost-Minimization Analysis of a Medical Record-based, Store and Forward and Provider-to-provider Telemedicine Compared to Usual Care in Catalonia: More Agile and Efficient, Especially for Users. *Int. J. Environ. Res. Public Health* **2020**, *17*, 2008. [CrossRef]

3. Lee, J.J.; English, J.C. Teledermatology: A Review and Update. *Am. J. Clin. Dermatol.* **2018**, *19*, 253–260. [CrossRef] [PubMed]
4. Dario, C.; Luisotto, E.; Dal Pozzo, E.; Mancin, S.; Aletras, V.; Newman, S.; Gubian, L.; Saccavini, C. Assessment of Patients' Perception of Telemedicine Services Using the Service User Technology Acceptability Questionnaire. *Int. J. Integr. Care* **2016**, *16*, 13–14. [CrossRef]
5. Livingstone, J.; Solomon, J. An assessment of the cost-effectiveness, safety of referral and patient satisfaction of a general practice teledermatology service. *Lond. J. Prim. Care (Abingdon)* **2015**, *7*, 31–35. [CrossRef]
6. Polinski, J.M.; Barker, T.; Gagliano, N.; Sussman, A.; Brennan, T.A.; Shrank, W.H. Patients' Satisfaction with and Preference for Telehealth Visits. *J. Gen. Intern. Med.* **2016**, *31*, 269–275. [CrossRef]
7. Rajda, J.; Seraly, M.P.; Fernandes, J.; Niejadlik, K.; Wei, H.; Fox, K.; Steinberg, G.; Paz, H.L. Impact of Direct to Consumer Store-and-Forward Teledermatology on Access to Care, Satisfaction, Utilization, and Costs in a Commercial Health Plan Population. *Telemed. e-Health* **2017**, *24*, 166–169. [CrossRef]
8. Vidal-Alaball, J.; Franch-Parella, J.; Lopez Seguí, F.; Garcia Cuyàs, F.; Mendioroz Peña, J. Impact of a Telemedicine Program on the Reduction in the Emission of Atmospheric Pollutants and Journeys by Road. *Int. J. Environ. Res. Public Health* **2019**, *16*, 4366. [CrossRef]
9. Paquette, S.; Lin, J.C. Outpatient Telemedicine Program in Vascular Surgery Reduces Patient Travel Time, Cost, and Environmental Pollutant Emissions. *Ann. Vasc. Surg.* **2019**, *59*, 167–172. [CrossRef]
10. Broens, T.H.; Huis in't Veld, R.M.; Vollenbroek-Hutten, M.M.; Hermens, H.J.; van Halteren, A.T.; Nieuwenhuis, L.J. Determinants of successful telemedicine implementations: A literature study. *J. Telemed. Telecare* **2007**, *13*, 303–309. [CrossRef]
11. Chau, P.Y.; Hu, P.J. Examining a model of information technology acceptance by individual professionals: An exploratory study. *J. Manag. Inf. Syst.* **2002**, *18*, 191–229. [CrossRef]
12. Wade, V.A.; Eliott, J.A.; Hiller, J.E. Clinician Acceptance is the Key Factor for Sustainable Telehealth Services. *Qual. Health Res.* **2014**, *24*, 682–694. [CrossRef] [PubMed]
13. Mounessa, J.S.; Chapman, S.; Braunberger, T.; Qin, R.; Lipoff, J.B.; Dellavalle, R.P.; Dunnick, C.A. A systematic review of satisfaction with teledermatology. *J. Telemed. Telecare* **2017**, *4*, 263–270. [CrossRef]
14. Weinstock, M.A.; Nguyen, F.Q.; Risica, P.M. Patient and referring provider satisfaction with teledermatology. *J. Am. Acad. Dermatol.* **2002**, *47*, 68–72. [CrossRef] [PubMed]
15. McFarland, L.V.; Raugi, G.J.; Reiber, G.E. Primary care provider and imaging technician satisfaction with a teledermatology project in rural Veterans Health Administration clinics. *Telemed. e-Health* **2013**, *19*, 815–825. [CrossRef]
16. MacNeill, V.; Sanders, C.; Fitzpatrick, R.; Hendy, J.; Barlow, J.; Knapp, M.; Rogers, A.; Bardsley, M.; Newman, S.P. Experiences of front-line health professionals in the delivery of telehealth: A qualitative study. *Br. J. Gen. Pract.* **2014**, *64*, 401–407. [CrossRef]
17. Devine, J. User Satisfaction and Experience with a Telemedicine Service for Diabetic Foot Disease in an Australian Rural Community. 2009. Available online: http://www.ircst.health.nsw.gov.au/__data/assets/pdf_file/0009/98397/Jenni_Devine_report.pdf (accessed on 20 April 2020).
18. Moffatt, J.J.; Eley, D.S. The reported benefits of telehealth for rural Australians. *Aust. Health Rev.* **2010**, *34*, 276. [CrossRef]
19. Klaz, I.; Wohl, Y.; Nathansohn, N.; Yerushalmi, N.; Sharvit, S.; Kochba, I.; Brenner, S. Teledermatology: Quality assessment by user satisfaction and clinical efficiency. *Isr. Med. Assoc. J.* **2005**, *7*, 487–490. [CrossRef]
20. Vidal-Alaball, J.; Peña, J.M.; Valmaña, G.S. Rural-Urban Differences in the Pattern of Referrals to an Asynchronous Teledermatology Service. *Int. Arch. Med.* **2018**, *11*, 1–5. [CrossRef]
21. Eedy, D.J.; Wootton, R. Teledermatology: A review. *Br. J. Dermatol.* **2001**, *4*, 696–707. [CrossRef]
22. Kolltveit, B.C.H.; Thorne, S.; Graue, M.; Gjengedal, E.; Iversen, M.M.; Kirkevold, M. Telemedicine follow-up facilitates more comprehensive diabetes foot ulcer care: A qualitative study in home-based and specialist health care. *J. Clin. Nurs.* **2018**, *27*, e1134–e1145. [CrossRef] [PubMed]
23. Baltaxe, E.; Cano, I.; Herranz, C.; Barberan-Garcia, A.; Hernandez, C.; Alonso, A.; Arguis, M.J.; Bescos, C.; Burgos, F.; Cleries, M.; et al. Evaluation of integrated care services in Catalonia: Population-based and service-based real-life deployment protocols. *BMC Health Serv. Res.* **2019**, *19*, 370. [CrossRef] [PubMed]
24. TiC Salut i Social. Mapa de Tendencias 2020. Available online: https://ticsalutsocial.cat/es/area/observatorio (accessed on 21 April 2020).

25. Seguí, F.L.; Vidal-Alaball, J.; Castro, M.S.; García-Altés, A.; Cuyàs, F.G. General Practitioners' Perceptions of Whether Teleconsultations Reduce the Number of Face-to-face Visits in the Catalan Public Primary Care System: Retrospective Cross-Sectional Study. *J. Med. Internet Res.* **2019**, *22*, 1–8. [CrossRef]
26. Seguí, F.L.; Walsh, S.; Solans, O.; Mas, C.A.; Ferraro, G.; García-Altés, A.; Cuyàs, F.G.; Salvador, L.; Carulla, J.V.A. Teleconsultation Between Patients and Healthcare Professionals in the Catalan Primary Care Service: Descriptive Analysis through Message Annotation in a Retrospective Cross-Sectional Study. *JMIR Prepr.* **2020**. Available online: https://www.jmir.org/preprint/19149 (accessed on 20 April 2020). [CrossRef]
27. Barbieri, J.S.; Nelson, C.A.; Bream, K.D.; Kovarik, C.L. Primary care providers' perceptions of mobile store-and-forward teledermatology. *Dermatol. Online J.* **2015**, *21*, 1–5.
28. Marchell, R.; Locatis, C.; Burgess, G.; Maisiak, R.; Liu, W.L.; Ackerman, M. Patient and Provider Satisfaction with Teledermatology. *Telemed. e-Health* **2017**, *8*, 640–680. [CrossRef]
29. Orruño, E.; Gagnon, M.P.; Asua, J.; Abdeljelil, A.B. Evaluation of teledermatology adoption by health-care professionals using a modified Technology Acceptance Model. *J. Telemed. Telecare* **2011**, *17*, 303–307. [CrossRef]
30. Vidal-Alaball, J.; Flores Mateo, G.; Garcia Domingo, J.L.; Marín Gomez, X.; Sauch Valmaña, G.; Ruiz-Comellas, A.; López Seguí, F.; García Cuyàs, F. Validation of a Short Questionnaire to Assess Healthcare Professionals' Perceptions of Asynchronous Telemedicine Services: The Catalan Version of the Health Optimum Telemedicine Acceptance Questionnaire. *Int. J. Environ. Public Health* **2020**, *17*, 2202. [CrossRef]
31. Davis, F.D. Perceived Usefulness, Perceived Ease of Use, and User Acceptance of Information Technology. *MIS Q.* **1989**, *13*, 319–340. [CrossRef]
32. Fernández, O.S.; Seguí, F.L.; Vidal-Aballl, J.; Simo, J.M.B.; Vian, O.H.; Cabo, P.R.; Hernandez, M.C.; Dominguez, C.O.; Reig, X.A.; Rodríguez, Y.D.; et al. Which characteristics of primary care doctors determine their use of teleconsultations in the catalan public Health system? A retrospective descriptive cross-sectional study (Preprint). *JMIR Med. Inform.* **2020**, *8*, e16484. [CrossRef]

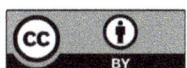

© 2020 by the authors. Licensee MDPI, Basel, Switzerland. This article is an open access article distributed under the terms and conditions of the Creative Commons Attribution (CC BY) license (http://creativecommons.org/licenses/by/4.0/).

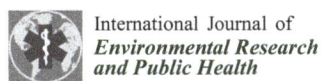

Article

Environmental and Patient Impact of Applying a Point-of-Care Ultrasound Model in Primary Care: Rural vs. Urban Centres

Francesc X Marín-Gomez [1,2,3,*], Jacobo Mendioroz Peña [1,2], Vicenç Canal Casals [4], Marcos Romero Mendez [5], Ana Darnés Surroca [6], Antoni Nieto Maclino [7] and Josep Vidal-Alaball [1,2]

[1] Health Promotion in Rural Areas Research Group, Institut Català de la Salut, 08272 Sant Fruitós de Bages, Spain; jmendioroz.cc.ics@gencat.cat (J.M.P.); jvidal.cc.ics@gencat.cat (J.V.-A.)
[2] Unitat de Suport a la Recerca de la Catalunya Central, Fundació Institut Universitari per a la Recerca a l'Atenció Primària de Salut Jordi Gol i Gurina, 08007 Barcelona, Spain
[3] Servei d'Atenció Primària Osona, Gerència Territorial de Barcelona, Institut Català de la Salut, 08500 Vic, Barcelona, Spain
[4] Centre d'Atenció Primària Vic Nord, Gerència Territorial de Barcelona, Institut Català de la Salut, 08500 Vic, Barcelona, Spain; vcanal.cc.ics@gencat.cat
[5] Centre d'Atenció Primària St. Quirze de Besora, Gerència Territorial de Barcelona, Institut Català de la Salut, 08580 Sant Quirze de Besora, Barcelona, Spain; mromerom.cc.ics@gencat.cat
[6] Centre d'Atenció Primària Manlleu, Gerència Territorial de Barcelona, Institut Català de la Salut, 08560 Manlleu, Barcelona, Spain; adarnes.cc.ics@gencat.cat
[7] Centre d'Atenció Primària Sta. Eugènia de Berga, Gerència Territorial de Barcelona, Institut Català de la Salut, 08507 Santa Eugènia de Berga, Barcelona, Spain; anieto.cc.ics@gencat.cat
* Correspondence: xmarin.cc.ics@gencat.cat

Received: 21 April 2020; Accepted: 7 May 2020; Published: 11 May 2020

Abstract: Motor vehicles are a major contributor to air pollution, and the exposure to this human-caused air pollution can lead to harmful health effects. This study evaluates the impact of the provision of point-of-care ultrasounds (POCUS) by primary care (PC) to avoid the patient's need to travel to a specialized service. The study estimates the costs and air pollution avoided during 2019. The results confirm that performing this ultrasound at the point of care reduces the emission of 61.4 gr of carbon monoxide, 14.8 gr of nitric oxide and 2.7 gr of sulfur dioxide on each trip. During the study, an average of 17.8 km, 21.4 min per trip and almost 2000 L of fuel consumed in a year were avoided. Performing POCUS from PC reduces fuel consumption and the emission of air pollutants and also saves time and money. Furthermore, only 0.3% of the scans had to be repeated by radiologists. However, more studies with more participants need to be done to calculate the exact impact that these pollution reductions will have on human health.

Keywords: point-of-care systems; ultrasonography; traffic-related pollution; primary care

1. Introduction

Over the last decade, numerous studies have shown that exposure to the current levels of human-caused air pollution can lead to a wide range of harmful health effects [1]. Current data makes it possible to give a rough estimate as to the number of health problems which can be directly attributed to air pollution in each territory and to detect the avoidable sources of such pollution. An assessment of the risks associated with human activities is an important tool for quantifying the current problem in terms of its size and how it is evolving, prior to being able to overcome such problems. Recent research shows that motor vehicles are a major contributor to air pollution [2] and suggest that harmful effects exist even at very low levels, with no clear evidence that there is a threshold below which pollution has no effects on people's health [3,4].

Several studies have analysed the environmental impact of the provision by primary care centres (PCCs) of various healthcare services, which up until now have been provided by hospitals or specialized services [5,6], thus avoiding the patient's need to travel to a specialized service [6–8]. However, the potential impact of conducting ultrasound scans in PCCs with regard to pollutant emissions has not previously been studied. At a time of growing interest in reducing the environmental impact of health-related activities [9], this study assesses the impact of conducting ultrasound scans in PCCs as a means to reduce the environmental footprint of this process. Nevertheless, the need for a medical test, such as an ultrasound, can be affected by geographical barriers, and often the distance which users need to travel can cause particular problems, especially for patients in rural communities or places where there is an insufficient number of doctors or deficiencies in the provision of health services [10,11].

Given these circumstances, in recent years ultrasound equipment has been introduced in PCCs to be used by a group of family medicine professionals with special training, fostering a programme of continuous training and an increasing volume of activity. For several years, Catalonia, alongside other autonomous communities, has been committed to equipping healthcare centres with ultrasound scanners and training their staff in how to use them. This study examines the model applied in the Central region of Catalonia, in Osona county, where for some years now [12] ultrasound equipment has been gradually introduced into primary care (PC), beginning with the centres which were the most willing to use them. During this time, the staff has received training in its usage.

This new ultrasound scan service means patients can visit their general practitioner (GP) to have their test done instead of having to go to the nearest radiology service in the county and waiting for an appointment. Although patients in urban areas live quite close to their referral hospital's radiology service, this type of service is especially valuable in rural areas where patients find it more difficult to reach the hospital [13]. As a result, the various professional bodies and groups which represent GPs support the use of ultrasound scans in a large number of clinical situations which form part of routine PC since it increases their ability to diagnose and treat cases, optimizing the use of referrals for diagnostic tests and reducing waiting times [14]. Furthermore, having such tests carried out in PC is well received by both users and healthcare professionals [15]. Nevertheless, few studies have been published which study this phenomenon in rural areas [16] and/or in PC [12], despite many scientific organisations offering training in this field.

In spite of the fact that the carrying out of ultrasound scans in PCCs may be seen as a novelty [17], Hahn et al. published a study examining the education and training received by family physicians more than 30 years ago [18], demonstrating that such programmes were cost-effective and provided quality care [19].

The potential for non-radiologists to perform ultrasound scans, what is known as the point-of-care ultrasound (POCUS) model [8], means the technique can actually form part of the consultation, giving it great potential for a timely evaluation and a speedy diagnosis. This in turn makes it highly appealing to GPs, who have increasingly undergone the necessary training to provide this service. The use of ultrasound scans at the patient's bedside is providing a speedy service to thousands of users [16], avoiding unnecessary travel to specialized services, while representing potential economic savings (environmentally beneficial) for each face-to-face consultation avoided.

Local air pollution and global climate change policies should work together to maximize the benefits of lowering air pollution levels. Evidence suggests that more in-depth cross-city studies have the potential to highlight best practices in both local and global terms [2]. Moreover, as a mobile business, the healthcare sector consumes countless liters of fossil fuels when patients and medical professionals travel to and from their appointments, to pick up prescriptions, or collect test results [20]. The healthcare sector, which has a special focus on health promotion, can thus reasonably be expected to have a moral obligation to set a good example. Ostrom argues that local initiatives are indeed the ones that have the greatest global impact [21]. Hence, potential local mitigation strategies relevant to the health sector are potentially transferable to other countries.

This study focused on the relatively unexplored use of POCUS as a health sector climate change mitigation and adaptation strategy, evaluating its different uses in rural and urban environments. Overall, this is an example of the growing concern of primary care centers with air pollution affecting their local communities.

2. Materials and Methods

This is a retrospective study using administrative data of patients who underwent an ultrasound examination in 2019 by one of the eight GPs of the five primary care centres (PCCs) belonging to the Catalan Institute of Health in Osona county. Of these five centres, two were urban and three rural.

The radiology referral service for all of the patients in the PCCs involved in the study was located in the capital of the region, Vic (Figure 1).

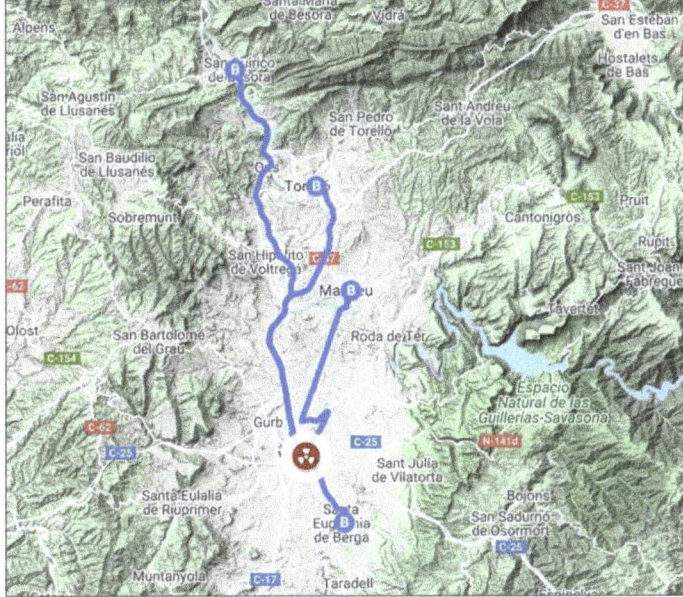

Figure 1. Map showing the primary care centres and their associated diagnostic imaging service in Osona.

This study employed the Primary Care Information System's [22] criteria to differentiate between urban and rural centres. It defines as rural those PCCs which have an assigned population density of less than 150 inhabitants/km^2 and less than 10,000 inhabitants [23].

Using the data regarding ultrasound scans, their impact on the journeys undertaken by users in their own vehicles was estimated in terms of the associated costs and the resulting reduction of air pollution. Distances avoided or not travelled were calculated in terms of return journeys from the PCC to the radiology referral service.

The reduction in the emissions of air pollution and greenhouse gases was calculated by multiplying the kilometres avoided by the corresponding emissions of each pollutant. The economic costs saved were derived from calculating the difference between the cost of traveling to the radiology referral service and that of traveling to the nearest PCC. Finally, the time saved was defined as the sum of the duration of the return journey to the radiology referral service. Data from Google Maps was used in order to calculate the distances travelled and the time saved on the journey using the existing road network. The search option "fastest route with the usual traffic" was employed in all instances. To calculate fuel consumption we used the average cost and consumption of a small family car, with fewer than three passengers with no luggage or additional luggage systems, being driven smoothly with an average fuel consumption of 6.9 L/km. The cost of fuel was calculated by averaging the cost of a liter of Gasoline SP95, Gasoline SP98, Diesel A, Diesel A+ and Biodiesel, which are the most commonly used fuels in motor vehicles. Road traffic emissions depend on many factors, such as the type of vehicle (passenger cars, light duty vehicles, heavy duty vehicles, mopeds and motorcycles), the speed at which they travel, the distance travelled, the type of fuel, the engine displacement and weight, the age of the vehicle and the technology it uses for the reduction of NO_x. In order to calculate the emissions for the study, it was considered that routes involving urban roads have an average speed of 30 km/h, secondary roads of 60 km/h, and that on main roads all vehicles travel at 120 km/h.

The main air pollutants analysed included NO_x, SO_x, O_3, CO, NH_3 and VOC. The emission of suspended particles (PM) which have a demonstrable impact on health was also calculated [24]. Particles smaller than 30 μm in diameter have an impact on the nose and throat, while those less than 10 μm, such as SO_2, NO_2 and ozone, have an impact on the trachea, bronchi and bronchioles. For these calculations, emission factors have been used according to the number of licensed vehicles in Catalonia in 2012 and the 2013 guide to calculating emissions of atmospheric pollutants [25]. Said guide is based on the COPERT 4 v10.0 software program which includes the emission factors described in the European Monitoring and Evaluation Programme (EMEP)/European Environment Agency (EEA) air pollutant emission inventory guidebook [26]. COPERT 4 v10.0 is a tool developed by Aristotle University of Thessaloniki and funded by the European Environment Agency [27].

The emission factor used in the study was an average emission factor which takes into account traffic for all types of road and is expressed in g/km. The calculation of emissions was carried out using the formula $E = M \times N \times EF$; where E is the emission of the pollutant (g), N is the number of vehicles, M is the distance travelled by the vehicle (km) and EF is the emission factor (g/km). The emission of air pollutants per km is shown in Table 1.

Table 1. Emission of pollutants specific to private vehicles (per passenger and per km).

Pollutant	Formula	Vehicle EF [1] (g/km)
Nitrogen oxides	NO_x	0.8287
Particles with a diameter of less than 10 μm	PM_{10}	0.0397
Particles with a diameter of less than 2.5 μm	$PM_{2.5}$	0.0339
Total particles	PM	0.0265
Carbon monoxide	CO	3.4391
Ammonia	NH_3	0.0201
Volatile organic compounds	VOC	0.31
Non-methane volatile organic compounds	NMVOC	0.2887
Methane	CH_4	0.0212
Nitrogen monoxide	NO	0.6666
Nitrogen dioxide	NO_2	0.1621
Nitrous oxide	N_2O	0.0058
Sulphur dioxide	SO_2	0.15

[1] EF: Emission Factor = Emissions (g)/number of vehicles × distance travelled (km). Source: 2013 guide to calculating emissions of atmospheric pollutants [25].

It was considered that an ultrasound scan conducted in a PCC avoided a face-to-face consultation with the radiology service when no subsequent face-to-face visit was made to the service in relation to the same type of ultrasound test in the three months following the ultrasound test conducted by the health centre [6,28].

Although the study focuses on the analysis of the environmental impact derived from the direct displacement of patients, to have a more complete picture we have included impact as a consequence of the mobility of professionals. There are multiple players who can participate in the ultrasound diagnostic process. Air pollution is a mixture of different pollutants and we cannot add up the risk for those pollutants. Epidemiological studies usually rely on a single marker of air quality. As in other previous studies [29], we have selected PM_{10} as the marker of air pollution. The population exposure to PM_{10} was represented by an average population-weighted concentration derived from PM10 concentration tables developed by local authorities.

A descriptive analysis of the different types of ultrasound scans conducted by the centres was carried out for the study according to whether the health centres were urban or rural, and by comparing those tests which required subsequent evaluation by the radiology referral service. The differences between centres were analysed based on the average cost per patient journey and on the average quantity of pollutants emitted in undertaking said journey. The data was processed and analysed using Microsoft Excel and SPSS 23.0 (SPSS Inc., Chicago, IL, USA) programs.

3. Results

An initial descriptive analysis of the study data shows that in 2019, the eight doctors who performed ultrasound scans in the Primary Care Centres (PCCs) in Osona county carried out a total of 1556 scans (Table 2). Almost half of the tests (48.5%) corresponded to abdominal ultrasound scans, more than a quarter to vesico-renal examinations and the remainder, in order of frequency, corresponded to ultrasound scans of the thyroid, soft tissue, joints and a small number of vascular ultrasounds. The average number of ultrasound scans, per professional, during the study year was 194.5 (42–449), with a standard deviation of up to 117.

Table 2. Types of ultrasound scans performed by the different primary care professionals according to whether they work in a rural or urban centre.

PCC Prof [1] n (%)	Abdomen	Joints	Soft Tissue	Thyroid	Vesico-Renal	Vascular	Total
P1	20 (47.6)			5 (11.9)	17 (40.5)		42 (2.7)
P2	102 (51.8)	14 (7.1)	8 (4.1)	13 (6.6)	60 (30.5)		197 (12.7)
P3	119 (43.8)	3 (1.1)		40 (14.7)	110 (40.4)		272 (17.5)
Urban	**241 (47.2)**	**17 (3.3)**	**8 (1.6)**	**58 (11.4)**	**187 (36.6)**		**511 (32.8)**
P4	52 (48.1)	2 (1.9)	9 (8.3)	13 (12.0)	32 (29.6)		108 (6.9)
P5	48 (35.0)	22 (16.1)	19 (13.9)	15 (10.9)	33 (24.1)		137 (8.8)
P6	56 (28.0)	27 (13.5)	48 (24.0)	10 (5.0)	56 (28.0)	3 (1.5)	200 (12.9)
P7	76 (50.3)	8 (5.3)	12 (7.9)	5 (3.3)	50 (33.1)		151 (9.7)
P8	282 (62.8)		17 (3.8)	65 (14.5)	85 (18.9)		449 (28.9)
Rural	**514 (49.2)**	**59 (5.6)**	**105 (10.0)**	**108 (10.3)**	**256 (24.5)**	**3 (0.3)**	**1045 (67.2)**
Total	**755 (48.5)**	**76 (4.9)**	**113 (7.3)**	**166 (10.7)**	**443 (28.5)**	**3 (0.2)**	**1556**

[1] PCC Prof: primary care centre professionals; We show in a bold format the grouped results of rural and urban centers' professionals.

Most of the ultrasound scans 1045/1556 (67.2%) were performed by doctors belonging to rural health centres, while 511/1556 (32.8%) were performed by doctors from urban centres.

The number of ultrasound scans performed according to the type of examination and characteristics of the centre (rural or urban) adjusted for the population served by the centre (population assigned to the centre * 10,000 inhabitants) showed an average of 229.7 tests for every 104 users assigned (SD 115.7) in rural centres and 108.6 (SD 56.4) in urban centres (Table 3). When comparing this rate according to the type of ultrasound scan, abdominal ultrasounds show a mean of 50.5 (SD 21.3) in urban centres vs. 117.2 (SD 27.7) for rural centres ($p = 0.06$).

Table 3. Ultrasound scan rate per inhabitant in rural vs. urban centres.

PCC Prof [1]	Abdomen	Type of Ultrasound Scan × 10^4 Inhabitants				Vascular	X̄ Total
		Joints	Soft Tissue	Thyroid	Vesico-Renal		
Urban centres	50.7	3.2	1.4	12.9	40.5		**108.6**
U1	65.7	1.4	0.0	21.3	60.1		148.5
U2	35.6	4.9	2.8	4.5	20.9		68.7
Rural centres	117.2	11.7	23.2	22.1	54.9	0.6	**229.7**
R1	138.6	35.2	52.6	25.7	102.1	1.8	356
R2	127.1	0.0	6.3	32.0	38.9		204.3
R3	85.9	0.0	10.7	8.6	23.6		128.9

[1] PCC Prof: primary care centre professionals; We show in a bold format the grouped results of rural and urban centers' professionals.

Of the total number of ultrasound scans performed, a total of 36 cases required a referral to a specialist radiology service for a face-to-face scan. Therefore, the percentage of face-to-face consultations avoided by conducting an ultrasound scan in a PCC was 97.7% (Table 4).

Table 4. Face-to-face consultations and consultations avoided by conducting ultrasound scans in primary care centres.

Ultrasound	Abdomen	Joints	Soft Tissue	Thyroid	Vesico-Renal	Vascular	Total
Type (n)	755	76	113	166	443	3	1556
2nd radiologist consult (n)	19	1	5	4	7		36
Avoided (%)	97.5	98.7	95.6	97.6	98.4	100	97.7

Table 5 shows the distance of the journeys avoided due to conducting ultrasound scans at PCCs and the time and cost savings of the journey in terms of unused fuel. The average round trip distance between a PCC and the radiology referral service was 17.8 km, with an average saving in travel time of 21.4 min. The journeys avoided during the year the study was conducted totaled 27,123 km, with a total saving of travel time of more than 22 days. Likewise, this meant a saving of 1872 L of fuel, with an associated total cost of €2658 per year.

Table 5. Reduction in journeys according to distance, time, fuel and cost.

Type PCT Saving	Average Number of Journeys Avoided *			Total of Journeys Avoided *		
	Rural (IC 95%)	Urban (IC 95%)	Total (IC 95%)	Rural	Urban	Total
Distance (km)	20.0 (19.1–20.8)	13.6 (12.6–14.5)	17.8 (17.2–18.5)	20,297.8	6825.2	27,123
Time (day:hour:min)	24.2 (23.5–24.9)	15.8 (14.7–16.9)	21.4 (20.8–22.1)	17:02:20	05:12:36	22:14:56
Fuel (L)	1.4 (1.3–1.4)	0.9 (0.9–1.0)	1.2 (1.2–1.3)	1400.5	470.9	1871.5
Cost (€)	2.0 (1.9–2.0)	1.3 (1.2–1.4)	1.7 (1.7–1.8)	1989.2	668.9	2658.1

* All nonparametric tests (Mann–Whitney U test) to determine if there were significant differences using rurality as an independent variable were significant ($p < 0.001$). Source: Cost of fuel in Spain [30].

If we focus on the health professionals' movements, the variations are minimal or non-existent since neither family doctors nor technicians or radiologists from specialized units changed their mobility. This was different in the case of maintenance staff in charge of installing, updating and maintaining the ultrasound scanners. The maintenance contract included the installation and comprehensive maintenance of the equipment (including those located in the specialized service and those located in primary care centres, as well as at least two preventive visits per year). Car journeys due to the maintenance of the devices accumulates a total of 10 annual trips in the case of ultrasound scanners located in primary care teams, and only two in the case of ultrasound scanners located in the specialized service. We do not have data relating to the travel costs to install and configure the devices for the first use, but this does not appear to be significant as they only involved one visit. Although it seems that the most used equipment requires the greatest amount of technical assistance, there is no evidence that more trips were needed during the year of the study.

Table 6 shows a breakdown of the reduction in air pollutant emissions. The total reduction in pollutants was equivalent to 92.7 kg of carbon monoxide, 22.3 kg of nitric oxide and 4 kg of sulphur dioxide per year. This represents an average reduction on each trip of 61.4 g of carbon monoxide, 14.8 g of nitric oxide and 2.7 g of sulphur dioxide.

Table 6. Reductions in the emissions of pollutant gases.

Pollutant	Average Emissions Per Journey * gr (IC 95%)			Total Emissions * (Total Journeys)		
	Total	U	R	Total	U	R
NO_x	14.8 (14.3–15.3)	11.2 (10.5–12.0)	16.5 (15.9–17.2)	22,328.8	5491	16,655.8
PM_{10}	0.7 (0.7–0.7)	0.5 (0.5–0.6)	0.8 (0.8–0.8)	912.5	223.4	680.1
$PM_{2.5}$	0.6 (0.6–0.6)	0.5 (0.4–0.5)	0.7 (0.6–0.7)	1070.8	264	798.8
PM	0.5 (0.5–0.5)	0.4 (0.3–0.4)	0.5 (0.5–0.6)	713.8	175.9	532.9
CO	61.4 (59.2–63.6)	46.7 (43.4–50.0)	68.6 (65.9–71.4)	92,664.7	22,786.5	69,120.2
NH_3	0.4 (0.3–0.4)	0.3 (0.3–0.3)	0.4 (0.4–0.4)	541.2	133.2	404
VOC	5.5 (5.3–5.7)	4.2 (3.9–4.5)	6.2 (5.9–6.4)	8353.1	2053.8	6230.3
NMVOC	5.2 (5.0–5.3)	3.9 (3.6–4.2)	5.8 (5.5–6.0)	7778.4	1912.4	5802
CH_4	0.4 (0.4–0.4)	0.3 (0.3–0.3)	0.4 (0.4–0.4)	571	140.7	426.3
NO	11.9 (11.5–12.3)	9.0 (8.4–9.7)	13.3 (12.8–13.8)	17,961.2	4416.7	13,397.5
NO_2	2.9 (2.8–3.0)	2.2 (2.0–2.4)	3.2 (3.1–3.4)	4367.6	1074.4	3258.3
N_2O	0.1 (0.1–0.1)	0.08 (0.07–0.08)	0.12 (0.11–0.12)	156.3	38,4.	116.5
SO_2	2.7 (2.6–2.8)	2.0 (1.9–2.2)	3.0 (2.9–3.1)	4041.5	993.8	3014.7

*All nonparametric tests (Mann–Whitney U test) to check if there were significant differences using rurality as an independent variable were significant ($p < 0.001$). Emissions are calculated in grams (gr) using formula in Table 1: number of vehicles × distance travelled × emission factor by pollutant.

As has already been observed when examining the fuel consumption and costs of the journeys avoided, as expected the reduction in pollutant emissions was also significantly higher (for all pollutants studied) in the journeys avoided from rural areas versus those originating from urban areas, given their greater average distance from the radiology referral service.

Demographic mortality data of the year 2019 was obtained from Catalonian Demographical Institute's (IDCAT) data, and the relative risk estimates (and 95% confidence intervals) for a 10 µg/m^3 PM10 increase were obtained from previous studies [31]. With 1426 deaths in 2019 from a total population of 153,000 inhabitants, by calculating the impact of reducing the average PM10 concentrations observed in the area (24.52 µg/m^3) to 20 µg/m^3 (recommended by WHO) and multiplying with the adjusted relative risk of 1.006 (1.004, 1.008) [30], we determined that reducing PM10 by an average of 4.52 µg/m^3 could avoid four (3–6) deaths per year. The study shows that the total amount of PM10 generated with the avoided journeys was only 0.00025 ug/m^3 per day which is not enough to prevent any deaths.

4. Discussion

This study analyses the impact that performing ultrasound scans in primary care centres has in terms of avoided journeys to specialized services, time saved, reduced fuel consumption and the consequent decrease in the emission of atmospheric pollutants. The rural and dispersed nature of most of the study centres highlights a greater effectiveness of the intervention in this field. The county in which the study was conducted has a population of 158,334 (160,464 registered residents), of which 54.89% are assigned to a rural health area with under 10,000 inhabitants and less than 150 inhabitants/km^2. From the patient's point of view, avoiding an unnecessary journey to the radiology service means, in addition to saving time, a reduction in fuel costs, while the same examination is performed in a manner which is similar to their own GP (primary care level).

This study joins others which show that when PCCs provide tests or services which until now have been offered exclusively by specialized units, it leads to a reduction in patient journeys and thus contributes to a significant reduction in the associated costs for users [32,33] in addition to a reduction in the emission of atmospheric pollutants [6,34]. According to data from the World Health Organization (WHO), air pollution in cities and rural areas is responsible for 4.2 million premature deaths per year due to exposure to particulate matter (PM) which causes cardiovascular and respiratory diseases and cancers [35]. Therefore, the reduction in emissions associated with the journeys shown to have been avoided would have a beneficial effect on the health of the population. In fact, the WHO has recently determined the environmental burden of diseases in each country based on selected risk factors including air pollution, and in the case of Spain the air pollution burden has been estimated to stand at 5800 deaths per year. This calculation assumes a reduction in the average urban levels of PM10 from 30 g/m^3 to 20 g/m^3, the average value of PM_{10} in the WHO's recent recommendations [36].

All factors in this study have been based on the mandatory reporting factors described in the EMEP/EEA air pollutant emissions inventory of the European Environment Agency [37]. Although carbon dioxide is a major factor in environmental pollution, it is not included in the inventory and has not been taken into account in the study as its inclusion could have altered reliability with respect to the calculations made with other factors that are in the EMEP/EEA inventory.

It should be noted that to facilitate the calculations made in the study and extrapolating from the most frequent case in the setting in which this study was conducted, the transport system used to make the journeys was taken to be a private, small family car with average fuel consumption. This study did not take into account any journeys which may have been made by public transport (very scarce or non-existent in certain rural populations), low or zero emission vehicles (hybrid and electric cars), or highly polluting vehicles (obsolete cars or towing a trailer).

Nonetheless, the present study has certain limitations. One being the fact that it is a retrospective study which does not allow us to obtain any information of interest such as data related to the loss of working hours and wages, the amount of stress related to driving, waiting times or additional costs such as parking charges. None of these costs are reflected in the current study. In addition, this study does not take into account factors which increase the cost of performing ultrasound scans in PCCs, such as the need to purchase equipment, the ongoing training of professionals, the additional time the professional needs to dedicate to conducting examinations or the possible increase in demand for ultrasound scans due to greater access to the test. The POCUS model could also lead to overdiagnosis if its use is not limited to the organs upon which the clinical suspicion that motivates the use is based.

One factor not assessed in the study, but which is of great interest, is the environmental impact generated by equipment wastage and consumable materials that might cause air and land pollution. Although this impact is not analysed in this study, we should also consider it in order to have a complete picture of the environmental impact. According to the purchasing department, the disposable materials relating to ultrasounds include gloves, disinfectant liquid, reel hand paper, a bunk bed, transducer covers and conductive gel. Among these materials, the only ones exclusive to ultrasounds are the conductive gel and the transducer covers (the rest are difficult to impute directly to the use of ultrasounds) [38]. The annual purchase of conductive gel for the radiology service was 713 units compared to 107 in primary care; 7776 transducer covers were purchased in the radiology service compared to 144 in primary care. Although the environmental impact of these wastes may be limited, it seems that there is a greater use of consumables and therefore a greater production of waste in the specialized services.

The study could also have evaluated other factors which affect the use of the POCUS model in primary care which go beyond the factors under investigation. Ultrasound scans performed using this model mean that any potential referrals can be optimised, minimizing uncertainty and ruling out certain diseases due to the equipment's high diagnostic precision. Ultrasound is an additional tool in the diagnosis process, but its use should be limited to certain clinical situations. Its use in the early detection of diseases prevalent in primary care ought to be appropriately evaluated [8].

5. Conclusions

This study confirms that the practice of conducting ultrasound scans in primary care reduces the environmental impact of atmospheric pollutants emitted by vehicles by avoiding the journeys which would have been necessary to carry out the scans by attending a specialized radiology service. The avoided journey results in savings of time and money for the user in addition to the reduction of fuel consumption and the emission of atmospheric pollutants. Other studies ought to analyse the potential impact of expanding the portfolio of primary care services on the potential savings in journeys made and their implications for the patients' work and personal life.

The increase in the number of POCUS programs, which has started to include the use of portable devices (hand-carried or hand-held ultrasounds) in patients' homes in rural and low income settings [39–42], ought to be seen as a new tool and part of a broader strategy to reduce emissions of air pollutants.

Earth pollution and climate change is a reality. The modern healthcare sector contributes towards this grave phenomenon and, at the same time, it is being affected by it. The present study was thus conducted to identify one of the multiple ways in which the health sector can contribute to prevent climate change. Private car travel is a major source of air pollution and Telemedicine has the potential to minimize it by reducing journeys [43]. Potential air pollutant savings are strongly associated with the number of users and appointments that can be replaced by teleconsultations or point-of-care visits. The benefits will depend on the amount, the distance and type of transportation replaced by those visits. Local health initiatives, as modest they are, could contribute to expand this new model of Green Health. Maybe the results of this study can contribute to extending the POCUS model, increasing its future environmental impact.

Author Contributions: Conceptualization, F.X.M.-G. and J.V.-A.; methodology, F.X.M.-G., J.V.-A. and J.M.P.; validation, F.X.M.-G., J.V.-A. and J.M.P.; formal analysis, F.X.M.-G.; investigation, F.X.M.-G.; resources, F.X.M.-G., V.C.C., M.R.M., A.D.S., A.N.M.; data curation, F.X.M.-G.; writing—original draft preparation, F.X.M.-G., J.V.-A. and J.M.P.; writing—review and editing, F.X.M-G. and J.V.-A. All authors have read and agreed to the published version of the manuscript.

Funding: This research received no external funding.

Acknowledgments: We would like to express our gratitude to the Unitat d'Investigació de Catalunya Central for their collaboration in conducting the study and to all those PHC professionals who registered the point-of-care ultrasounds from their primary care centers in Osona county. The study was carried out within the framework of the PROSAASU research group.

Conflicts of Interest: The authors declare no conflict of interest.

References

1. De Keijzer, C.; Agis, D.; Ambrós, A.; Arévalo, G.; Baldasano, J.M.; Bande, S. The association of air pollution and greenness with mortality and life expectancy in Spain: A small-area study. *Environ. Int.* **2017**, *99*, 170–176. [CrossRef]
2. Slovic, A.D.; de Oliveira, M.A.; Biehl, J.; Ribeiro, H. How Can Urban Policies Improve Air Quality and Help Mitigate Global Climate Change: A Systematic Mapping Review. *J. Urban Health* **2016**, *93*, 73–95. [CrossRef] [PubMed]
3. Lepeule, J.; Laden, F.; Dockery, D.; Schwartz, J. Chronic Exposure to Fine Particles and Mortality: An Extended Follow-up of the Harvard Six Cities Study from 1974 to 2009. *Environ. Health Perspect* **2012**, *120*, 965–970. [CrossRef] [PubMed]

4. Laden, F.; Schwartz, J.; Speizer, F.E.; Dockery, D.W. Reduction in Fine Particulate Air Pollution and Mortality. *Am. J. Respir. Crit. Care Med.* **2006**, *173*, 667–672. [CrossRef] [PubMed]
5. Alshqaqeeq, F.; Amin Esmaeili, M.; Overcash, M.; Twomey, J. Quantifying hospital services by carbon footprint: A systematic literature review of patient care alternatives. *Resour. Conserv. Recycl.* **2020**, *154*. [CrossRef]
6. Vidal-Alaball, J.; Franch-Parella, J.; Lopez Seguí, F.; Garcia Cuyàs, F.; Mendioroz Peña, J. Impact of a Telemedicine Program on the Reduction in the Emission of Atmospheric Pollutants and Journeys by Road. *Int. J. Environ. Res. Public Health* **2019**, *16*, 4366. [CrossRef]
7. Oliveira, T.C.; Barlow, J.; Gonçalves, L.; Bayer, S. Teleconsultations reduce greenhouse gas emissions. *J. Health Serv. Res. Policy* **2013**, *18*, 209–214. [CrossRef]
8. Calvo Cebrián, A.; López García-Franco, A.; Short Apellaniz, J. Modelo Point-of-Care Ultrasound en Atención Primaria: ¿herramienta de alta resolución? *Atención Primaria* **2018**, *50*, 500–508. [CrossRef]
9. Hensher, M. Incorporating environmental impacts into the economic evaluation of health care systems: Perspectives from ecological economics. *Resour. Conserv. Recycl.* **2020**, *154*. [CrossRef]
10. Bradford, N.K.; Caffery, L.J.; Smith, A.C. Telehealth services in rural and remote Australia: A systematic review of models of care and factors influencing success and sustainability. *Rural Remote Health* **2016**, *16*, 3808.
11. Jetty, A.; Moore, M.A.; Coffman, M.; Petterson, S.; Bazemore, A. Rural Family Physicians Are Twice as Likely to Use Telehealth as Urban Family Physicians. *Telemed. J. E. Health* **2018**, *24*, 268–276. [CrossRef] [PubMed]
12. Esquerrà, M.; Roura Poch, P.; Masat Ticó, T.; Canal, V.; Maideu Mir, J.; Cruxent, R. Ecografía abdominal: Una herramienta diagnóstica al alcance de los médicos de familia. *Atención Primaria* **2012**, *44*, 576–583. [CrossRef] [PubMed]
13. Nilam, J.S.; Robert, A.; Pierre, K. *Point of Care Ultrasound E-book*; Elsevier Saunders: Amsterdam, The Netherlands, 2014.
14. Lindgaard, K.; Riisgaard, L. Validation of ultrasound examinations performed by general practitioners. *Scand J. Prim. Health Care* **2017**, *35*, 256–261. [CrossRef] [PubMed]
15. Díaz Rodríguez, N. La ecografía en Atención Primaria. *Semer Med. Fam.* **2002**, *28*, 376–384. [CrossRef]
16. Mengarelli, M.; Nepusz, A.; Kondrashova, T. A Comparison of Point-of-Care Ultrasonography Use in Rural Versus Urban Emergency Departments Throughout Missouri. *Mo Med.* **2018**, *115*, 56–60.
17. Gillman, L.M.; Kirkpatrick, A.W. Portable bedside ultrasound: The visual stethoscope of the 21 stcentury. *Scand J. Trauma Resusc. Emerg. Med.* **2012**, *20*. [CrossRef]
18. Hahn, R.G.; Roi, L.D.; Ornstein, S.M.; Rodney, W.M.; Garr, D.R.; Davies, T.C. Obstetric ultrasound training for family physicians. Results from a multi-site study. *J. Fam. Pract* **1988**, *26*, 553–558.
19. Hahn, R.G.; Ho, S.; Roi, L.D.; Bugarin-Viera, M.; Davies, T.C.; Rodney, W.M. Cost-effectiveness of office obstetrical ultrasound in family practice: Preliminary considerations. *J. Am. Board Fam. Pract.* **1988**, *1*, 33–38.
20. Stott, R.; Godlee, F. What should we do about climate change? *BMJ* **2006**, *333*, 983–984. [CrossRef]
21. Ostrom, E. A Polycentric Approach for Coping with Climate Change (English). In *Policy Research Working Paper*; World Bank: Washington, DC, USA, 2009.
22. Fina Avilés, F.; Méndez, L.; Coma, E.; Medina, M. Sistema de Información de los Servicios de Atención Primaria (SISAP). La Experiencia 2006–2009 de l'Institut Català de la Salut. Available online: https://www.researchgate.net/publication/33544050_Sistema_de_Informacion_de_los_Servicios_de_Atencion_Primaria_La_experiencia_2006-2008_del_Institut_Catala_de_la_Salut (accessed on 10 May 2020).
23. Domínguez Amorós, M.; Monllor Rico, N.; Simó Solsona, M. *Món rural i joves. Realitat juvenil i Polítiques de Joventut als Municipis Rurals de Catalunya. Estudis 31*; Secretaria de Joventut de la Generalitat de Catalunya: Barcelona, Spain, 2010.
24. Sherman, J.D.; MacNeill, A.; Thiel, C. Reducing Pollution From the Health Care Industry. *JAMA* **2019**. [CrossRef]
25. Generalitat de Catalunya. *Guia de càlculs D'emisions de Contaminants a L'atmosfera 2013*. Available online: http://mediambient.gencat.cat/ca/05_ambits_dactuacio/atmosfera/emissions_industrials/inventaris-emissions-atm/guia-de-calcul-demissions/ (accessed on 10 May 2020).
26. European Environment Agency. *EMEP/EEA Air Pollutant Emission Inventory Guidebook 2019: Technical Guidance to Prepare National Emission Inventories (3.B Manure Management)*; Publications office of the European Union: Luxemburg, 2019.

27. Aristotle University Thessaloniki. COPERT 4 v10.0 n.d. Available online: http://www.emisia.com/copert/ (accessed on 10 May 2020).
28. Vidal-Alaball, J.; Garcia Domingo, J.L.; Garcia Cuyàs, F.; Mendioroz Peña, J.; Flores Mateo, G.; Deniel Rosanas, J. A cost savings analysis of asynchronous teledermatology compared to face-to-face dermatology in Catalonia. *BMC Health Serv. Res.* **2018**, *18*, 1–6. [CrossRef]
29. Pérez, L.; Sunyer, J.; Künzli, N. Estimating the health and economic benefits associated with reducing air pollution in the Barcelona metropolitan area (Spain). *Gac. Sanit* **2009**, *23*, 287–294. [CrossRef] [PubMed]
30. Cost of fuel in Spain. Available online: https://www.dieselogasolina.com (accessed on 1 January 2020).
31. Anderson, H.; Atkinson, R.; Peacock, J.; Marston, L.; Konstantinou, K. *Meta-Analysis of Time-Series Studies and Panel Studies of Particulate Matter (PM) and Ozone (O_3)*; WHO Regional Office for Europe: Copenhagen, Denmark, 2004; pp. 1–68.
32. Wootton, R.; Bahaadinbeigy, K.; Hailey, D. Estimating travel reduction associated with the use of telemedicine by patients and healthcare professionals: Proposal for quantitative synthesis in a systematic review. *BMC Health Serv. Res.* **2011**, *11*, 185. [CrossRef] [PubMed]
33. Whetten, J.; Montoya, J.; Yonas, H. ACCESS to Better Health and Clear Skies: Telemedicine and Greenhouse Gas Reduction. *Telemed J. E. Health* **2019**, *25*, 960–965. [CrossRef] [PubMed]
34. Wootton, R.; Tait, A.; Croft, A. Environmental aspects of health care in the Grampian NHS region and the place of telehealth. *J. Telemed. Telecare* **2010**, *16*, 215–220. [CrossRef] [PubMed]
35. World Health Organization (WHO). Ambient (Outdoor) air Quality and Health 2018. Available online: https://www.who.int/en/news-room/fact-sheets/detail/ambient-(outdoor)-air-quality-and-health/ (accessed on 10 May 2020).
36. WHO (World Health Organization). Country profiles of Environmental Burden of Disease. 2009. Available online: https://www.who.int/quantifying_ehimpacts/national/countryprofile/spain.pdf?ua=1 (accessed on 10 May 2020).
37. European Parliament and Council. DIRECTIVE (EU) 2016/2284 OF THE EUROPEAN PARLIAMENT AND OF THE COUNCIL of 14 December 2016 on on the reduction of national emissions of certain atmospheric pollutants, amending Directive 2003/35/EC and repealing Directive 2001/81/EC. *Off. J. Eur. Union.* **2016**, *344*, 1–31.
38. Salmon, M.; Salmon, C.; Bissinger, A.; Muller, M.M.; Gebreyesus, A.; Geremew, H. Alternative ultrasound gel for a sustainable ultrasound program: Application of human centered design. *PLoS ONE* **2015**, *10*, e0138400. [CrossRef]
39. Minardi, J.; Davidov, D.; Denne, N.; Haggerty, T.; Kiefer, C.; Tillotson, R. Bedside ultrasound: Advanced technology to improve rural healthcare. *W V Med. J.* **2013**, *109*, 28–33.
40. Sippel, S.; Muruganandan, K.; Levine, A.; Shah, S. Review article: Use of ultrasound in the developing world. *Int. J. Emerg. Med.* **2011**, *4*, 72. [CrossRef]
41. Becker, D.M.; Tafoya, C.A.; Becker, S.L.; Kruger, G.H.; Tafoya, M.J.; Becker, T.K. The use of portable ultrasound devices in low- and middle-income countries: A systematic review of the literature. *Trop. Med. Int. Health* **2016**, *21*, 294–311. [CrossRef]
42. Clevert, D.A.; Schwarze, V.; Nyhsen, C.; D'Onofrio, M.; Sidhu, P.; Brady, A.P. ESR statement on portable ultrasound devices. *Insights Imaging* **2019**, *10*. [CrossRef]
43. Holmner, A.; Rocklöv, J.; Ng, N.; Nilsson, M. Climate change and eHealth: A promising strategy for health sector mitigation and adaptation. *Glob. Health Action* **2012**, *5*, 1–10. [CrossRef] [PubMed]

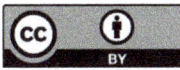

© 2020 by the authors. Licensee MDPI, Basel, Switzerland. This article is an open access article distributed under the terms and conditions of the Creative Commons Attribution (CC BY) license (http://creativecommons.org/licenses/by/4.0/).

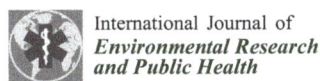
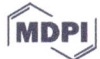

Article

The Antecedents of Poor Doctor-Patient Relationship in Mobile Consultation: A Perspective from Computer-Mediated Communication

Mengling Yan [1], Hongying Tan [1,*], Luxue Jia [1] and Umair Akram [2]

[1] School of Economics and Management, Beijing University of Posts and Telecommunications, Beijing 100876, China; emilyatpku@126.com (M.Y.); jialx2302@163.com (L.J.)
[2] Guanghua School of Management, Peking University, Beijing 100871, China; akram.umair88@pku.edu.cn
* Correspondence: tanhy@bupt.edu.cn

Received: 24 February 2020; Accepted: 8 April 2020; Published: 9 April 2020

Abstract: This study aims to understand the underlying reasons for poor doctor-patient relationships (DPR). While extant studies on antecedents of poor DPR mainly focus on the offline context and often adopt the patients' perspective, this work focuses on the mobile context and take both doctors' and mobile consultation users' perspectives into consideration. To fulfill this purpose, we first construct a theoretical framework based on the Computer-Mediated Communication (CMC) literature. Then we coded 592 doctor-user communication records to validate and elaborate the proposed theoretical model. This work reveals that characteristics of mobile technologies pose potential challenges on both doctors' and patients' information providing, informative interpreting, and relationship maintaining behaviors, resulting in 10 and 6 types of inappropriate behaviors of doctors and users, respectively, that trigger poor DPR in the mobile context. The findings enrich the research on online DPR and provide insights for improving DPR in the mobile context.

Keywords: poor doctor-patient relationship; healthcare consultation; mobile context; computer-mediated communication

1. Introduction

The emerging use of mobile medical consultation in China has propelled the establishment of doctor-patient relationships (DPRs) in the mobile context. DPR relies on mutual familiarity, trust, and interaction between physicians and patients during healthcare planning [1], and is essential for developing superior healthcare services. Given its significance, ample attention has been paid to exploring the antecedents and outcomes of DPR [1–4]. With the wide application of mobile medical consultation in China, people are allowed to interact with doctors to make inquiries and obtain medical information through computer-mediated communication [4,5]. Through this service, the scenes where DPR is established are extended from the offline context to the mobile context. In addition, mobile medical consultation service offers medical information not only for patients but also for other users who are not necessarily patients. To avoid confusion, we use the term "user(s)" when discussing DPR in a mobile context.

Compared to the rapid increase of mobile medical consultation users, perceptions towards mobile DPR is less optimistic. According to a related industry report, more than 40% of doctors have reported that they consider the DPR to be tense in a mobile context [6]. Hao and Zhang [7] found that 12% of users made negative comments on the treatment effect, and 9% made negative comments on the service attitude of doctors on a Chinese mobile consultation platform. Poor DPR not only impairs users' health conditions at the individual level [8] but also causes serious social problems at the society level [9].

Extant research on mobile healthcare service is emerging, but studies that aim at uncovering the underlying reasons for poor DPRs in the mobile context are still lacking. The majority of previous research tends to focus on the positive experience brought about by mobile healthcare services, such as user satisfaction [10] and the adoption or continuous usage of mobile technology [3,11]. However, the experience of dissatisfied participants is largely ignored. The negative experience is also worth noting because understanding the complaints guide practitioners to improve service quality [8]. Although a few studies have paid attention to the dissatisfying experience of mobile healthcare services, they tend to interpret the experience only from the perspective of users [8,12]. While these studies are insightful, a single perspective from users is not adequate, because they missed the perception of doctors which is considered quite different from that of users [13,14].

These two literature gaps (namely lacking studies on dissatisfying experience of mobile healthcare services and lacking dual perspectives from both users and doctors) might partly be attributed to the mainstream research method in the healthcare field. Most studies rely on questionnaires and interviews to collect subjective ratings about mobile healthcare services, such as Akter et al. (2013) [15], Deng et al. (2015) [16], and Wu et al. (2018) [17]. The collected responses are usually inaccurate since respondents are rating events that happened at an earlier time. Besides, it is difficult to match responses from doctors and patients via questionnaires.

This work aims to uncover the underlying reasons for poor DPR from dual perspectives of both doctors and users in mobile medical consultation service. To achieve our goals, we first reviewed the literature on Computer-Mediated Communication (hereafter, CMC) in search of theoretical accounts for the poor DPR in the mobile context. The CMC literature focuses on the influence of the features of CMC on communication processes, which enables us to understand the potential negative impacts that CMC brings to doctor-user communication. As a result, the CMC literature guides us to identify the underlying reasons and mechanisms of poor DPR in the mobile context [18].

Next, we conducted an in-depth qualitative analysis based on objective communication records collected from a leading Chinese mobile healthcare application, Chunyu Doctor, to validate and refine the theoretical accounts. Chunyu Doctor is a commercial mobile consultation platform that connects users who search for medical information and doctors who work in public hospitals in China. On this platform, doctors are free to define their service prices and can earn legal income by providing consultation services for users. Meanwhile, users can pay a fee to consult doctors and make service evaluations after the consultation. Users can consult doctors either by telephone or by texts and pictures, but the latter is more frequently adopted in practice. This mobile platform is chosen due to the following two reasons. First, founded in 2011, Chunyu Doctor was among the first to start a mobile consultation service in China. By the end of 2017, it had accumulated 125 million users and 500 thousand physicians and conducted more than 330 thousand consultations per day, which allows us to get access to a large number of real communication records. Second, Chunyu Doctor provides users with a service evaluation system, in which a user can rate the service as "satisfied", "general" or "dissatisfied". Analyzing communication records rated as "dissatisfied" is helpful to discern potential problems in mobile consultation from both users' and doctors' perspectives.

The findings of this work contribute to the theorizing and understanding of DPR in the mobile context by offering theoretical accounts from the perspective of CMC. We also shed light on effective ways to improve users' or doctors' satisfaction towards mobile healthcare service. Both users and doctors are suggested to change their expectations and interaction habits to better adapt to the features of mobile communication.

2. Theoretical Background

To understand the key antecedents of poor DPR in the mobile context, we first reviewed the CMC literature to summarize the features of CMC and their potential negative impacts on communication. Then, we narrowed down our discussion on the relationships among CMC, doctor-user communication, and DPR in the mobile context, and proposed a theoretical framework that explains the antecedents of poor DPR in the mobile context.

2.1. Features of Computer-Mediated Communication

Computer-Mediated-Communication (CMC) refers to communication-based on computers and the internet, such as e-mail, web messaging systems, online forums, and mobile applications [19,20].

Abundant studies have examined the features and differences between traditional face-to-face communication and CMC [21]. Based on an in-depth literature review, we identified four features of CMC, namely connectivity, text-based communication, asynchronism, and anonymity. Connectivity refers to the fact that users can initiate or participate in online interaction regardless of time and space limits [22]. Text-based communication refers to the fact that the majority of communication is delivered through texts, lacking audio or visual clues [20]. The asynchronous nature of the media implies that there is a time delay during the communication [23,24]. Admittedly, as technologies keep upgrading, voice, picture messages and even synchronous video communication are also supported by CMC, but they are still used in relatively low frequency. Finally, anonymity refers to the fact that CMC enables users to hide his or her real identity by using a screen name, which is considered as the most remarkable difference between CMC and traditional offline communication.

CMC brings both positive and negative impacts on the communication process. In Table 1, we draw on extant studies and summarize the potential positive and negative impacts that CMC may have on users' online communication behaviors. In this study, we apply CMC in the mobile medical consultation context and focus on the potential negative impacts.

Table 1. The potential positive and negative impacts of each CMC feature on online activities.

CMC Features	Potential Positive Impacts	Potential Negative Impacts
Connectivity	• Transcend traditional time and space limitation, provide easy access to online information [25,26]	• Increased workload for doctors [18] • Information overloading [27] • Conflicting information [14]
Text-based communication	• Easy documentation and clear description of symptoms and instructions [23]	• Higher-level cognitive effort compared to audio and visual communication [28] • Lack of intimacy and weak at relationship development [20,29]
Asynchronism	• Transcend traditional time and space limitation [25] • Less interrupting [18] • Flexible thinking time [30]	• Hard to ensure timely response [31] • Cause misunderstanding
Anonymity	• Encourage expression [32,33]	• Easy engender negative emotion and misconduct online [34]

2.2. A Computer-Mediated Communication Perspective on Poor DPR

DPR refers to the collaborative and affective bond between doctors and patients [35]. Satisfaction has been proved to be a critical determinant of DPR [2,36]. For the patient, patient satisfaction significantly increases the likelihood of the patient returning to the doctor for treatment. If the patient's needs are met during the service, there will be fewer complaints and medical disputes, which contributes to positive DPR [4]. For the doctor, doctor satisfaction can increase doctors' work enthusiasm and promote the willingness to establish a friendly relationship with patients [36]. In summary, satisfaction is a key driver for improving DPR for both doctors and patients. Accordingly, unsatisfactory service experience will lead to poor DPR for both doctors and patients [14].

Effective doctor-patient communication is essential to realize satisfactory service and maintain harmonious DPR [5,37]. On the contrary, undesirable doctor-user communication can cause poor DPR [14]. Extant studies consensus on the use of informational and emotional dimensions to depict the communication processes between doctors and patients [1,17,38]. Informational-oriented communication, also termed as task-focused communication [38,39], refers to communication on medical information provision and interpretation. To be more specific, the informational communication can be divided into information providing and information interpreting [14,40]. Emotional-oriented communication, also termed as socio-emotion-focused communication [38,41], refers to communication on the identification and response of emotional cues. Emotional-oriented communication is conducive to meeting both doctors' and users' emotional needs and maintaining a friendly relationship [41]. Both informational-oriented and emotional-oriented communication are two-way communications between doctors and users.

When the medical environment shifts from the traditional face-to-face context to the mobile context, the features of the medium that supports doctor-patient communication have also changed [18,42,43]. While traditional face-to-face medical communication relies on synchronous communication with language tones and facial or body cues, mobile communication relies on text-based asynchronous communication [18]. According to media synchronicity theory, features of media determine the media capabilities in supporting information transmission and information processing and further determine the communication outcomes [40]. Therefore, there are reasons to believe that the features of CMC will impact the doctor-user communication process and further impact DPR in mobile consultation.

Based on the above arguments, we propose a theoretical model (as is shown in Figure 1), aiming at explaining the antecedents of poor DPR in the mobile context. The key arguments of this model are: (1) Features of CMC create barriers for information providing, information interpreting and relationship maintaining for both doctors and users during the two-way communication, and (2) the undesirable doctor-user communication caused by features of CMC leads to poor DPR that is manifested by doctors' and users' dissatisfaction.

While this preliminary framework sheds light upon the logical relationships between CMC features, doctor-patient communication, and DPR, it also reveals several directions for further exploration: 1) it is unclear what representative information providing, information interpreting, and relationship maintaining behaviors of doctors and users lead to poor DPR, and 2) it is unclear how limitations of CMC account for these behaviors. As a result, this preliminary theoretical framework provides initial answers to our research question and guides our data analysis to answer the remaining questions.

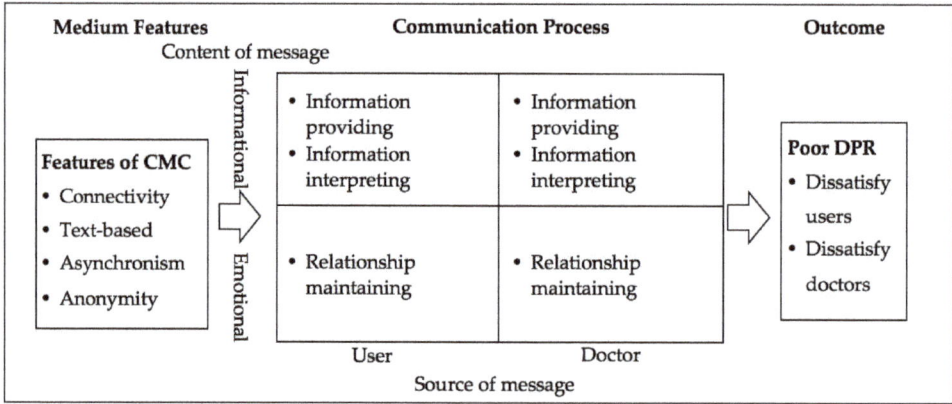

Figure 1. Theoretical framework.

3. Research Method

To empirically validate and elaborate our proposed theoretical framework, this work employs netnography, or internet-based ethnography, as the qualitative research method [41,44,45]. The study proceeded in three steps: (1) developing a preliminary coding plan based on the CMC literature (as is shown in Figure 1), (2) downloading and coding objective communication records as well as comments that are rated as "dissatisfied" by users in the selected mobile application; and (3) analyzing the data to identify representative interaction behaviors from users' and doctors' perspectives. The detailed steps of data collection, data analysis, and data interpretation are shown in Figure 2.

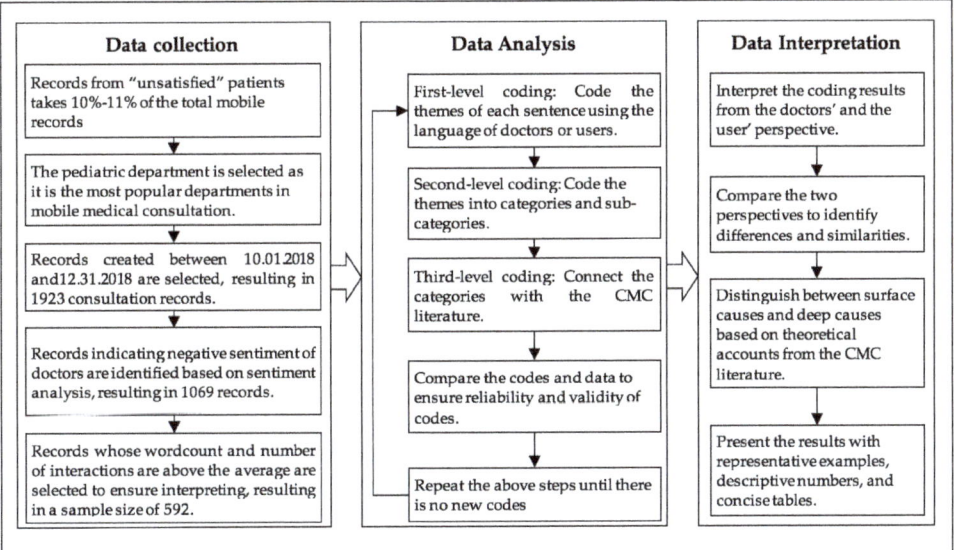

Figure 2. The methodology roadmap.

3.1. Data Collection

Mobile consultation service allows users to chat with professional and experienced doctors in real-time by sending messages with texts and photos. The electronic medical records of patient-doctor communication during the online consultation process are mainly text-based. Therefore, communication records between doctors and users are valuable materials that worth analyzing. Researchers can analyze these communication records from the perspectives of both users and doctors, and gain an insight into the online patient-doctor communication process.

The communication records used in this study were collected from Chunyu Doctor. We analyzed the communication records that were rated as "dissatisfied" by users on the platform. A Java-based program was developed to automatically download the communication records between doctors and users. On average, consultation records that are labeled "dissatisfied" by users take 10%-11% of the total records. In total, we have downloaded 1923 "dissatisfied" interaction threads between 633 doctors and 1923 users from October 1st, 2018 to December 31st, 2018 in the pediatric department. The period was selected because this quarter of the year is reported to have the highest average monthly user activity in Chunyu Doctor [46]. The pediatric department was selected due to two reasons. On the one hand, pediatrics is the most frequently visited department in mobile consultation due to the shortage of pediatricians in offline hospitals. On the other hand, collecting data from pediatric is conducive to reflecting poor DPR in mobile consultation, because users in the pediatric department are usually the guardians of patients rather than patients themselves. And guardians who have strong feelings for their loved children are more likely to have conflicts with doctors [47]. The "dissatisfied" consultation records represent users' dissatisfactory experience. Additional steps were taken to screen records that reflect doctors' dissatisfactory experience. To be more specific, we used a widely applied Python-based program of Chinese sentiment analysis to obtain the sentiment score of all words generated by the doctor in each dialog. The accuracy of this program is tested as 0.8277 [48]. Through the analysis, results show that the mean value and the variance of doctors' sentiment in 1923 records are -0.0642 and 0.1645 respectively. Records that score in the range of -1 to 0 indicate potential negative emotions of doctors. Based on this analysis, the research team manually went through all the selected records to ensure accurate identification, resulting in a sample size of 1069 records. Finally, to rule out the possibility that poor DPR is a result of insufficient communication, we selected communication records with word counts and the number of interactions during the communication above the average. As a result, a total of 592 detailed consultation threads from 358 doctors were collected for analysis. In the final sample, the total Chinese characters amount to 166,985, the average word count is 282.07, an average number of interactions for each communication thread is 33.24.

3.2. Data Analysis

To analyze the text-based communication records, qualitative analysis is considered appropriate [12,14,41,49,50]. Specifically, using netnography and coding skills from the qualitative analysis [51], the qualitative data analysis proceeded in the following four steps.

First, first-level coding. This is also referred to as open coding in classic qualitative analysis, where topics are generated from words or sentences of the original material [51]. Researchers of this study coded each line of communication records as well as user' comments after the consultation experience using the language of doctors or users. To ensure the validity and reliability of qualitative coding, three researchers read and coded the original communication records independently. After each of their initial coding was completed, they go through all the coding results and discuss different opinions through in-depth discussion until they reached consensus.

Second, second-level coding. This is also referred to as axial coding in classic qualitative analysis, where topics are consolidated and abstracted to categories and sub-categories based on comparison and contrast [51]. Usually, the categories and sub-categories may appropriate the terms and phrases from the literature. As a result, first-level codes in our study were further classified into informational and emotional dimensions. Through this step, doctors' information-related behaviors and emotion-related behaviors that cause users' dissatisfaction, as well as users' information-related behaviors and emotion-related behaviors that cause doctors' dissatisfaction, are obtained.

Third, Third-level coding. This is also referred to as selected coding in classic qualitative analysis, where categories are connected to tell a logical story of the intended phenomenon [51]. We counted the frequencies of each identified category and selected categories with high frequencies to form the complete model that explains the antecedents of poor DPR in the mobile context. Based on these selected categories, challenges of mobile technologies identified using the CMC literature and interaction behaviors of doctors and users identified in the communication records are connected. Specifically, each of the researchers tried to understand the underlying reasons behind doctors' and users' mobile misbehaviors by referring to the CMC features identified by the CMC literature. To ensure the validity and reliability of the classification, three researchers conduct this step independently and converge opinions through in-depth discussion.

Forth, developing coding schemes. Based on the above three steps, we developed a coding schemes, and use this coding scheme to code subsequent consultation records. To ensure the reliability and validity of the codes, different researchers repeat the above coding steps and compare the codes and data to reach a converged opinion. The above coding steps repeat until there are no new themes, categories, or sub-categories that are generated to explain the original data.

4. Findings

4.1. The Users' Perspective

By adopting the users' perspective, we identified 10 representative types of doctor behaviors, as is shown in Table 2. In the following, we introduce quantitative coding results and representative behaviors of doctors in terms of the information providing, information interpreting, and relationship maintaining categories.

Table 2. Antecedents of poor DPR from the users' perspective.

Category	Subcategory	Percentage	Description
Barriers in information providing	Lack of etiology analysis	6.42%	The doctor fails to explain the etiology for the user.
	Lack of diagnostic evidence	18.92%	The doctor fails to provide the user with sufficient evidence for diagnosis.
	Lack of operational advice	16.22%	The doctor fails to give the user explicit operational instructions.
	Ambiguous answer	25.00%	The doctor's answer is ambiguous.
Barriers in information interpreting	Ignoring information	3.04%	The doctor ignores the information provided by the user, such as symptoms.
	Irrelevant answer	3.38%	The answer provided by the doctor cannot answer the question asked by the user.
Barriers in relationship maintaining	Delayed reply	26.69%	The doctor is not able to respond to the user in time.
	Lack of initiative	10.81%	The doctor fails to provide relevant information actively.
	Lack of emotional comport	5.74%	The doctor lacks emotional comfort for the user.
	Unfriendly attitude	13.18%	The doctor is impatient and unfriendly

4.1.1. Barriers for Doctors in Information Providing

That doctors fail to provide accurate and adequate medical information for users over mobile consultation is a major reason that causes users' dissatisfaction. Nowadays, users of mobile medical services require richer information to understand their physical conditions and make reasonable medical decisions [7]. They not only require information about the treatment suggestions, but also require information about why they become sick, how to treat the disease, and why the doctor makes a specific diagnosis. However, in the mobile context, text-based and asynchronous communication makes it more difficult for doctors to reply to every message from users. Specifically, doctors may fail to explain etiology, diagnostic evidence, and fail to offer clear and effective suggestions, which leaves users' information-related needs unmet. As a result, users complain during their communication with doctors or in their service comments, such as "the doctor didn't explain the causes of my disease", "I'm not clear about how he makes this diagnosis", or "the advice is not detailed enough". Of all our codes for the doctors' behaviors from the users' perspective, the percentages of codes indicating lacking etiology analysis, lacking diagnostic evidence, lacking operational advice and ambiguous answers account for 6.42%, 18.92%, 16.22% and 25.00% of the dissatisfying conversations respectively.

Here we provide an example for lacking etiology analysis. A user consulted a doctor on the causes of his child's symptoms. The doctor diagnosed the symptoms as viral infections and gave drug recommendations. The user inquired again about the etiology, but the doctor ignored the user's question and gave advice on medication again. The user then complained, "I'm asking you about the causes of the disease, doctor. You only tell me what medicine to eat".

Users also frequently complain about a lack of diagnostic evidence during mobile consultation. Users sometimes ask their doctors, "how did you make your judgment?", "why did you choose this medicine over that one?", or "how did you come to the treatment plan?'. The doctor usually repeated his suggestions, ignored users' questions, or replied "it is too complex to explain to you".

Lacking actionable advice is another type of behavior frequently complained by the users. Sometimes, due to limited diagnostic clues or mild symptoms, doctors may suggest continuous observation without any actionable advice. Many users find this suggestion unacceptable and evaluate the mobile consultation service as dissatisfactory. Actionable advice creates a sense of security because users feel they can do something to prevent the disease from worsening [16]. Moreover, actionable advice is consistent with users' offline consultation expectations. Most users decide to go to offline hospitals only when they have severe symptoms. As a result, most users get actionable advice from their doctors [52]. When users extend their offline expectations to the mobile consultation service, lacking actionable advice may easily cause dissatisfaction.

Ambiguous answers may cause dissatisfaction of users. Doctors sometimes provide general rather than customized suggestions to users due to limited diagnostic clues, time constraints, or simply because they ignore the specific requirements of users. An example of an ambiguous answer is shown in the following. A user described the symptoms of his child to a doctor, and the doctor answered, "that may be bacterial infection". Then the user asked again, "what are the causes?". The doctor said, "not sure. Many factors can cause infection". The user made a negative comment and complained "Too vague! The doctor didn't give explicit answers".

4.1.2. Barriers for Doctors in Information Interpreting

In mobile consultation, doctors sometimes overlook information provided by users or provide irrelevant answers to users' questions. This is in part because the asynchronism feature of CMC increases the difficulties of reading and interpreting information during the consultation. As a result, users feel their needs are neglected. Of all our codes for the doctors' behaviors from the users' perspective, the percentages of codes indicating doctors' ignoring information provided by users and irrelevant answers are 3.04% and 3.38% respectively.

A typical example showing doctors ignore information provided by users is described in the following. A user told the doctor that his child had allergic rhinitis last year and then he described the symptoms that the child had. The doctor replied, "it must be the symptoms of rhinitis". The user complained that the doctor only repeated the information provided in his symptom description.

Doctors sometimes provide irrelevant answers because they fail to understand users' intentions. Here we provide an example for this case. A user asked his doctor "what is the harm of low fever?". The doctor skipped this question and constantly asked "what is the temperature? Are there any symptoms?" As a result, the user complained, "I just want to know the harm of low fever. Why not answer this question straightway?".

4.1.3. Barriers for Doctors in Relationship Maintaining

Representative behaviors that fail to meet users' emotional needs include delayed response, lack of initiatives, lack of emotional comfort, and being unfriendly, each takes 26.69%, 10.81%, 5.74%, and 13.18% respectively in our coding for the doctors' behaviors from the users' perspective.

During mobile consultation, doctors' delayed response is a prominent issue that causes dissatisfaction of users. Asynchronous communication makes it difficult to guarantee the timeliness of doctors' replies in mobile consultation. If doctors fail to respond to users' questions promptly, users will feel neglected, disrespected and are not willing to establish a good relationship with their doctors [14]. Our data analysis reveals that when the mobile conversation is temporarily stopped due to doctors' delayed response, users may complain, "I've waited for so long", "I am very worried, can you hurry up to reply my questions", or "your response is too slow".

Doctors are coded as "lack of initiatives" when they fail to provide additional information that is usually closely related to the questions asked by their users. For example, a doctor asked about what medicine the user was currently taking. After receiving the users' reply, the doctor typed, "this medicine contains suspected carcinogen". Since the doctor failed to provide choices or precautions during the conversation, the user felt very anxious and rated "dissatisfied" in the end. Typical complaints from users include "the doctor merely answers the questions that I ask, but not provide any additional information", "cherish your words like gold", or "the doctor talks as squeezing the toothpaste".

Lacking emotional comfort is also a common phenomenon that causes dissatisfaction of users in mobile consultation. Doctors' emotional comfort has a strong effect on alleviating users' negative emotions [41]. However, due to the lack of visual and auditory cues, doctors cannot effectively perceive the negative emotions of users and omit to express emotional comfort. For example, a user expressed his worry and anxiety about his child's condition, but the doctor neglected the negative emotion and just put forward another question as a response. The user made a negative comment, "professional, but also so indifferent".

Negative comments about doctors' unfriendly attitude frequently happened. During mobile communication, doctors may use a strong tone or words, express the impatient mood, or use rhetorical questions, which makes users feel uncomfortable. As a result, users may complain like "too fierce", "bad service attitude", "not friendly at all". Here we provide an example. When a user asked the doctor a question that he did not understand, the doctor replied, "I don't need to repeat the question that I have explained! Haven't I made myself clear?". The user complained that "that's terrible. I just ask a question, while he answers me like a teacher teaches a student".

4.2. The Doctors' Perspective

By adopting the doctors' perspective, we identified 6 representative types of user behaviors, as is shown in Table 3. In the following, we introduce the results of quantitative coding and the representative information providing, information interpreting, and relationship maintaining behaviors of users.

Table 3. Antecedents of poor DPR from the doctors' perspective.

Category	Subcategory	Percentage	Description
Barriers in information providing	Lack of diagnostic clues	6.76%	The user fails to provide adequate or accurate diagnostic clues for the doctor
Barriers in information interpreting	Insufficient medical knowledge	4.39%	The medical knowledge of the user is inadequate to interpret or understand the suggestions from the doctor
	Conflicting opinions	1.01%	The user has difficulty in understanding the doctor's advice due to different opinions with their doctors.
Barriers in relationship maintaining	Distrust towards the information	13.51%	The user doubts the correctness and reliability of the information provided by the doctor.
	Distrust towards the identity	3.38%	The user doubts whether the doctor's identity is real or authorized
	Personal remark	11.82%	The user expresses dissatisfaction in a bad tone

4.2.1. Barriers for Users in Information Providing

Users' failure to provide accurate or adequate medical information to their doctors through mobile consultation is a common cause of doctors' dissatisfaction. In traditional offline consultations, doctors acquire diagnostic clues through observation and examination. But in mobile consultations, medical clues, such as symptoms, prior medical treatment experience, and medicine usage, can only be provided by the users. However, due to the lack of professional knowledge, it is difficult for users to select useful medical information for doctors. Sometimes, they even provide a conflicting description or refuse to provide the information to assist the diagnosis. As a result, doctors complain during mobile consultation services, such as "why not answer my questions", "no picture to assist my judgment", or "I can't understand your description". Of all our codes for the users' behavior from the doctors' perspective, the percentage of codes indicating inadequate and vague diagnostic clues is 6.76%.

Here we provide an example of failing to provide adequate clues. A user consulted a doctor on the causes of his child's symptoms. The doctor replied, "it is hard to say, I can tell you based on a laboratory test, but it is hard to judge by naked eyes". The user complained, "You are telling me nothing". The doctors replied, "you did not even provide me a picture, you just keep sending me questions".

4.2.2. Barriers for Users in Information Interpreting

During mobile consultations, users sometimes fail to understand the questions or suggestions offered by their doctors because they lack adequate medical knowledge or hold divergent medical opinions with their doctors. As a result, even though doctors spend much time repeating their opinions or explaining medical principles, users misunderstand their doctors' suggestions. Of all our codes for the users' behavior from the doctors' perspective, the percentages of codes indicating users' lacking adequate medical knowledge and holding conflicting opinions with their doctors are 4.39% and 1.01% respectively.

Here is an example that lacking adequate medical knowledge causes poor DPR. A doctor recommended formula milk to a mother because her child was diagnosed with milk protein allergy. Formula milk was suggested since it is easier for a child with dyspepsia to digest. However, this recommendation stimulated a strong objection from the mother. She said, "why not feed him with breast milk? He can't get better with the formula milk. Are you kidding me!" Although the doctor had repeated the detailed medical principle to the mother, she still posted a negative evaluation of the doctor's service. The doctor replied, "as a doctor, I recommend based on my knowledge and the condition of my patients".

Information interpretation issues caused by conflicting opinions also appear in our codes. Some users stick to their inherent opinions that are formed in their prior experience [52]. This "confidence" sometimes leads to users' difficulties in information interpretation. Conflicting opinions between traditional Chinese medical science and western medical science sometimes caused poor DPR. For example, the doctor made a diagnosis with western medical science, while the user tried to interpret the result from the perspective of Chinese medical knowledge. A user asked, "is that caused by the coldness of the body?" The doctor answered, "we are not talking about the same thing". This is special in the Chinese context where traditional Chinese medical science co-exists with western medical science. Another example is the conflicting opinions about the treatment. For example, the doctor offered a treatment plan, but the user thought that taking medicine had unavoidable harm and asked for more conservative treatment. The doctor answered, "this treatment is necessary and you should follow doctors' advice."

4.2.3. Barriers for Users in Relationship maintaining

During mobile consultation, users sometimes doubt the information offered by doctors, causing tense DPR from the doctors' perspective. Users in the mobile era no longer rely on information from a single doctor. Instead, they search the internet, consult other doctors, and compare the information they collected from multiple sources and multiple times. Once there is conflicting information, the users tend to explicitly express their distrust towards their doctors during doctor-user communication. For example, users said, "I disagree with you", "you might be wrong, I consulted multiple doctors and received conflicting recommendations", or "no, I hear that ... while you said that ... ". In response, some doctors said during the interaction, "why do you distrust my opinion?". Of all our codes for the users' behavior from the doctors' perspective, the percentage of codes indicating that users doubt the information provided by their doctors is 13.51%.

Sometimes, when there are divergent opinions, users even doubt the identity of their doctors. Different from the traditional offline context, the sense of authority and security used to associate with doctors is weakened in the mobile context. Moreover, users have less tolerance and understanding when their doctors make mistakes. In our codes, some users wrote, "I doubt whether you are a registered doctor", "are you a real doctor/ an intern/a robot", or "you're not professional, I know it better than you". As a result, doctors replied to these comments like "I've been working for 5 years", "interns are not allowed to register for this service", or "you are too rude". Of all our codes for the users' behaviors from the doctors' perspective, the percentage of codes indicating that users doubt the identity of doctors is 3.38%.

In more extreme cases, users vent their negative emotions by giving personal remarks towards their doctors. For example, some users wrote, "I think you are a quack" or "why don't you go elsewhere and sell your quack medicine to others". As a result, during the interaction with these users, doctors replied by writing "please mind your tone", "please do not use terrible words", "show some respect", or "you show no respect to me". Of all our codes for the users' behaviors from the doctors' perspective, the percentage of codes indicating that users give personal remarks towards their doctors is 11.82%.

5. Discussion

This study discusses the impact of mobile technologies on DPR and pays special attention to the antecedents of poor DPR during mobile medical consultation. Figure 3 summarizes our key findings.

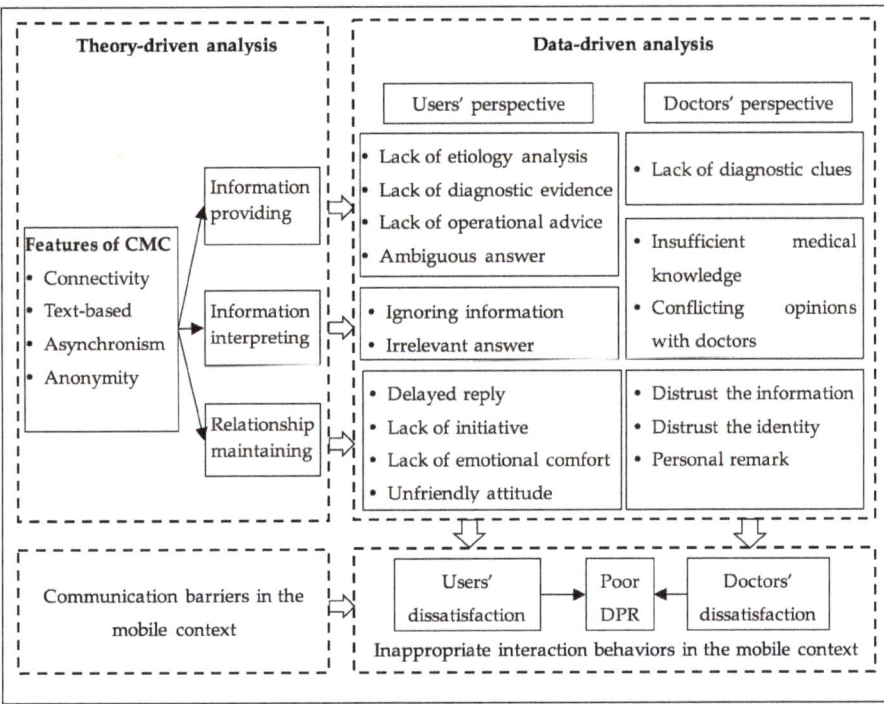

Figure 3. Antecedents of poor DPR in the mobile medical context.

First, inappropriate information providing, information interpreting and relationship maintaining behaviors of doctors and users are the direct causes of poor DPR in mobile consultation. From the perspective of users, mobile technologies have the potential to empower users with more medical knowledge and greater decision power over their health conditions [12]. However, their doctors fail to provide adequate support to realize the potential, which leads to user dissatisfaction and poor DPR. In specific, we find that some doctors fail to provide the etiology analysis, diagnostic basis, clear operational advice, or targeted answers to users' questions. Moreover, some doctors ignore users' emotional needs during communication and fail to provide a timely reply, an active inquiry, emotional comfort and/or a friendly service attitude to their worried users. From the doctors' perspective, we find that some users fail to provide adequate or accurate diagnostic clues for their doctors, and some others fail to interpret the advice correctly due to limited medical knowledge or conflicting medical opinions. Moreover, we highlight that the emotional needs of doctors have been overlooked during doctor-user communication. Although doctors expect trust, respect, and understanding from users [18], they are susceptible to doubts and even personal remarks from users. These inappropriate communication behaviors directly lead to the dissatisfaction of doctors and users in mobile consultation services.

Second, doctor-user communication is compromised by CMC, which is the underlying cause of poor DPR in mobile consultation. The connectivity feature of mobile applications might lead to increased workload for doctors or information conflicting and overloading for users. Accordingly, for doctors, an overwhelming amount of workload may reduce the amount of time that doctors spend on each user, which may result in inadequate information providing and information interpreting.

Meanwhile, users are more likely to be exposed to conflicting medical information, which might weaken their trust towards their doctors [14].

Features of text-based communication and asynchronism create barriers in medical information providing, information interpreting, and relationship maintaining behaviors for both users and doctors. For users, it is difficult to provide sufficient diagnostic clues to their doctors via texts and pictures. Moreover, lacking visual clues of doctors may weaken users' trust toward their doctors. For doctors, lacking visual clues and asynchronous communication increase the difficulty to diagnose and interpret users' symptoms, increase the time cost to provide a medical suggestion and increase the difficulty of perceiving users' emotion [33,34].

The misbehaviors of users along the relationship maintaining dimension can be partly explained by the anonymity nature of mobile communication. In anonymous communication, people are more inclined to express negative emotions towards others compared to face-to-face communication because of reduced social presence [53]. Therefore, in mobile consultation users are more likely to an overt and explicit expression of negative emotions, which leads to poor DPR.

5.1. Theoretical Implications

Our findings have the following three theoretical implications:

First, this study extends existing studies on poor DPR by integrating both doctors' and users' perspectives. The majority of existing studies tend to investigate DPR only from users' perspectives, such as Um et al. (2018) [8] and Zhang et al. (2018) [12], ignoring the significance of interpreting DPR from dual perspectives of users and doctors. Mobile consultation transforms the traditional doctor-dominated relationship to a more equal and reciprocal relationship [36,54], which emphasizes the importance of taking doctors' experience into account to understand DPR. By discerning causes of poor DPR for both doctors and users, this study provides a more comprehensive understanding of DPR in the mobile context.

Second, this research contributes to existing knowledge on the causes of poor DPR in the mobile context by elaborating on both direct and underlying causes of poor DPR. Existing studies mainly ascribe poor DPR to observed behaviors, such as long waiting hours, no treatment plan and impatience [7,14], which fails to explore the underlying reasons for these behaviors. By drawing on the theoretical perspective of CMC and by conducting a qualitative study on a leading Chinese mobile medical platform, this study not only highlights representative misbehaviors of doctors and users as the direct causes of poor DPR but also identifies CMC limitations as the underlying reasons.

Last but not least, by comparing the traditional face-to-face consultation with CMC medical communication, this study extends the current mobile health studies by identifying the unique but dark side of mobile health services. Even though mobile health services are becoming extensively popular in recent years, the unique settings of mobile medical consultation make it difficult to further improve user satisfaction. By distinguishing the potential challenges of the mobile healthcare services, this study provides a brand-new perspective to explain user satisfaction, that is to explain user satisfaction from the mobile context itself, rather than from the interaction process.

5.2. Practical Implications

Our findings also provide practical implications for doctors, users and mobile consultation application developers. Doctors are suggested to provide more support for users to take part in their medical decisions. In specific, besides diagnostic results, more and more users regard the diagnostic process, evidence, advice, and etiology as additional information to make a medical decision. When doctors overlook or refuse to follow up on these information needs, users often, but not always, feel dissatisfied. In the meanwhile, doctors are suggested to understand and respond to users' emotional needs in mobile consultation service. For example, doctors should try their best to guarantee timely responses, make explanations or ask for understanding when responses have been delayed.

Users are suggested to acknowledge the limitation of mobile consultation service, and adjust their behaviors and expectation to cope with the potential challenges brought by mobile-mediated doctor-user communication. To be more specific, users should offer adequate, accurate, and relevant medical information on their initiatives to help doctors to understand their physical conditions and emotional needs. Moreover, expressing understanding and respect is helpful for users to build friendly relationships with their doctors.

Mobile consultation applications developers are supposed to optimize product designs by developing more effective tools to facilitate effective communication between doctors and users. For example, provide a template to instruct users to provide the required information for the diagnosis such as symptoms, examination reports, and medication use. The list of the required information help doctors collect users' information conveniently and avoid repeated inquiries. Response templates are also helpful for doctors to provide detailed and standard medical information. Other useful implications for developers may include monitoring users' waiting time during consultations to avoid users' negative feelings and giving appropriate reminders to physicians when necessary.

This study has several limitations, but it also points out several future directions. First, it is hard to capture doctors' feelings and opinions in communication records. Although we adopt measures to screen records that can reflect doctors' negative emotions, more effective methods of reflecting doctors' feelings and evaluations are needed. Future studies are encouraged to use questionnaires or interviews to collect data from doctors, to supplement existing qualitative second-hand data and further discover potential problems from the doctors' perspective. Second, to simplify the data analysis process, this study restricts doctor-user communication in one consultation. DPR stems from a long-term experience of care and counseling. Future research can consider the evolving characteristics of DPR and uncover the evolutionary process of poor DPR in the mobile context.

6. Conclusions

Mobile healthcare service has substantially changed the way people obtain medical service. Nevertheless, the majority of extant studies have focused on the potential positive impact and paid limited attention to potential challenges. We can refine the mobile consultation service and take better advantage of mobile technology by focusing on these potential challenges. This study uncovers the underlying reasons for poor DPR in mobile healthcare consultation services by taking both doctors' and users' perspectives into account. Drawing on the CMC literature, we identified the potential challenges brought by mobile technologies on the information providing, information interpreting, and relationship maintaining processes during doctor-user communication. Meanwhile, by analyzing the objective mobile communication records between doctors and users with qualitative methods, we identified representative misbehaviors of both doctors and users that cause poor DPR in the mobile context. We conclude that doctors and users' inappropriate behaviors are the direct causes of poor DPR and limitations of mobile communication are the primary underlying cause of poor DPR in mobile consultation.

Author Contributions: Conceptualization, M.Y. and H.T.; methodology, M.Y., H.T., and L.J.; software, M.Y., H.T., and L.J.; validation, H.T., L.J., and U.A.; formal analysis, M.Y., H.T., and L.J.; resources, H.T.; data curation, M.Y., H.T., and L.J.; writing—original draft preparation, M.Y., H.T., and L.J.; writing—review and editing, M.Y., H.T., L.J., and U.A.; visualization, M.Y. and H.T.; supervision, M.Y., H.T., and U.A.; project administration, M.Y. and H.T.; funding acquisition, M.Y. and H.T. All authors have read and agreed to the published version of the manuscript.

Funding: This research was funded by Humanities and Social Sciences of the Ministry of Education Foundation [grant number 18YJC630221], Beijing University of Posts and Telecommunications Excellent Ph.D. Students Foundation [grant number CX2019234], and National Natural Science Foundation of China [grant numbers 71874018, 71772017]. The funders had no role in the design of the study; in the collection, analyses, or interpretation of data; in the writing of the manuscript, or in the decision to publish the results.

Conflicts of Interest: The authors declare no conflict of interest. The funders had no role in the design of the study; in the collection, analyses, or interpretation of data; in the writing of the manuscript, or in the decision to publish the results.

References

1. Liu, C.-F.; Tsai, Y.-C.; Jang, F.-L. Patients' Acceptance towards a Web-Based Personal Health Record System: An Empirical Study in Taiwan. *Int. J. Environ. Res. Public Health* **2013**, *10*, 5191–5208. [CrossRef]
2. Shaw, B.R.; Han, J.Y.; Hawkins, R.P.; James, S.; McTavish, F.; Gustafson, D.H. Doctor–patient relationship as motivation and outcome: Examining uses of an interactive cancer communication system. *Int. J. Med. Inform.* **2017**, *76*, 274–282. [CrossRef]
3. Tang, Y.; Yang, Y.-T.; Shao, Y.-F. Acceptance of Online Medical Websites: An Empirical Study in China. *Int J. Environ. Res. Public Health* **2019**, *16*, 943. [CrossRef]
4. Liang, C.; Gu, D.; Tao, F.; Jain, H.K.; Zhao, Y.; Ding, B. Influence of mechanism of patient-accessible hospital information system implementation on doctor–patient relationships: A service fairness perspective. *Inf. Manag.* **2017**, *54*, 57–72. [CrossRef]
5. Zhang, X.; Guo, X.; Lai, K.H.; Yi, W. How does online interactional unfairness matter for patient–doctor relationship quality in online health consultation? The contingencies of professional seniority and disease severity. *Eur. J. Inf. Syst.* **2019**, *28*, 336–354. [CrossRef]
6. iResearch. Report on the Demand of Doctors in China's Online Medical Market. 2016. Available online: http://report.iresearch.cn/report/201609/2650.shtml (accessed on 29 September 2016).
7. Hao, H.; Zhang, K. The voice of Chinese health consumers: A text mining approach to web-based physician reviews. *J. Med. Internet Res.* **2016**, *18*, 108–119. [CrossRef]
8. Um, K.H.; Lau, A.K.W. Healthcare service failure: How dissatisfied patients respond to poor service quality. *Int. J. Oper. Prod. Manag.* **2018**, *38*, 1245–1270. [CrossRef]
9. Zhou, M.; Zhao, L.; Campy, K.; Wang, S. Changing of China's health policy and Doctor–Patient relationship. *Health Policy Technol.* **2017**, *6*, 358–367. [CrossRef]
10. Gu, D.; Yang, X.; Li, X.; Jain, H.K.; Liang, C. Understanding the Role of Mobile Internet-Based Health Services on Patient Satisfaction and Word-of-Mouth. *Int. J. Environ. Res. Public Health* **2018**, *15*, 1972. [CrossRef]
11. Mein Goh, J.; Gao, G.; Agarwal, R. The creation of social value: Can an online health community reduce rural–urban health disparities? *MIS Q.* **2016**, *40*, 1–22.
12. Zhang, W.; Deng, Z.; Hong, Z.; Evans, R.D.; Ma, J.; Zhang, H. Unhappy Patients Are Not Alike: Content Analysis of the Negative Comments from China's Good Doctor Website. *J. Med. Internet Res.* **2018**, *20*, 35–49. [CrossRef]
13. Sewitch, M.J.; Abrahamowicz, M.; Dobkin, P.L.; Tamblyn, R. Measuring Differences Between Patients' and Physicians' Health Perceptions: The Patient–Physician Discordance Scale. *J. Behav. Med.* **2003**, *26*, 245–264. [CrossRef]
14. Atanasova, S.; Kamin, T.; Petri, G. The benefits and challenges of online professional-patient interaction: Comparing views between users and health professional moderators in an online health community. *Comput. Human Behav.* **2018**, *83*, 106–118. [CrossRef]
15. Akter, S.; D'Ambra, J.; Ray, P. Development and validation of an instrument to measure user perceived service quality of mHealth. *Inf. Manag.* **2013**, *50*, 181–195. [CrossRef]
16. Deng, Z.; Liu, S.; Hinz, O. The health information seeking and usage behavior intention of Chinese consumers through mobile phones. *Inf. Technol. People* **2015**, *28*, 405–423. [CrossRef]
17. Wu, T.; Deng, Z.; Zhang, D.; Buchanan, P.R.; Zha, D.; Wang, R. Seeking and using intention of health information from doctors in social media: The effect of doctor-consumer interaction. *Int. J. Med. Inform.* **2018**, *105*, 106–113. [CrossRef]
18. Lee, S.A.; Zuercher, R.J. A current review of doctor–patient computer-mediated communication. *J. Commun. Healthc.* **2017**, *10*, 22–30. [CrossRef]
19. Ang, C.S.; Talib, M.A.; Tan, K.A.; Tan, J.P.; Yaacob, S.N. Understanding computer-mediated communication attributes and life satisfaction from the perspectives of uses and gratifications and self-determination. *Comput. Hum. Behav.* **2015**, *40*, 20–29. [CrossRef]
20. Lewandowski, J.; Rosenberg, B.D.; Parks, M.J.; Siegel, J.T. The effect of informal social support: Face-to-face versus computer-mediated communication. *Comput. Hum. Behav.* **2011**, *27*, 1806–1814. [CrossRef]
21. Bae, M. The effects of anonymity on computer-mediated communication: The case of independent versus interdependent self-construal influence. *Comput. Hum. Behav.* **2016**, *55*, 300–309. [CrossRef]

22. Rains, S.A. A meta-analysis of research on formal computer-mediated support groups: Examining group characteristics and health outcomes. *Hum. Commun. Res.* **2010**, *35*, 309–336. [CrossRef]
23. Andreassen, H.K.; Trondsen, M.; Kummervold, P.E.; Gammon, D.; Hjortdahl, P. Patients who use e-mediated communication with their doctor: New constructions of trust in the patient-doctor relationship. *Qual. Health Res.* **2006**, *16*, 238–248. [CrossRef]
24. Ho, S.M.; Lowry, P.B.; Warkentin, M.; Yang, Y.; Hollister, J.M. Gender deception in asynchronous online communication: A path analysis. *Inf. Process. Manag.* **2017**, *53*, 21–41. [CrossRef]
25. Adrianson, L. Gender and computer-mediated communication: Group processes in problem solving. *Comput. Hum. Behav.* **2001**, *17*, 71–94. [CrossRef]
26. Wright, K.B.; Bell, S.B. Health-related support groups on the Internet: Linking empirical findings to social support and computer-mediated communication theory. *J. Health Psychol.* **2003**, *81*, 39–54. [CrossRef]
27. Borowitz, S.M.; Wyatt, J.C. The origin, content, and workload of e-mail consultations. *JAMA* **1998**, *280*, 1321–1324. [CrossRef]
28. Colvin, J.; Chenoweth, L.; Bold, M.; Harding, C. Caregivers of older adults: Advantages and disadvantages of Internet-based social support. *Fam. Relat.* **2004**, *53*, 49–57. [CrossRef]
29. Riordan, M.A.; Kreuz, R.J. Emotion encoding and interpretation in computer-mediated communication: Reasons for use. *Comput. Hum. Behav.* **2010**, *26*, 1667–1673. [CrossRef]
30. Angeli, C.; Schwartz, N.H. Differences in electronic exchanges in synchronous and asynchronous computer-mediated communication: The effect of culture as a mediating variable. *Interact. Learn. Environ.* **2016**, *24*, 1109–1130. [CrossRef]
31. Katz, S.J.; Moyer, C.A.; Cox, D.T.; Stern, D.T. Effect of a Triage-based E-mail System on Clinic Resource Use and Patient and Physician Satisfaction in Primary Care: A Randomized Controlled Trial. *J. Gen. Intern. Med.* **2003**, *18*, 736–744. [CrossRef]
32. Joinson, A.N. Self-disclosure in computer-mediated communication: The role of self-awareness and visual anonymity. *Eur. J. Soc. Psychol.* **2001**, *31*, 177–192. [CrossRef]
33. Patt, M.R.; Houston, T.K.; Jenckes, M.W.; Sands, D.Z.; Ford, D.E. Doctors who are using e-mail with their patients: A qualitative exploration. *J. Med. Internet Res.* **2003**, *5*, 1–23. [CrossRef]
34. Tidwell, L.C.; Walther, J.B. Computer-mediated communication effects on disclosure, impressions, and interpersonal evaluations: Getting to know one another a bit at a time. *Hum. Commun. Res.* **2010**, *28*, 317–348. [CrossRef]
35. Eveleigh, R.M.; Muskens, E.; van Ravesteijn, H.; van Dijk, I.; van Rijswijk, E.; Lucassen, P. An overview of 19 instruments assessing the doctor-patient relationship: Different models or concepts are used. *J. Clin. Epidemiol.* **2012**, *65*, 10–15. [CrossRef]
36. Fuertes, J.N.; Anand, P.; Haggerty, G.; Kestenbaum, M.; Rosenblum, G.C. The Physician–Patient Working Alliance and Patient Psychological Attachment, Adherence, Outcome Expectations, and Satisfaction in a Sample of Rheumatology Patients. *Behav. Med.* **2015**, *41*, 60–68. [CrossRef]
37. Teutsch, C. Patient-doctor communication. *Med. Clin. North Am.* **2003**, *87*, 1115–1145. [CrossRef]
38. Ong, L.; De Haes, J.; Hoos, A.; Lammes, F. Doctor-patient communication: A review of the literature. *Soc. Sci. Med.* **1995**, *40*, 908–918. [CrossRef]
39. Pian, W.; Song, S.; Zhang, Y. Consumer health information needs: A systematic review of measures. *Inf. Process. Manag.* **2020**, *57*, 102077. [CrossRef]
40. Dennis, A.; Fuller, R.; Valacich, J. Media, tasks, and communication processes: A theory of media synchronicity. *MIS Q. Manag. Inf. Syst.* **2008**, *32*, 575–600. [CrossRef]
41. Liang, B.; Scammon, D.L. E-Word-of-Mouth on health social networking sites: An opportunity for tailored health communication. *J. Consum. Behav.* **2011**, *10*, 322–331. [CrossRef]
42. Motamarri, S.; Akter, S.; Ray, P.; Tseng, C.L. Distinguishing " mHealth" from Other Healthcare Services in a Developing Country: A Study from the Service Quality Perspective. *Commun. Assoc. Inf. Syst.* **2014**, *34*, 669–692. [CrossRef]
43. Zhang, X.; Yan, X.; Cao, X.; Sun, Y.; Chen, H.; She, J. The role of perceived e-health literacy in users' continuance intention to use mobile healthcare applications: An exploratory empirical study in China. *Inf. Technol. Dev.* **2018**, *24*, 198–223. [CrossRef]
44. Kozinets, R.V. The field behind the screen: Using netnography for marketing research in online communities. *J. Mark. Res.* **2002**, *39*, 61–72. [CrossRef]

45. Murthy, D. Digital Ethnography: An Examination of the use of new technologies for social Research. *Sociology* **2008**, *42*, 837–855. [CrossRef]
46. Analysys. Annual Comprehensive Analysis of Internet Healthcare in China 2018. 2018. Available online: https://www.analysys.cn/article/analysis/detail/20018737 (accessed on 1 December 2018).
47. Burt, J.; Abel, G.; Elmore, N.; Lloyd, C.; Benson, J.; Sarson, L.; Carluccio, A.; Campbell, J.; Elliott, M.N.; Roland, M. Understanding negative feedback from South Asian patients: An experimental vignette study. *BMJ Open* **2016**, *6*, e011256. [CrossRef]
48. Octacon. Chinese Sentiment Analysis. 2018. Available online: https://github.com/octacon/bixin (accessed on 10 June 2018).
49. Montini, T.; Noble, A.A.; Stelfox, H.T. Content analysis of patient complaints. *Int. J. Qual. Health Care* **2008**, *20*, 412–420. [CrossRef]
50. Liu, C.; Uffenheimer, M.; Nasseri, Y.; Cohen, J.; Ellenhorn, J. "But His Yelp Reviews Are Awful!": Analysis of General Surgeons' Yelp Reviews. *J. Med. Internet Res.* **2019**, *21*, e11646. [CrossRef]
51. Saldana, J. *The Coding Manual for Qualitative Researchers*, 3rd ed.; SAGE Publications Ltd.: London, UK, 2009.
52. Zhang, X.; Guo, X.; Lai, K.-h.; Yin, C.; Meng, F. From offline healthcare to online health service: The role of offline healthcare satisfaction and habits. *J. Electron. Commer. Res.* **2017**, *18*, 138–154.
53. Derks, D.; Fischer, A.H.; Bos, A.E. The role of emotion in computer-mediated communication: A review. *Comput. Hum. Behav.* **2008**, *24*, 766–785. [CrossRef]
54. Guo, S.; Guo, X.; Fang, Y.; Vogel, D. How Doctors Gain Social and Economic Returns in Online Health-Care Communities: A Professional Capital Perspective. *J. Manag. Inf. Syst.* **2017**, *34*, 487–519. [CrossRef]

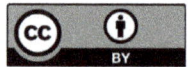

© 2020 by the authors. Licensee MDPI, Basel, Switzerland. This article is an open access article distributed under the terms and conditions of the Creative Commons Attribution (CC BY) license (http://creativecommons.org/licenses/by/4.0/).

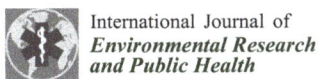

Article

Contextualising the 2019 E-Cigarette Health Scare: Insights from Twitter

Wasim Ahmed [1,*], Xavier Marin-Gomez [2,3] and Josep Vidal-Alaball [2,4]

1. Newcastle University Business School, Newcastle University, 5 Barrack Rd, Newcastle upon Tyne NE1 4SE, UK
2. Health Promotion in Rural Areas Research Group, Gerència Territorial de la Catalunya Central, Institut Català de la Salut, 08272 Sant Fruitós de Bages, Spain; xmarin.cc.ics@gencat.cat (X.M.-G.); jvidal.cc.ics@gencat.cat (J.V.-A.)
3. Servei d'Atenció Primària d'Osona, Gerència Territorial de la Catalunya Central, Institut Català de la Salut, 08500 Vic, Spain
4. Unitat de Suport a la Recerca de la Catalunya Central, Fundació Institut Universitari per a la recerca a l'Atenció Primària de Salut Jordi Gol i Gurina, 08272 Sant Fruitós de Bages, Spain
* Correspondence: wasim.ahmed@newcastle.ac.uk

Received: 19 February 2020; Accepted: 26 March 2020; Published: 26 March 2020

Abstract: A health scare can be described as a campaign that attempts to alert the public of a particular substance or activity that can lead to a negative effect on health. A recent health scare to emerge relates to the health hazards associated with the use of e-cigarettes, which has caused widespread debate, which peaked towards the end of 2019. Health scares need to be studied in the context in which they occur, and one method of studying them is through social media. This paper identifies two key topics of discussion on Twitter, which consisted of pro-vaping and anti-vaping views. The paper then identifies influential users, frequently occurring words, hashtags, and websites related to this time period in order to gain insight into e-cigarette perceptions. The paper then reviews current scientific evidence and develops a flowchart for the general public, which can be used to for public reassurance and guidance.

Keywords: electronic nicotine delivery systems; social media; smoking; twitter

1. Introduction

Electronic cigarettes or e-cigarettes are handheld battery operated devices that heat liquid and deliver an aerosol that simulates smoking. They may also be referred to as electronic nicotine delivery systems (ENDS) in certain literature. In conjunction with the increased use of these devices [1], a health concern has emerged linking the use of e-cigarettes with pulmonary illness [2–4]. The Centers for Disease Control and Prevention (CDC) and the U.S. Food and Drug Administration (FDA) are investigating a multistate outbreak of lung injury associated with the use of e-cigarette or vaping products [5,6]. All of this information is generating widespread debate, which we can be framed as a health scare [7,8] similar to other scares such as the current COVID-19 scare, as well as the H1N1 virus (swine flu), trans fats, Ebola, and the mobile phone usage health scare [9,10]. Health scares can be described as campaigns that attempt to alert the public of a particular substance or activity that can lead to a negative effect on health [11].

Tobacco can be traced back thousands of years and was grown as a crop from around 5000–3000 BC, led by the communities in the Andes, South America (Ram, Nathan, Balraj, 2017). Native Americans would cultivate and smoke tobacco for medicinal and ceremonial purposes. Tobacco eventually spread around other continents and eventually all around the world [12]. Henceforth, it had many thousands of years to become ingrained within human culture and society. In the early years of the

20th Century, cigarette and nicotine marketing through print, television, and radio only helped to boost sales. In recent years, and after the dangers of traditional forms of smoking, e-cigarettes have risen in popularity.

The tobacco industry is argued to be one of the most profitable and deadly industries that exists with cigarette retail values in 2013 hitting $ 722 billion and there being 5.7 trillion cigarettes in circulation [12]. In today's digital world, it is possible for consumers and the general public to offer their views and opinions across social media platforms. One of the most open platforms to converse about public health is Twitter, where it is also possible to extract tweets for academic research purposes. Previous research has utilised Twitter to identify public views, key discussions, content, and stakeholders related to health scares [13–15]. Twitter can be used to study and understand the context of the current e-cigarette health scare. Twitter is an important platform to study because it has the potential to shape mainstream news because tweets can be embedded in online news stories, as well as highlighted in traditional media (such as TV or radio), amplifying their reach. Health scares need to be studied in the context in which they occur, and one method of studying them is through the use of Twitter [10,16]. This is because Twitter provides citizens with a platform that permits the rapid sharing of public views and opinions and allows these views to become viral and highly shared, regardless of their factual truth; henceforth, this is an important and significant area to study. Moreover, the debate around the safety of e-cigarettes is likely to be of interest to a wide variety of stakeholders.

Our study sought to examine an influential time-point related to e-cigarettes from 2019 when there was a heightened interest in e-cigarette safety. We identified a gap in knowledge as no previous empirical work has conducted an analysis of Twitter data related to this time point. Moreover, this is an important topic to study because it aims to build an understanding of how social media may play a role in the global dissemination of amateur and unfounded speculation against accepted medical research. This type of research is increasingly important, as we find medical studies being socially challenged by various social media networks at an increasing rate. We utilised a mix of social network, automated text, and link analysis in order to identify network structures, influential users, the most utilised words, and hashtags.

We sought to address the following research questions:

1. What was the overall shape of the network structure on Twitter related to the e-cigarette debate?
2. What key themes and/or topics emerged when Twitter users conversing about e-cigarettes on Twitter?
3. Who were the key stakeholders, and what types of content were they sharing on Twitter related to the e-cigarette debate?

A further objective of the study was to review existing literature in order to develop a flowchart for consumers to assess the safety of e-cigarettes by analysing public views from Twitter and by drawing up current advice from health authorities and domain experts. This flowchart is likely to be of interest to consumers and public health agencies across the world.

2. Methods

We retrieved data from Twitter using NodeXL related to the time when the first study was published linking cancer and vaping in mice. NodeXL utilises the Search Application Programming Interface (AP)I. We retrieved data using the keywords "ecigarette" OR "e-cig" OR "ecig" OR "vaping", and we were able to retrieve a sufficient amount of tweets. The tweets in the network were tweeted over the 17 h, 37 min period from Monday, 07 October 2019, at 21:20 Coordinated Universal Time (UTC), to Tuesday, 08 October 2019, at 14:58 UTC. The graph represents a network of 14,912 Twitter users.

We utilised social network analysis, which is an established method of studying social media content, and a complete overview of network shapes and structures can be found elsewhere [17]. Within our network graph, there was an edge for each "replies-to" relationship in a tweet, an edge for each "mentions" relationship in a tweet, and a self-loop edge for each tweet that was not a "replies-to" or "mentions". The graph was directed, and vertices were grouped by cluster using the Clauset–Newman–Moore cluster algorithm. The graph was laid out using the Harel–Koren fast multiscale layout algorithm.

3. Results

3.1. Social Network Analysis of Study Linking Cancer and Vaping Published Research (October 2019)

Figure 1 below shows a social network analysis of tweets from early October 2019, which relates to a time period when the first academic study was published linking vaping to cancer in mice. Figure 2 is zoomed into Group 2 and labels the influential users within the group. From group 3 onwards we have abbreviated the word 'Group' to 'G'.

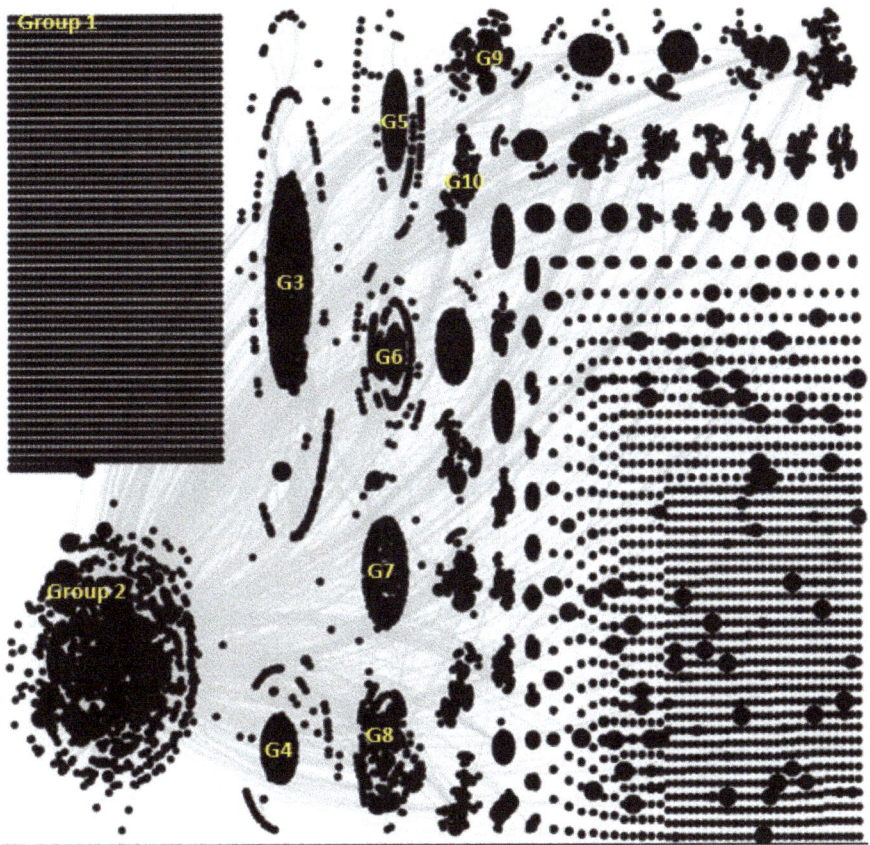

Figure 1. Tweets related to e-cigarettes in October 2019.

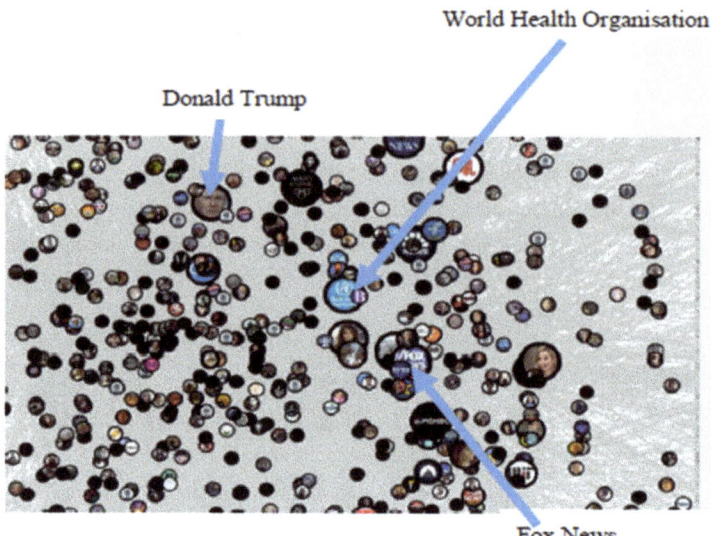

Figure 2. Zooming into Group 2.

The network graph highlights that there were different clusters of discussion taking place on Twitter during this time with two large groups and several smaller groups indicating a number of communities that had emerged related to this topic. The ten largest groups were labelled. There was also a sizeable isolates group (Group 1), which indicated that a number of Twitter users were tweeting about e-cigarettes without mentioning or replying to other Twitter users. In Figure 2, we zoom into Group 2 in which discussions were formed around a number of influential user accounts such as President Donald Trump, the World Health Organisation, and Fox News. Alongside this network graph, we were also able to identify the most frequently used words, hashtags, websites, and most influential users in the network, which are described below.

3.2. Most Frequently Occurring Words

Table 1 below displays the most frequently occurring words during this time period. It highlights that mentions of e-cigarettes were made in conjunction with the scientific work that linked them to cancer.

Table 1. Most frequently occurring words.

Words	No.
vaping	15,452
cancer	5181
cigarettes	4034
mice	3377

The most frequently occurring words in Group 1 are displayed in Table 2 below. Here, it can also be seen that many of these words centred on the news story linking vaping to cancer.

Table 2. Most frequently occurring words in Group 1.

Words	No.
vaping	2177
cigarettes	373
lung	315
cancer	310

The most frequently occurring words in Group 2 (the second largest cluster of Twitter users) are highlighted in Table 3 below. It is important to note that the word-count numbers listed above would also contain hashtags that used those words.

Table 3. Most frequently occurring words in Group 2.

Words	No.
vaping	3452
# vaping	1163
# wevapewevote	1054
# vapeban	807

These words in Group 2 highlighted the polarisation on Twitter as certain hashtags were against the idea of any restrictions on vaping by governments, and Twitter users expressed this through the use of the hashtag "#wevapewevote", whereas those against e-cigarettes would use hashtags such as "#vapeban".

3.3. Most Frequently Occurring Hashtags

The most frequently occurring hashtags overall are summarized in Table 4 below. These hashtags highlighted division and polarisation on Twitter as some hashtags related to campaigns against vaping such as "vapeban", whereas other hashtags such as "wevapewevote" were pro-vaping. There were more Twitter users using pro-vaping based hashtags than against them.

Table 4. Most frequently occurring hashtags.

Words	No.
vaping	1459
wevapewevote	515
vape	424
vapeban	391

3.4. Most Frequently Occurring Websites

The top URL shared on Twitter during this time was entitled "Lung Damage From Vaping Resembles Chemical Burns, Report Says" published in the New York Times (n = 341) [18]. The other URLs consisted of an article by the Consumer News and Business Channel (CNBC) (n = 229) titled Researchers find e-cigarettes cause lung cancer in mice in first study tying vaping to cancer. Further websites also appeared such as an article titled Expert reaction to study on ecig vapour and cancer in mice, which was published by the Science Media Centre (n = 124). Interestingly, the article contained reactions from two professors with expertise in tobacco research, and both noted that the study linking e-cigarettes and cancer to mice was potentially seriously flawed in its relevance for human vapers. Another article titled Juul Is Sued by School Districts That Say Vaping Is a Dangerous Drain on Their

Resources published by the New York Times was also shared ($n = 88$). These results are summarized in Table 5 below.

Table 5. Most frequently occurring hashtags.

Title	Publisher	No.
Lung Damage From Vaping Resembles Chemical Burns, Report Says	New York Times	341
Researchers find e-cigarettes cause lung cancer in mice in first study tying vaping to cancer	CNBC	229
Expert reaction to study on ecig vapour and cancer in mice	Science Media Centre	124
Juul Is Sued by School Districts That Say Vaping Is a Dangerous Drain on Their Resources published	New York Times	88

3.5. Influential Users Ranked by Betweenness Centrality

Influential users were ranked by the betweenness centrality algorithm using NodeXL. Influential users consisted of CNBC, which had 3.3 million followers, and the news anchor of Columbia Broadcasting System's (CBS) Nightly Business Report, who had 31.3 thousand followers. The reason for the prominence of CNBC was because they had published an article on October 7th titled *'Researchers find e-cigarettes cause lung cancer in mice in first study tying vaping to cancer'*. A citizen who tweeted the study and noted the findings of the study for the reason for "not following trends" received over 400 retweets and 1.8 thousand likes also became influential and had 6.1 thousand followers. The user was characterizing e-cigarettes as a societal trend with dissent towards those who were using e-cigarettes. A user replied to this tweet indicating that the fear around e-cigarettes seemed irrational when traditional e-cigarettes were still being sold. Other influential accounts consisted of The Centres for Disease Control (CDC) with 1.24 million followers who tweeted about cases of lung damage of users of mostly illicit e-cigarettes containing the Tetrahydrocannabinol (THC), and Gregory Conley, with 18.1 thousand followers, who is a tobacco harm-reduction advocate and supporter of e-cigarettes who was tweeting at this time. Table 6 below provides a summary of the influential users in the network.

Table 6. Influential users ranked by betweenness centrality.

Rank	Influential User Account	Followers
1	CNBC	3.3 million followers
2	Anchor of CBS's Nightly Business Report	31.3 thousand followers
3	The Centres for Disease Control	1.24 million
4	Citizen	6.1 thousand followers
5	Gregory Conley	18.1 thousand followers

3.6. Pro-Vaping and Anti-Vaping Themes

Much of the content around this time related to Twitter users sharing the news story linking vaping and cancer in mice. Furthermore, our tweet clustering, word, and hashtag analysis revealed two further main themes taking place within the overall network related to Twitter users who were, broadly speaking, either pro-vaping or anti-vaping. In order to confirm this finding, we utilised content analysis to categorize tweets until thematic saturation occurred, and we found two additional main themes related to pro-vaping or anti-vaping views.

Twitter users who were supporting vaping tweeted how using vaping products had helped them stop smoking and also highlighted how the current issue around vaping was very specific to certain illicit types of vaping products that contained Tetrahydrocannabinol (THC). Arguments were also made towards vaping serving a function in harm-reduction as it was comparably safer than smoking.

Twitter users against vaping requested for people to stop using e-cigarettes and for tougher legalisation on vaping products. Below, we provide anonymized tweets related to these two main themes.

3.7. Pro-Vaping Tweet Extracts

There were a number of Twitter users who would share their own positive personal experiences of using e-cigarette devices:

"I was a heavy smoker for many decades and knew I'd be dead in my 50 s and never get a chance to see my grandchildren. But then 5 years ago I started to use e-cigarettes and I may be able to see my grandchildren now"

Other Twitter users were concerned about the increased focus on younger people using e-cigarettes:

"The dangers of vaping and youth is completely overblown! Car crashes are actually the leading cause of death in younger people"

There were also Twitter users who noted the dangers of cigarettes compared to e-cigarettes:

"Right then, they will ban e-cigs because it causes deaths, but regular cigarettes don't seem to be a problem, lol!"

There were also Twitter users who criticised the study linking cancer and vaping:

"If they re-ran the study and compared vaping and real cigarettes then vaping would be the safer alternative! #vapingsavedmylife"

In the above tweet extract, the user employed the hashtag "vapingsavedmylife", which was used by Twitter users to indicate the life-saving potential of vaping.

3.8. Anti-Vaping Tweet Extracts

There were also Twitter users who called for people to quit vaping:

"Please stop vaping! – read this news story Lung Damage From Vaping Resembles Chemical Burns, Report Says"

Other Twitter users called for parents to inform their children that e-cigarettes were unsafe:

"Let your children know that vaping is NOT SAFE, doesn't matter what their friends say, they've been brainwashed by big Tobacco!"

There were also a number of general comments noting that e-cigarette use was likely to be dangerous:

"I am not a medical professional, but most likely that vaping is not good for you"

Another Twitter user noted:

"I used to smoke 50 cigarettes a day and managed to just quit, that's the best way to quit. Vaping is not safe."

From the tweet extracts above, we can see that there was a diverse range of views and comments noting that e-cigarettes were unsafe.

4. Discussion

This study showed the effects of a research study linking cancer in mice to vaping on Twitter. The study was tweeted by several mainstream media outlets and dominated discussions of e-cigarettes on Twitter. The study, however, was questioned by several experts as they noted that the study conducted on mice could not be generalised to humans. Our study highlighted the impact of academic research on Twitter when it is disseminated through the mainstream media. The publication of the study caused great concern over the safety of e-cigarettes on Twitter, and users of the platform were quick to point out that e-cigarettes were still a much safer alternative to traditional smoking. For instance, health authorities such as the National Health Service in the United Kingdom still noted that e-cigarettes contained a fraction of the risk when compared to that of traditional cigarettes [19]. However, the publication of the study linking cancer to mice may have incorrectly been interpreted and understood by some members of the public who would now believe that e-cigarettes were just as unsafe and/or more unsafe when compared to traditional tobacco based cigarettes. Current advice provided by Centers for Disease Control [20–22] notes that e-cigarettes are likely to be safer than smoking traditional cigarettes. Our recommendation to health authorities is to offer guidance to the public in order for citizens to make informed decisions about whether e-cigarettes are safe to consume. A key aspect of assessing whether vaping is safe depends on whether an individual is already engaged in using traditional cigarettes and/or rolled tobacco products. However, information disseminated to consumers around the safety of e-cigarettes can be confusing and vague. Moreover, we found that Twitter users tended to be unsure about the safety of e-cigarettes. Henceforth, based on a review of the literature and the advice provided by the Centers for Disease Control, the National Health Service (NHS), and Cancer Research UK [20–22], we developed a flowchart, as shown in Figure 3, that could be utilised by consumers and medical professionals when making a decision about whether e-cigarettes are likely to be safe or unsafe based on their circumstances.

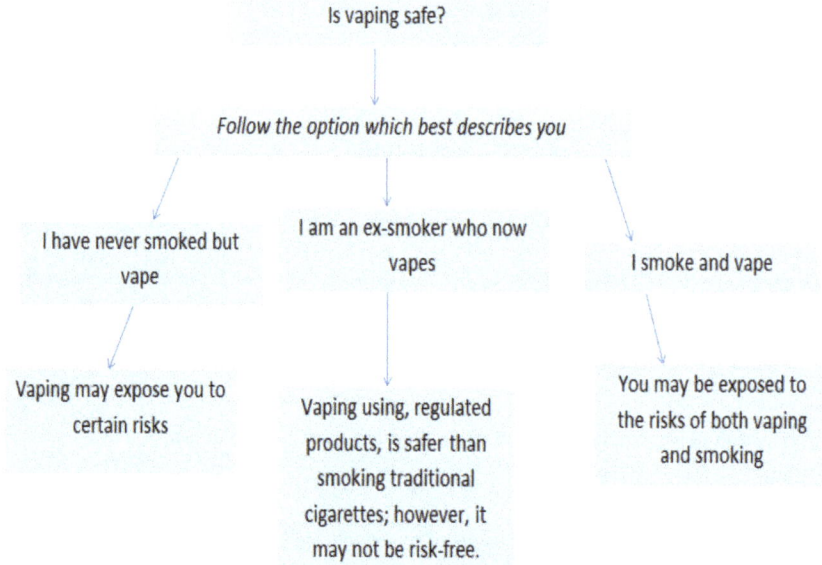

Figure 3. Flowchart based on current by Centers for Disease Control, the NHS, and Cancer Research UK [20–22].

By analysing public comments on Twitter, we were able to identify potential points of confusion by consumers, and combining our results with that of current medical advice led to the development of the flowchart above. Social media may be a source of information for a subset of the population, and it is important to analyse this information from a public health surveillance perspective. Our findings can also be contrasted with previous empirical work in this area. A study published in 2018 [23] conducted an analysis of e-cigarette discussions on Twitter from 2012 to 2015, which examined the reasons for using such devices. The study found that one of the most popular reasons for using e-cigarettes was to quit traditional cigarettes, and Twitter users were positive towards e-cigarette devices. Moreover, they found that 43% of Twitter users were able to give up traditional cigarettes, which demonstrated the potential of e-cigarettes for smoking cessation. The findings of this study were similar to our present study, which also found that there was a sizeable "pro-vaping" community on Twitter. A further study [24] published in 2014 looked at a specific case study containing tweets for and against public health policy related to the Chicago Department of Public Health. This study also found pro- and anti-e-cigarette views such as that they promote smoking cessation, but also that they are harmful and foster nicotine addiction. A further study in the United Kingdom [25] surveyed 3538 current and 579 recent smokers in November and December 2012. It was also found that there were mixed views among the public about whether e-cigarettes were more or less harmful than traditional cigarettes, with a number of citizens unsure of their safety at the time. These results further highlight the need for easy-to-understand guidance for consumers, and our flowchart developed above will be of interest to health authorities.

5. Conclusions

This paper conducted an analysis of current debates surrounding e-cigarette usage on Twitter. We identified two main themes that arose, which were either based on pro-vaping or anti-vaping views, and this method has been utilised in previous research [26]. Our work adds to the body of literature demonstrating the potential of Twitter for health research [27]. We then developed a flowchart, by reviewing existing literature, which can be used to inform public health information dissemination. A limitation of our study is that we examined only English-language tweets, which may have led to more tweets from English-speaking countries such as the United States and the United Kingdom. Furthermore, there may have been some tweets not related to e-cigarettes in the dataset.

Author Contributions: Conceptualization, W.A.; investigation, X.M.-G. and J.V.-A. All authors have read and agreed to the published version of the manuscript.

Funding: This research received no external funding

Conflicts of Interest: The authors declare no conflict of interest.

References

1. Brożek, G.M.; Jankowski, M.; Lawson, J.A.; Shpakou, A.; Poznański, M.; Zielonka, T.M.; Klimatckaia, L.; Loginovich, Y.; Rachel, M.; Gereová, J.; et al. The Prevalence of Cigarette and E-Cigarette Smoking among Students in Central and Eastern Europe—Results of the YUPESS Study. *Int. J. Environ. Res. Public Health* **2019**, *16*, 2297. [CrossRef]
2. Layden, J.E.; Ghinai, I.; Pray, I.; Kimball, A.; Layer, M.; Tenforde, M.; Navon, L.; Hoots, B.; Salvatore, P.P.; Elderbrook, M.; et al. Pulmonary Illness Related to E-Cigarette Use in Illinois and Wisconsin—Preliminary Report. *N. Engl. J. Med.* **2019**, *382*, 903–916. [CrossRef]
3. Christiani, D.C. Vaping-Induced Lung Injury. *N. Engl. J. Med.* **2019**, 1–2. [CrossRef]
4. Gotts, J.E.; Jordt, S.E.; McConnell, R.; Tarran, R. What are the Respiratory Effects of E-cigarettes? *BMJ* **2019**, *366*, l5275. [CrossRef] [PubMed]
5. Centers for Disease Control and Prevention. Severe Pulmonary Disease Associated with Using E-Cigarette Products. 2019; Emergency Preparedness and Response. Available online: https://emergency.cdc.gov/han/han00421.asp (accessed on 10 October 2019).
6. Centers for Disease Control and Prevention. Outbreak of Lung Injury Associated with E-Cigarette Use, or Vaping. 2019; Smoking & Tobacco Use. Available online: https://www.cdc.gov/tobacco/basic_information/e-cigarettes/severe-lung-disease.html#map-of-reported-cases (accessed on 10 October 2019).

7. Kaplan, S.; Richtel, M. The Mysterious Vaping Illness That's 'Becoming an Epidemic'. *The New York Times*, 31 August 2019.
8. Richtel, M. Another Patient Has Died From Lung Disease After Vaping. *The New York Times*, 4 September 2019.
9. Mesch, G.S.; Schwirian, K.P.; Kolobov, T. Attention to the media and worry over becoming infected: The case of the Swine Flu (H1N1) Epidemic of 2009. *Sociol. Health Illn.* **2013**, *35*, 325–331. [CrossRef]
10. Towers, S.; Afzal, S.; Bernal, G.; Bliss, N.; Brown, S.; Espinoza, B.; Jackson, J.; Judson-Garcia, J.; Khan, M.; Lin, M.; et al. Mass media and the contagion of fear: The case of Ebola in America. *PLoS ONE* **2015**, *10*, 1–13. [CrossRef]
11. Hooker, C. Health scares: Professional priorities. *Health* **2010**, *14*, 3–21. [CrossRef]
12. Ram, D.S.; Nathan, R.J.; Balraj, A. Purchase Factors for Products with Ineslastic demand: A Study on Tobacco Sector. *J. Eng. Appl. Sci.* **2017**, *12*, 1754–1761.
13. Stefanidis, A.; Vraga, E.; Lamprianidis, G.; Radzikowski, J.; Delamater, P.L.; Jacobsen, K.H.; Pfoser, D.; Croitoru, A.; Crooks, A. Zika in Twitter: Temporal Variations of Locations, Actors, and Concepts. *JMIR Public Health Surveill.* **2017**, *3*, e22. [CrossRef] [PubMed]
14. Ahmed, W.; Bath, P.A.; Sbaffi, L.; Demartini, G. Novel insights into views towards H1N1 during the 2009 Pandemic: A thematic analysis of Twitter data. *Health Inf. Libr. J.* **2019**, *36*, 60–72. [CrossRef] [PubMed]
15. Oyeyemi, S.O.; Gabarron, E.; Wynn, R. Ebola, Twitter, and misinformation: A dangerous combination? *BMJ* **2014**, *349*, 14–15. [CrossRef] [PubMed]
16. Yagahara, A.; Hanai, K.; Hasegawa, S.; Ogasawara, K. Relationships among tweets related to radiation: Visualization using co-occurring networks. *J. Med. Internet Res.* **2018**, *20*. [CrossRef] [PubMed]
17. Smith, M.A.; Rainie, L.; Himelboim, I.; Shneiderman, B. Mapping Twitter Topic Networks: From Polarized Crowds to Community Clusters. *Pew Res. Cent.* **2014**, *20*, 1–57.
18. Butt, Y.M.; Smith, M.L.; Tazelaar, H.D.; Vaszar, L.T.; Swanson, K.L.; Cecchini, M.J.; Boland, J.M.; Bois, M.C.; Boyum, J.H.; Froemming, A.T.; et al. Pathology of Vaping-Associated Lung Injury. *N. Engl. J. Med.* **2019**, *381*, 1780–1781. [CrossRef]
19. National Health Service. E-Cigarettes. Vapes. 2019. Smokefree. Available online: https://www.nhs.uk/smokefree/help-and-advice/e-cigarettes (accessed on 3 December 2019).
20. Centers for Disease Control and Prevention. In *Electronic Cigarettes (E-Cigarettes)*; 2020; Smoking & Tobacco Use. Available online: https://www.cdc.gov/tobacco/basic_information/e-cigarettes/index.htm (accessed on 19 February 2020).
21. National Health Service. Using E-Cigarettes to Stop Smoking. 2020. Available online: https://www.nhs.uk/live-well/quit-smoking/using-e-cigarettes-to-stop-smoking/ (accessed on 18 February 2020).
22. Cancer Research UK, E-Cigarette Safety. Available online: https://www.cancerresearchuk.org/health-professional/awareness-and-prevention/e-cigarette-hub-information-for-health-professionals/safety (accessed on 18 February 2020).
23. Ayers, J.W.; Leas, E.C.; Allem, J.P.; Benton, A.; Dredze, M.; Althouse, B.M.; Cruz, T.B.; Unger, J.B. Why do people use electronic nicotine delivery systems (electronic cigarettes)? A content analysis of Twitter, 2012–2015. *PLoS ONE* **2017**, *12*, e0170702. [CrossRef]
24. Harris, J.K.; Moreland-Russell, S.; Choucair, B.; Mansour, R.; Staub, M.; Simmons, K. Tweeting for and against public health policy: Response to the Chicago Department of Public Health's electronic cigarette Twitter campaign. *J. Med Internet Res.* **2014**, *16*, e238. [CrossRef]
25. Hitchman, S.C.; Brose, L.S.; Brown, J.; Robson, D.; McNeill, A. Associations between e-cigarette type, frequency of use, and quitting smoking: Findings from a longitudinal online panel survey in Great Britain. *Nicotine Tob. Res.* **2015**, *17*, 1187–1194. [CrossRef]
26. Ahmed, W. Public health implications of #ShoutYourAbortion. *Public Health* **2018**, *163*, 35–41.
27. Zhang, Z.; Ahmed, W. A comparison of information sharing behaviours across 379 health conditions on Twitter. *Int. J. Public Health* **2019**, *64*, 431–440. [CrossRef] [PubMed]

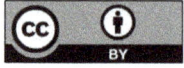

© 2020 by the authors. Licensee MDPI, Basel, Switzerland. This article is an open access article distributed under the terms and conditions of the Creative Commons Attribution (CC BY) license (http://creativecommons.org/licenses/by/4.0/).

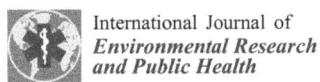

Article

Validation of a Short Questionnaire to Assess Healthcare Professionals' Perceptions of Asynchronous Telemedicine Services: The Catalan Version of the Health Optimum Telemedicine Acceptance Questionnaire

Josep Vidal-Alaball [1,2,3,*], Gemma Flores Mateo [4,*], Josep Lluís Garcia Domingo [3], Xavier Marín Gomez [1,2], Glòria Sauch Valmaña [1,2], Anna Ruiz-Comellas [1,5], Francesc López Seguí [6,7] and Francesc García Cuyàs [8]

1. Health Promotion in Rural Areas Research Group, Gerència Territorial de la Catalunya Central, Institut Català de la Salut, 08272 Sant Fruitós de Bages, Spain; xmarin.cc.ics@gencat.cat (X.M.G.); gsauch.cc.ics@gencat.cat (G.S.V.); aruiz.cc.ics@gencat.cat (A.R.-C.)
2. Unitat de Suport a la Recerca de la Catalunya Central, Fundació Institut Universitari per a la Recerca a l'Atenció Primària de Salut Jordi Gol i Gurina, 08272 Sant Fruitós de Bages, Spain
3. Department of Economics and Business, Universitat de Vic-Universitat Central de Catalunya, 08500 Vic, Spain; jlgarcia@uvic.cat
4. Unitat d'anàlisi i Qualitat, Xarxa Sanitària i Social de Santa Tecla, 43003 Tarragona, Spain
5. Centre d'Atenció Primària Sant Joan de Vilatorrada, Gerència Territorial de la Catalunya Central, Institut Català de la Salut, 08250 Sant Joan de Vilatorrada, Spain
6. TIC Salut Social–Generalitat de Catalunya, 08005 Barcelona, Spain; flopez@ticsalutsocial.cat
7. CRES&CEXS–Universitat Pompeu Fabra, 08002 Barcelona, Spain
8. Hospital Sant Joan de Déu, Digital Care Research Group, Universitat de Vic-Universitat Central de Catalunya, 08500 Vic, Spain; francesc.garcia@umedicina.cat
* Correspondence: jvidal.cc.ics@gencat.cat (J.V.-A.); gfloresm@xarxatecla.cat (G.F.M.); Tel./Fax: +34-936-93-00-40 (J.V.-A.)

Received: 14 February 2020; Accepted: 24 March 2020; Published: 25 March 2020

Abstract: Telemedicine is both effective and able to provide efficient care at a lower cost. It also enjoys a high degree of acceptance among users. The Technology Acceptance Model proposed is based on the two main concepts of ease of use and perceived usefulness and is comprised of three dimensions: the individual context, the technological context and the implementation or organizational context. At present, no short, validated questionnaire exists in Catalonia to evaluate the acceptance of telemedicine services amongst healthcare professionals using a technology acceptance model. This article aims to statistically validate the Catalan version of the EU project Health Optimum telemedicine acceptance questionnaire. The study included the following phases: adaptation and translation of the questionnaire into Catalan and psychometric validation with construct (exploratory factor analysis), consistency (Cronbach's alpha) and stability (test–retest) analysis. After deleting incomplete responses, calculations were made using 33 participants. The internal consistency measured with the Cronbach's alpha coefficient was good with an alpha coefficient of 0.84 (95%, CI: 0.79–0.84). The intraclass correlation coefficient was 0.93 (95% CI: 0.852–0.964). The Kaiser–Meyer–Olkin test of sampling showed to be adequate (KMO = 0.818) and the Bartlett test of sphericity was significant (Chi-square 424.188; gl = 28; $p < 0.001$). The questionnaire had two dimensions which accounted for 61.2% of the total variance: quality and technical difficulties relating to telemedicine. The findings of this study suggest that the validated questionnaire has robust statistical features that make it a good predictive model of healthcare professional's satisfaction with telemedicine programs.

Keywords: telemedicine; questionnaires and surveys; validation studies; health personnel

1. Introduction

Although at present there is no clear consensus as to the economic impact of telemedicine [1,2], recent evidence has shown it can be effective, provide efficient care at a lower cost [3–7] and enjoy a high degree of acceptance among users. Moreover, telemedicine reduces journeys by road and therefore decreases the environmental impact of atmospheric pollutants emitted by vehicles [8]. Published studies have already provided some insights as to the acceptance drivers. Eddy et al. reported high patient satisfaction with teledermatology and amongst physicians, although this satisfaction was higher in primary care doctors than in dermatologists [9]. McKoy et al. used questionnaires to assess the acceptance of a teledermatology service and reported that 82% of users saw it as a valid alternative to face-to-face consultations [10]. In another qualitative study using semi-structured interviews with 32 healthcare professionals, MacNeill et al. showed mixed points of view: while it was broadly welcomed by nursing staff, some primary care physicians were worried that telemedicine could increase their workload and it could potentially undermine their professional autonomy [11]. A comprehensive systematic review recently published by Mounessa et al. reported that patients and healthcare providers were in general highly satisfied with the two types of telemedicine: store-and-forward and real time telemedicine [11]. Whilst all the studies provided valuable inputs to help understand the complex heterogeneous effect of the participants' acceptance of new healthcare models, it is of the utmost importance that any published evidence uses validated questionnaires to perform reliable and comprehensive evaluations [12].

The Technology Acceptance Model (TAM) proposed by Davis (1989) [11] is based on the two main concepts of ease of use and perceived usefulness, and comprises three dimensions: the individual context, the technological context and the implementation or organizational context. Based on his benchmark, studies have adapted their methodology to create validated questionnaires. For example, Orruño et al. (2011) evaluated teledermatology adoption by healthcare professionals using a modified 33-item version of this model grouped into eight theoretical dimensions. The Cronbach's alpha for each theoretical variable and internal consistency of the questionnaire reported good results which suggest the proposed questionnaire is a valid tool for assessing acceptance in this setting [13].

In the REgioNs of Europe WorkINg toGether for HEALTH (RENEWING HEALTH) project, Kidholm et al. reviewed the scientific literature to find questionnaires used in European telemedicine projects to assess the stakeholders' perceptions. One such questionnaire was used in the EU project Health Optimum (Delivery OPTIMisation through telemedicine) [14,15]. This questionnaire for healthcare professionals includes eight general questions irrespective of their medical specialty and focuses on the physicians' perception of the quality of the telemedicine service, their convenience, technical and other difficulties and potential effects on the health of the patients using the service (see Appendix A). The questionnaire was not validated and although it does not strictly use the TAM, it adopts some of its dimensions. An easy-to-answer questionnaire increases the response rate but no other short validated questionnaire using the TAM to assess healthcare professionals' perceptions of asynchronous telemedicine services was found.

Whilst the Catalan Ministry of Health is putting a lot of effort into developing telemedicine, the degree of acceptance of these tools has yet to be investigated using validated questionnaires.

It is not possible to deploy telehealth services without first carrying out a thorough assessment of practitioner's perceptions of their usefulness, a factor which is critical in fostering their deployment in public and private healthcare systems. Brief questionnaires are preferable as a means to improve response rates as studies using long questionnaires based on the TAM have reported low response rates [16,17]. For these reasons, the aim of our study is the statistical validation of the Catalan version of the EU project Health Optimum telemedicine acceptance questionnaire.

2. Methods

2.1. Likert Scale

The original questionnaire used an incomplete Likert scale with an even number of answers to the questions, while it is recommended that questionnaires use an odd number of answers [18]. Furthermore, there were more positive options than negative in the first two questions. We decided to add an extra possible response to the first four questions in order to have an odd number of options and therefore obtain a complete Likert scale.

2.2. Translation into Catalan and Data Collection

To achieve the higher content validity, a translated and back-translated methodology was used [19,20]. The original English version of the questionnaire (Appendix A) was translated into Catalan independently by two authors who are native Catalan speakers and who are both proficient in English. An agreed Catalan version of the questionnaire was obtained following several drafts (Appendix B).

In order to validate the new Catalan version of the Health Optimum questionnaire, the Google Forms tool was used to send it to primary healthcare professionals in the Catalan central region who had used telemedicine services in the past. WhatsApp health professional groups were used to disseminate the questionnaire. Members were asked to answer the questionnaire and to resend it to other potential respondents. The twitter account of the principal investigator (@jvalaball, >10K followers) was also used for further dissemination. Additional information regarding the respondents' basic characteristics was added to the questionnaire: age, sex and professional role and the kind of telemedicine services available in the Catalan central region which they had used (teledermatology, teleulcers or teleaudiometries). Non health professionals were asked not to answer the questionnaire.

The questionnaire called "Questionnaire to assess healthcare professionals' perceptions of asynchronous telemedicine services" (Qüestionari per avaluar la percepció dels professionals sanitaris amb els serveis de telemedicina asíncrona) had 8 questions with a complete Likert scale of 5 answers the first 4 questions and 3 answers the last 4 questions. It was first sent at the beginning of April 2018 and it was closed 3 d later. It was resent 2 weeks later, asking participants to answer it again in order to check for consistency. The questionnaire was closed definitively 5 d later. Completing the questionnaire was considered as an indication of consent to participate in the study. The study protocol was approved by the University Institute for Primary Care Research (IDIAP) Jordi Gol Health Care Ethics Committee (Code P16/046).

2.3. Scale Level Descriptive Analysis

Following Argimon et al.'s methodology [21], we have assessed the variability in responses to the questionnaire calculating the average and the standard deviation (SD) and calculated the frequencies to check for floor and ceiling effects [22]. These effects are important as they can influence the validity, reliability and responsiveness of a questionnaire and they are used to check the percentage of participants with very low and very high scores. We have taken this effect to exist when 15% or more of the responses are found in the higher or lower values [23].

We checked the discriminating capacity of the items using the discriminative rate, which compares the responses in the two extreme groups (individuals who have obtained a total score below the 33rd percentile and individuals who have scored above the 66th percentile). Discriminative rates above 0 indicate discriminating capacity of the items [22].

2.4. Internal Consistency

The internal consistency of the Catalan version of the Health Optimum questionnaire was tested using Cronbach's alpha. This statistical test checks for the degree of common information that share the items of a scale of measurement. It is an average of the variances between the variables that are part of a scale. Values of α above 0.7 indicate an appropriate internal consistency [22].

2.5. Temporal Stability—Reliability

To check for the intra-observer stability of our questionnaire, a test–retest methodology was used. Its reliability was calculated with intraclass correlations (ICC) between the scores at Time 1 and Time 2 at the individual item level. Intraclass correlation coefficients over 0.75 are considered good and over 0.90 excellent [22].

2.6. Factor Analysis

Factor analysis was used to simplify the information given by a correlation matrix to make it more easily interpretable [23]. To check for the appropriate conditions to perform a factor analysis we have used 2 methods: the Kaiser–Meyer–Olkin test and the Bartlett sphericity test. The first ranges from 0 to 1, with a value lower than 0.5 indicating that it is inappropriate to do the analysis. A significant result of the Bartlett sphericity test ($p < 0.05$) indicates that it is pertinent to make a factor analysis. To check for the number of different dimensions of the questionnaire, 3 different criteria were used: (1) Kaiser rule which selects the number of factors with a value greater than 1; (2) the percentage of explained variance which is determined by the accumulated percentage of variation extracted in each factor (varimax rotation with Kaiser's normalization was used to simplify the number of dimensions); (3) a scree plot which graphically represents the number of factors or dimensions extracted, we retained the factors or components to the left of the inflection point on the graph [23].

The statistical programs STATA version 15/SE and SPSS v23 (SPSS Inc., Chicago, IL, USA) were used for these statistical analyses. Results were considered significant with $p < 0.05$.

3. Results

3.1. Test–Retest

Although 212 responses were received, only 37 individuals responded to the questionnaire twice as required. After checking the response times, we found four respondents that although responded twice to the questionnaire, didn't wait the necessary minimum two weeks period between the responses. After excluding these other four respondents, calculations were made using 33 participants: 24/33 were women (72%) and their average age was 50.9 (SD: 8.87) years. Among them, 24/33 (72%) were family physicians, 2/33 were nurses (6%), 1/33 was a dermatologist (3%) and 4/33 (12%) had other specialties.

The internal consistency measured with the Cronbach's alpha coefficient showed none of the items significantly altered the consistency of the instrument. The overall alpha coefficient was 0.84 (95%, CI: 0.79–0.84). Table 1 shows the alpha coefficient for each of the eight items in the questionnaire. With respect to temporal stability, the intraclass correlation coefficient value stands at 0.93 (95% CI: 0.852–0.964), thus showing excellent reliability of the test.

Table 1. Psychometric validation.

Questionnaire's Items	Descriptive Statistics		Item Parameter Estimates			Reliability	
	Mean	Standard Deviation	IDI [1]	Ceiling Effect (%)	Floor Effect (%)	Item-Correlation	Cronbach Alpha
1. Global quality [a]	3.51	0.85	1.24	8.3	1.4	0.79	0.79
2. Technical quality [a]	3.47	0.87	1.13	5.6	2.8	0.75	0.80
3. Clinical quality [a]	3.01	0.86	1.40	2.8	0.7	0.73	0.81
4. Convenience [a]	3.67	0.89	1.36	16.0	1.4	0.75	0.80
5. Health effects [b]	2.68	0.61	0.54	75.7	-	0.56	0.83
6. Technical difficulties [b]	2.03	0.56	0.59	-	-	0.67	0.81
7. Organizational difficulties [b]	2.10	0.57	0.60	-	-	0.64	0.82
8. Future use [b]	2.53	0.51	0.51	-	-	0.54	0.84

[1] IDI: Item Discrimination Index, [a] Items scored on a 5-point response scale ranging from 1 "very dissatisfied" to 5 "very satisfied"; [b] Items scored on a 3-point response scale.

3.2. Descriptive Analysis of the Items

All discriminative rates were above zero and, for the first four questions, they were above one. The highest discrimination item was Item 3, "Clinical quality" (discrimination index = 1.40), and the lowest discrimination item was Item 8, "Future use" (0.51). Table 1 describes the average score for each group and the discrimination index of each of the eight items in the questionnaire.

The lowest ceiling effect score was for Item 3 "Clinical quality" and the highest score was for Item 5, "Health effects". Furthermore, two out of five items were above the ceiling-effect criterion of 15%.

3.3. Exploratory Factor Analysis

The Kaiser–Meyer–Olkin test of sampling was adequate (KMO = 0.818) and the Bartlett test of sphericity was significant (Chi-square 424.188; gl = 28; $p < 0.001$), indicating that the items were appropriate for a factor analysis. Two factors emerged with an eigenvalue greater than one (Table 2). The factor with questions about the quality of telemedicine technology (Items 1–5) was named Quality. The other factor contained items relating to technical difficulties in telemedicine (Items 6–8) and was named Difficulties. The two constructs together accounted for 61.2% of total variance, all factor loadings being higher than 0.40. Figure 1 shows the scree plot representing the number of dimensions extracted.

Table 2. Exploratory factor analysis (EFA): data on commonalities of items, item loadings in Factor 1 and Factor 2.

Questionnaire Items	Factor 1	Factor 2	Communalities (h^2)
1. Global quality [a]	0.712	0.430	0.692
2. Technical quality [a]	0.526	0.571	0.603
3. Clinical quality [a]	0.785	0.234	0.671
4. Convenience [a]	0.827	0.201	0.722
5. Health effects [a]	0.670	-	0.450
6. Technical difficulties [b]	0.154	0.836	0.722
7. Organizational difficulties [b]	-	0.870	0.763
8. Future use [b]	0.281	0.441	0.274
Eigenvalues	3.76	1.14	
Average variance explained (%)	47.04	14.21	
Cronbach's α reliability	0.830	0.672	

Extraction method, principal component analysis, rotation method, varimax with Kaiser normalization; rotation converged in three iterations. Factors: [a] Quality, [b] Difficulties.

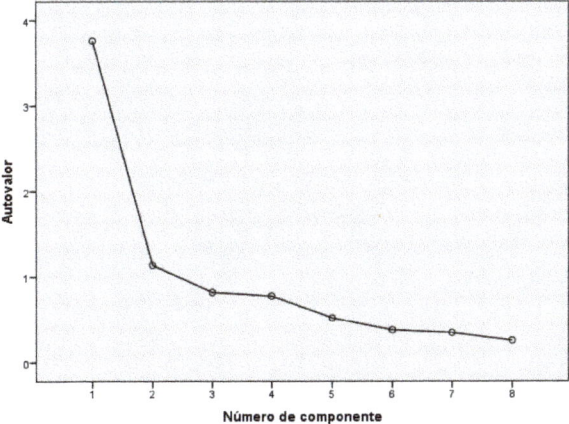

Figure 1. Scree plot.

These results show that the Catalan version of the Health Optimum questionnaire to assess practitioner's perceptions of telemedicine tools is statistically robust.

4. Discussion

The validation of the telemedicine questionnaire for healthcare professionals showed good reliability and an acceptable level of validity. Two questions suffered from the ceiling effect which limit the validity, but all the questions had discriminative rates above zero, higher for the first four questions, showing that all the questions had a discriminative capacity. We could increase the response options to the items to help optimize their discriminative power, but this would reduce the comparability of the scores with the original questionnaire.

The internal consistency was good, with Cronbach's alpha coefficients for the overall questionnaire and Factor 1 above 0.80. The Cronbach's alpha coefficient was slightly below the acceptable cut-off for Factor 2 (0.67). The low number of items included in the second factor may contribute to this finding. These results are slightly worse than the one reported by Argimon et al. using a similar methodology [24]. The ceiling effect was found in two questions, though this was not measured in the English original version, meaning that we are unable to conclude that it is an intrinsic characteristic of the questionnaire or a weakness in the Catalan translation.

Our results show that the Catalan version of the Health Optimum questionnaire is a robust tool for assessing healthcare professional's satisfaction with a telemedicine program. All the questions presented a positive discrimination rate, especially Item 3, "Clinical quality". This means that the questionnaire is clearly able to distinguish the clinical quality of a telemedicine program.

The results show that it was adequate to perform the factor analysis and showed that the questionnaire had two dimensions, which accounts for 61.2% of the total variance: one concerning the quality of the telemedicine technology and another about technical difficulties relating to telemedicine.

The questionnaire will be useful to evaluate healthcare professionals' perceptions of the growing number of different asynchronous telemedicine programs available in Catalonia as well as allowing comparisons between them to inform which characteristics make them more accepted by professionals [25].

Limitations

This study has several limitations. The pilot questionnaire was distributed to healthcare professionals via WhatsApp healthcare professional groups asking them to only answer if they had used a telemedicine program in the past. As the questionnaire was anonymous we can not verify whether they had in fact used these programs and we are unable to be sure that the questionnaire was not distributed to other individuals who are unrelated to healthcare professions. The number of respondents (33) was small compared to other studies [24], nevertheless this number was suficient to validate the questionnaire.

5. Conclusions

The Catalan version of the Health Optimum telemedicine acceptance questionnaire has been validated with this study showing robust statistical features that make it a quality tool to assess healthcare professional's satisfaction with telemedicine programs. As the validation was not performed looking at a specific telemedicine program, the validated questionnaire is potentially valid for any telemedicine program.

Author Contributions: Conceptualization, J.V.-A., G.F.M., J.L.G.D. and G.S.V.; Data curation, J.V.-A.; Formal analysis, J.V.-A., G.F.M. and F.L.S.; Investigation, J.V.-A.; Methodology, G.F.M. and J.L.G.D.; Project administration, J.V.-A. and F.G.C.; Resources, X.M.G.; Supervision, J.V.-A. and J.L.G.D.; Validation, F.L.S.; Visualization, A.R.-C.; Writing—original draft, J.L.G.D., G.S.V. and F.G.C.; Writing—review and editing, J.V.-A., G.F.M., X.M.G., A.R.-C. and F.L.S. All authors have read and agreed to the published version of the manuscript.

Funding: This research received no external funding.

Acknowledgments: This study was conducted with the support of the Secretary of Universities and Research of the Department of Business and Knowledge at the Generalitat de Catalunya.

Conflicts of Interest: The authors declare no conflict of interest.

Appendix A Original EU Project Health Optimum Telemedicine Acceptance Questionnaire

1. How do you rate the overall quality of the telemedicine consultation?

   1. Excellent
   2. Good
   3. Fair
   4. Poor

2. How would you rate the technical quality of the telemedicine consultation?

   1. Excellent
   2. Good
   3. Fair
   4. Poor

3. How do you rate the quality of care delivered by the telemedicine service when compared to the quality of traditional care?

   1. Better
   2. About the same
   3. Not as good
   4. Not sure

4. Were you comfortable during the telemedicine consultation?

   1. Yes, very comfortable
   2. Yes, somewhat comfortable
   3. No, somewhat uncomfortable
   4. No, very uncomfortable

5. Do you feel that the telemedicine consultation service may influence the health status of your patients?

   1. Improved health
   2. No change
   3. Negative effects on health

6. Did you experience technical difficulties that might affect the quality of care delivered by the telemedicine service?

   1. Not at all
   2. Sometimes
   3. Often

7. Did you experience organisational or other difficulties that might affect the quality of care delivered by the telemedicine service?

   1. Not at all
   2. Sometimes
   3. Often

8. Would you continue to use the telemedicine service?

1. Yes, in the same way as the service has be deployed
2. Yes, but with improvements
3. No

Appendix B Catalan Version of the Questionnai

1. Com qualificaries la qualitat global de les consultes de telemedicina?

   1. Excel·lent
   2. Bona
   3. Normal
   4. Regular
   5. Dolenta

2. Com qualificaries la qualitat tècnica de les consultes de telemedicina?

   1. Excel·lent
   2. Bona
   3. Normal
   4. Regular
   5. Dolenta

3. Com qualificaries la qualitat assistencial proporcionada pels serveis de telemedicina comparant-la amb la qualitat de l'atenció habitual?

   1. Molt millor
   2. Millor
   3. Igual
   4. Pitjor
   5. Molt pitjor

4. Et sents còmode durant les consultes de telemedicina?

   1. Sí, molt còmode
   2. Sí, bastant còmode
   3. Ni còmode, ni incòmode
   4. No, bastant incòmode
   5. No, molt incòmode

5. Creus que els serveis de telemedicina poden influir en l'estat de salut dels teus pacients?

   1. Sí, poden millorar la seva salut
   2. No, no canvien la seva salut
   3. Sí, poden tenir efectes negatius en la seva salut

6. Has experimentat dificultats tècniques que poden haver afectat la qualitat de l'atenció proporcionada pels serveis de telemedicina?

   1. No, mai
   2. Alguns cops
   3. Sovint

7. Has experimentat dificultats de tipus organitzatiu o d'altres dificultats que poden haver afectat la qualitat de l'atenció proporcionada pels serveis de telemedicina?

   1. No

2. Algunes vegades
3. Sovint

8. Continuaràs utilitzant els serveis de telemedicina?

1. Sí, igual que ara
2. Sí, però amb millores
3. No

References

1. NICE. *National Institute for Health and Care Excellence Evidence Standards Framework for Digital*; NICE: London, UK, 2019.
2. World Health Organization. *WHO Guideline: Recommendations on Digital Interventions for Health System Strengthening*; WHO: Genev, Switzerland, 2019.
3. Delgoshaei, B.; Mobinizadeh, M.; Mojdekar, R.; Afzal, E.; Arabloo, J.; Mohamadi, E. Telemedicine: A systematic review of economic evaluations. *Med. J. Islamic Repub. Iran* **2017**, *31*, 754–761. [CrossRef]
4. Langabeer, J.R.; Champagne-Langabeer, T.; Alqusairi, D.; Kim, J.; Jackson, A.; Persse, D.; Gonzalez, M. Cost-benefit analysis of telehealth in pre-hospital care. *J. Telemed. Telecare* **2017**, *23*, 747–751. [CrossRef] [PubMed]
5. Vidal-Alaball, J.; Garcia Domingo, J.L.; Garcia Cuyàs, F.; Mendioroz Peña, J.; Flores Mateo, G.; Deniel Rosanas, J.; Sauch Valmaña, G. A cost savings analysis of asynchronous teledermatology compared to face-to-face dermatology in Catalonia. *BMC Health Serv. Res.* **2018**, *18*, 650. [CrossRef] [PubMed]
6. Van Der Heijden, J.P.; De Keizer, N.F.; Bos, J.D.; Spuls, P.I.; Witkamp, L. Teledermatology applied following patient selection by general practitioners in daily practice improves efficiency and quality of care at lower cost. *Br. J. Dermatol.* **2011**, *165*, 1058–1065. [CrossRef] [PubMed]
7. Bashshur, R.L.; Shannon, G.W.; Tejasvi, T.; Kvedar, J.; Gates, M. The Empirical Foundations of Teledermatology: A Review of the Research Evidence. *Telemed. Health* **2015**, *21*, 10–27. [CrossRef] [PubMed]
8. Vidal-Alaball, J.; Franch-Parella, J.; Lopez Segui, F.; Garcia Cuyàs, F.; Mendioroz Peña, J. Impact of a Telemedicine Program on the Reduction in the Emission of Atmospheric Pollutants and Journeys by Road. *Int. J. Environ. Res. Public Health* **2019**, *16*, 4366. [CrossRef] [PubMed]
9. Eedy, D.J.; Wootton, R. Teledermatology: A review. *Br. J. Dermatol.* **2001**, *4*, 696–707. [CrossRef] [PubMed]
10. McKoy, K.C.; DiGregorio, S.; Stira, L. Asynchronous Teledermatology in an Urban Primary Care Practice. *Telemed. J. Health* **2004**, *10*, S-70–S-80.
11. MacNeill, V.; Sanders, C.; Fitzpatrick, R.; Hendy, J.; Barlow, J.; Knapp, M.; Rogers, A.; Bardsley, M.; Newman, S.P. Experiences of front-line health professionals in the delivery of telehealth: A qualitative study. *Br. J. Gen. Pract.* **2014**, *64*, 401–407. [CrossRef] [PubMed]
12. Thijssing, L.; Tensen, E.; Jaspers, M. Patient's Perspective on Quality of Teleconsultation Services. *Stud. Health Technol. Inf.* **2016**, *228*, 132–136.
13. Orruño Aguado, E.; Gagnon, M.P.; Asua, J.; Abdeljelil, A. Ben Evaluation of teledermatology adoption by health-care professionals using a modified Technology Acceptance Model. *J. Telemed. Telecare 2011* **2011**, *17*, 303–307. [CrossRef] [PubMed]
14. Kidholm, K.; Nielsen, A.D.; Prior, R. *REgioNs of Europe WorkINg toGether for HEALTH*; European Comission: Brussells, Belgium, 2011.
15. Momentum Health Optimum. Available online: http://www.telemedicine-momentum.eu/health-optimum-dk/ (accessed on 15 January 2020).
16. Asua, J.; Orruño Aguado, E.; Reviriego, E.; Gagnon, M.P. Healthcare professional acceptance of telemonitoring for chronic care patients in primary care. *BMC Med. Inform. Decis. Mak.* **2012**, *12*, 139. [CrossRef] [PubMed]
17. Gagnon, M.P.; Orruño Aguado, E.; Asua, J.; Abdeljelil, A.B.; Emparanza Knör, J. Using a Modified Technology Acceptance Model to Evaluate Healthcare Professionals' Adoption of a New Telemonitoring System. *Telemed. Health* **2012**, *18*, 54–59. [CrossRef] [PubMed]
18. Jamieson, S. Likert Scale, in *Encyclopædia Britannica*. Available online: https://www.britannica.com/topic/Likert-Scale (accessed on 20 March 2018).

19. Beaton, D.E.; Bombardier, C.; Guillemin, F.; Ferraz, M.B. Guidelines for the process of cross-cultural adaptation of self-report measures. *Spine* **2000**, *25*, 3186–3191. [CrossRef] [PubMed]
20. Guillemin, F.; Bombardier, C.; Beaton, D. Cross-cultural adaptation of health-related quality of life measures: Literature review and proposed guidelines. *J. Clin. Epidemiol.* **1993**, *46*, 1417–1432. [CrossRef]
21. Argimon-Pallàs, J.M.; Flores Mateo, G.; Jiménez-Villa, J.; Pujol-Ribera, E.; Foz, G.; Bund-Vidiella, M.; Juncosa, S.; Fuentes-Bellido, C.M.; Pérez-Rodríguez, B.; Margalef-Pallarès, F.; et al. Study protocol of psychometric properties of the Spanish translation of a competence test in evidence based practice: The Fresno test. *BMC Health Serv. Res.* **2009**, *9*, 37. [CrossRef]
22. Ware, J.E.; Gandek, B. Methods for testing data quality, scaling assumptions, and reliability: The IQOLA Project approach. *J. Clin. Epidemiol.* **1998**, *51*, 945–952. [CrossRef]
23. Rattray, J.; Jones, M.C. Essential elements of questionnaire design and development. *J. Clin. Nurs.* **2007**, *16*, 234–243. [CrossRef] [PubMed]
24. Argimon-Pallàs, J.M.; Flores Mateo, G.; Jiménez-Villa, J.; Pujol-Ribera, E. Psychometric properties of a test in evidence based practice: The Spanish version of the Fresno test. *BMC Med. Educ.* **2010**, *10*, 45. [CrossRef] [PubMed]
25. TiC Salut i Social. Mapa de Tendencias|TIC Salut Social. Available online: https://ticsalutsocial.cat/es/area/observatorio/ (accessed on 28 February 2020).

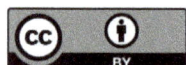

© 2020 by the authors. Licensee MDPI, Basel, Switzerland. This article is an open access article distributed under the terms and conditions of the Creative Commons Attribution (CC BY) license (http://creativecommons.org/licenses/by/4.0/).

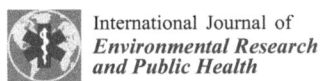
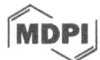

Article

A Cost-Minimization Analysis of a Medical Record-based, Store and Forward and Provider-to-provider Telemedicine Compared to Usual Care in Catalonia: More Agile and Efficient, Especially for Users

Francesc López Seguí [1,2], Jordi Franch Parella [3], Xavier Gironès García [3], Jacobo Mendioroz Peña [4,5], Francesc García Cuyàs [6], Cristina Adroher Mas [6], Anna García-Altés [7] and Josep Vidal-Alaball [4,5,*]

1. TIC Salut Social, Catalan Ministry of Health, 08005 Barcelona, Spain; francesc.lopez@cmail.cat
2. CRES&CEXS, Pompeu Fabra University, 08003 Barcelona, Spain
3. Faculty of Social Sciences, Universitat de Vic-Universitat Central de Catalunya, 08242 Manresa, Spain; jfranch@umanresa.cat (J.F.P.); XGirones@umanresa.cat (X.G.G.)
4. Health Promotion in Rural Areas Research Group, Gerència Territorial de la Catalunya Central, Institut Català de la Salut, 08272 Sant Fruitós de Bages, Spain; jmendioroz.cc.ics@gencat.cat
5. Unitat de Suport a la Recerca de la Catalunya Central, Fundació Institut Universitari per a la recerca a l'Atenció Primària de Salut Jordi Gol i Gurina, 08272 Sant Fruitós de Bages, Spain
6. Sant Joan de Déu Hospital, Catalan Ministry of Health, 08950 Barcelona, Spain; fgarciac@sjdhospitalbarcelona.org (F.G.C.); cadroher@sjdhospitalbarcelona.org (C.A.M.)
7. Agency for Healthcare Quality and Evaluation of Catalonia (AQuAS), Catalan Ministry of Health, 08003 Barcelona, Spain; agarciaaltes@gencat.cat
* Correspondence: jvidal.cc.ics@gencat.cat

Received: 23 January 2020; Accepted: 17 March 2020; Published: 18 March 2020

Abstract: Background: Telemedicine (interconsultation between primary and hospital care teams) has been operating in the counties of Central Catalonia Bages, Moianès and Berguedà since 2011, specializing in teledermatology, teleulcers, teleophthalmology and teleaudiometries. For the period until the end of 2019, a total of 52,198 visits were recorded. Objective: To analyze the differential costs between telemedicine and usual care in a semi-urban environment. Methodology: A cost-minimization evaluation, including direct and indirect costs from a societal perspective, distinguishing healthcare and user's costs, was carried out over a three-month period. Results: Telemedicine saved € 780,397 over the period analyzed. A differential cost favorable to telemedicine of about € 15 per visit was observed, with the patient being the largest beneficiary of this saving (by 85%) in terms of shorter waiting times and travel costs. From the healthcare system perspective, moving the time spent in a hospital care consultation to primary care is efficient in terms of the total time devoted per patient. In social terms and in this context, telemedicine is more efficient than usual care. Conclusion: Allowing users to save time in terms of consultation and travel is the main driver of interconsultation between primary and hospital care savings in a semi-urban context. The telemedicine service is also economically favorable for the healthcare system, enabling it to provide a more agile service, which also benefits healthcare professionals.

Keywords: cost analysis; health technology assessment; provider-to-provider telemedicine; telehealth; economic analysis

1. Introduction

Telemedicine nowadays coexists alongside conventional healthcare in most healthcare systems [1]. Although systematic reviews of its economic impact suggest that, for the time being, it is not suited to widespread implementation in all specialties and contexts [2,3], recent studies suggest that it is cost-effective in fields such as emergency medicine, cardiology, the management of diabetes and ophthalmology [4–11].

In Catalonia, the integration of the health information systems between primary care and specialized care allows for a fluid telemedicine-based case management. This implies relatively low coordination costs among different health specialties and incentivizes the use of these tools by health providers. Furthermore, the availability of information on healthcare activities provides an excellent opportunity to evaluate their impacts. To this end, this study case includes four telemedicine specialties (teledermatology, teleulcers, teleophthalmology and teleaudiometries) which are currently conducted in the Catalan public healthcare system, Central Catalonia Health Region. This includes the counties of Bages, Moianès and Berguedà, located in a large, mainly rural area, which also includes two major cities (Manresa and Berga) with an overall population of approximately 230,000 inhabitants.

A cost-minimization analysis performed in the same setting for the specific case of teledermatology [12] showed social savings of approximately €11.4 per visit, which have an impact, especially on users (77% of the total amount saved) as opposed to the healthcare system (23%). This is due to the size of the reduction in the commuting time and travel costs, which is especially significant in rural settings, a thesis which has been backed up by subsequent research [13]. Nevertheless, the study evaluated a short time period (teledermatology in 2016) and did not take into account other indirect costs such as the time spent by caregivers. In this context, the objective of the study is to broaden evidence on the economic impact of telemedicine with respect to usual care including other types of telemedicine (teleulcers, teleophthalmology and teleaudiometries) using a cost-minimization analysis from a societal perspective, including all feasible and significant direct and indirect costs.

2. Methodology

2.1. Service Description

The four studied telemedicine programs all operate in a similar manner: the primary care physician or nurse (salaried staff employed by the Catalan public healthcare system) uploads a file (such as a photograph) to the patient's electronic health record together with their clinical notes; hospital specialists access the patient's electronic health record, view the images and suggest treatment or an action plan; the primary care physician or nurse reviews the instructions and makes a phone call to the patient to give them the results of the consultation; if the specialist has any doubts, they can ask the primary care professional to arrange a face-to-face consultation with the patient (Figure 1). In other words, we can describe the process as medical record-based, store and forward and provider-to-provider asynchronous telemedicine between primary and hospital care. The Catalan healthcare system, which provides publicly financed universal health coverage, is free at the point of access, and thus, no fee is charged for the either face-to-face visits or the telemedicine service. We will assume that a telemedicine consultation avoids a face-to-face referral if it does not result in a referral for the same matter within the following 3 months. It has been shown that this telemedicine setting reduces waiting lists while improving access to GPs [14].

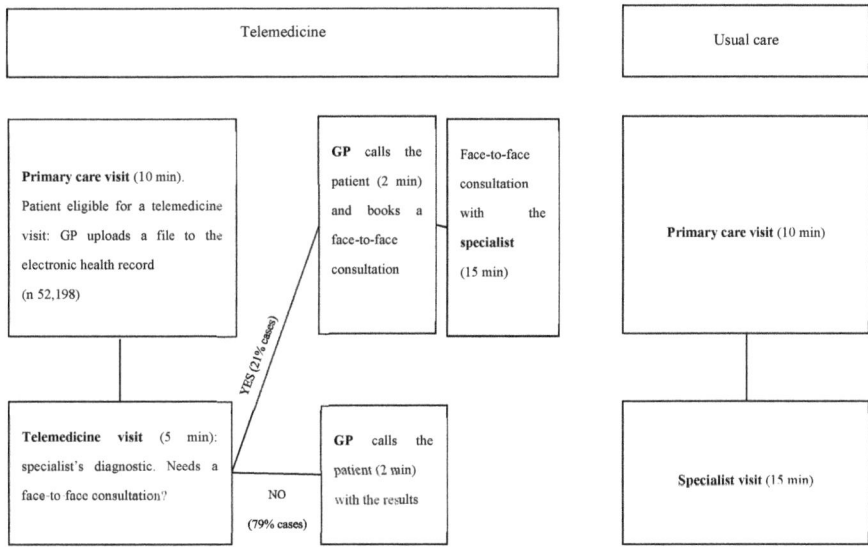

Figure 1. Patient flow: telemedicine vs. usual care.

2.2. Study Type

A cost-minimization analysis was carried out over a three-month period using a societal perspective. Direct costs (healthcare costs corresponding to time spent by professionals and users during visits and travel expenses by users) and indirect costs (patient and caregiver's time) were included. No staff training or equipment costs were included (practitioners used pre-existing devices), since they were not subject to the analyzed interventions. The cost estimate is based on 2019, a year which showed a higher number of telemedicine visits. A sensitivity analysis was carried out increasing the baseline costs. Calculations were performed using a Google Drive spreadsheet. The study was approved by the Ethical Committee for Clinical Research at the Foundation University Institute for Primary Health Care Research Jordi Gol i Gurina (registration number P19/182-P).

2.3. Direct Costs

The Catalan Institute of Health provided anonymized individual data regarding all 52,198 telemedicine consultation services performed during the period November 2011–November 2019. This dataset contains information on a case-by-case basis on the source and destination of every type of telemedicine service and whether it avoided a subsequent face-to-face visit or not. As Table 1 shows, all telemedicine services result in high face-to-face savings, ranging from 72% to 88% of the queries received.

Table 1. Number of telemedicine visits and % of face-to-face visits saved, per type.

Type of Telemedicine	Number of Visits	Face-to-Face Visits Saved (%)
Teledermatology	40,658	77.7
Teleophthalmology	1180	72.1
Teleaudiometries	9823	86.2
Teleulcers	537	88.5
Total (weighted average)	52,198	(79.3)

In order to calculate the derived potential societal savings, differential costs attributable to the time spent by practitioners and citizens using telemedicine and usual care were taken into account. From the healthcare system point of view, the savings resulting from this form of intervention are based on the reduction of case management time. Whereas in usual care, the time spent on a face-to-face visit with a hospital care professional is 15 minutes, it is calculated that telematic monitoring of the case reduces the time to 5 minutes, redirecting the case back to the primary care professional, who calls the patient for approximately 2 minutes and closes the case, if applicable. If the specialist has any doubts, they can ask the primary care professional to book the patient for a face-to-face consultation (15 minutes). It was taken into account that, although in the teledermatology, teleophthalmology and teleaudiometry services, a primary care doctor is the one who makes the referral, in the case of teleulcers, a (primary and hospital care) nurse reviews the images and sends a reply. Baseline wages are used, according to standard labor agreements, for medical and nursing professionals in primary and hospital care. Travel costs (private car expenses) are calculated using the average travel distance (the methodology is described below) and the baseline price per kilometer.

2.4. Indirect Costs

Productive time (commuting to the hospital) lost by patients and caregivers was considered. The user also benefits from greater agility in the resolution of the case, reducing waiting time, as well as in terms of travel time to a hospital consultation (Hospitals in Manresa and Berga). Employing the methodology used by Vidal-Alaball et al. 2019 [13], through a combination of the R 3.6.1 software (The R Foundation for Statistical Computing, Vienna, Austria), a Google Maps API and the information from each of the user's Primary Care Team (as a proxy for the user's place of residence), together with the referral hospital, a very accurate calculation of the total number of kilometers and time of journeys saved by the intervention was obtained (Figure 2). Therefore, the sample saved 893,820 kilometers (21.58 km per case, for the round trip) and 16,812 hours (25 minutes per case) of travel. The costs to users (patient and caregiver) have been calculated by multiplying travel and consultation time by the average salary/hour.

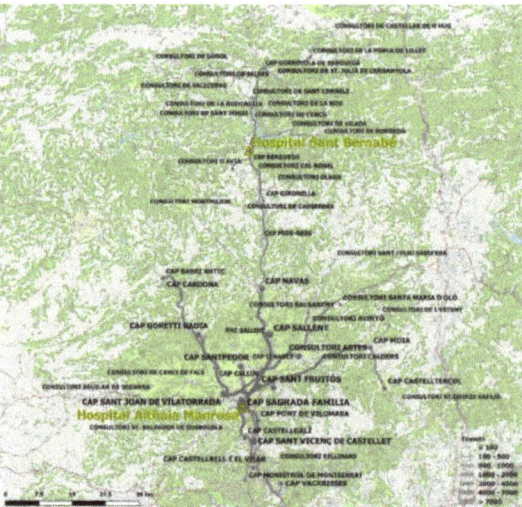

Figure 2. Origin and destination (either Hospital Sant Bernabé in Berga or Althaia Xarxa Assistencial Universitària in Manresa) of telemedicine visits avoided. The thickness of the line corresponds to the number of journeys saved.

Also, according to an aggregate analysis of the users' profiles, it can be observed that the average age of a telemedicine service user is 52, with a standard deviation of 23, suggesting the heterogeneity of the beneficiary profile. If we assume that people aged over 65 (34% of the total sample) and under 16 (8%) require the company of a caregiver during their visits, this means that we have to add the indirect impact in terms of opportunity costs of the time spent by caregivers in 42% of the cases analyzed.

The nature of each type of cost is shown in Table 2.

Table 2. Direct and indirect costs, for users and for the healthcare system.

	Direct Costs	Indirect Costs
Users	Travel costs	Time spent by caregiversTravel time
Healthcare system	GP's timeNurse's time	

Finally, Table 3 shows the parameters which were considered when making calculations and their corresponding sources: the hourly wages of professionals, the price per kilometer, the opportunity cost of the user, the total number of visits (saved), consultation time with the specialist with and without telemedicine, the primary care professional's phone call time, and average time and distance for users. The results are shown for both perspectives (i.e., healthcare system and user).

Table 3. Calculation parameters.

	Concept	Amount	Source
Costs (€)	Wage/h primary care doctor	24.60	ICS [15]
	Wage/h primary care nurse	17.68	
	Wage/h hospital doctor	22.46	UCH [16]
	Wage/h hospital nurse	16.53	
	Travel cost per km	0.25 *	Own
	Average time value (patient and caregiver)	13.36	SAIT [17]
Variables observed	Total number of visits	52,198	Own
	Number of visits saved	41,402	
	TeleUlcers number of visits	537	
	TeleUlcers number of visits saved	472	
	Not teleUlcers number of visits	51,661	
	Not teleUlcers number of visits saved	40,930	
	Minutes with specialist in face-to-face visit	15 *	
	Minutes with specialist in teleconsultation	5 *	
	Minutes in primary care visit	2 *	
	Average travel distance km	21.58	R + Google API
	Average travel time	0.4	R + Google API

* For the comparability between studies, the baseline scenario takes the same parameter as in Vidal-Alaball et al. [12].

3. Results

Table 4 shows the results of calculating the societal savings (distinguishing between those of the healthcare system and of the users) from the use of telemedicine in comparison to usual care. While the cost of making phone calls is exclusive to the telemedicine program (€ 42,675), there is a reduction in the time spent by hospital staff. Despite the fact that 21% result in a face-to-face visit, and that the salary per hour is higher in the context of primary care than in hospital care, the consultation time of 79% of cases was reduced by 8 minutes, implying savings in relation to usual care, where all visits are face to face and 15 minutes, for a professional time equivalent to € 154, 542 for the sample under analysis.

Table 4. Differential costs between telemedicine and usual care (in €).

	Concept	Telemedicine	Usual Care	Difference
Healthcare system's costs	Primary care staff phone call	42,675		42,675
	Hospital staff	137,805	292,347	−154,542
Users' costs(patient and caregiver)	Consultation time	62,240	247,565	−185,325
	Travel time	962	318,957	−317,995
	Travel cost (private car)	58,244	223,455	−165,211
	Total	301,926	1082,324	−780,397
	Total per patient	5.78	20.73	−14.95

Regarding patients, while also taking into account cases where telemedicine is ineffective in avoiding a face-to-face visit, there is a saving on consultation and travel time of € 185,325 and € 317,995 respectively. These two parameters take into account the assumption that 42% of the cases had to be accompanied in face-to-face visits. In terms of fuel, the difference between the cost of telemedicine and usual care is € 165,211, calculated as the result of subtracting the product of the average travel distance per case (21 km) by the cost/km (€ 0.25) by the number of cases that have avoided a face-to-face visit (41,402, totaling € 223,455) and the equivalent cost from telemedicine visits that have not avoided a face-to-face visit (€ 58,244). Thus, the total of the costs and differential savings for the different types of telemedicine is approximately € 780,397 (a saving of € 15 per visit).

Sensitivity Analysis: An Even More Favorable Scenario for Telemedicine

In order to comparatively evaluate the results, a maximum estimate of the sensitivity analysis is included by varying some of the assumptions (Table 5). This second scenario increases the costs included in Table 3 by 20%: the patient travel time and that of their possible companion (assuming that the actual time is not wholly shown in Google Maps, but that there are transaction costs derived from going to pick up the car, looking for a parking space, attending the consultation or waiting for the patient's turn), the travel cost (measured in €/km, assuming that it could be increased with respect to the evaluation performed for teledermatology [12]) and the hourly wages of medical professionals (assuming that the real cost may be closer to the company cost, rather than the actual remuneration received by the health professionals). The results of this scenario show that the savings increase by approximately 8%, i.e., as much as € 17 per visit and continue to be mostly favorable for the user (85%). A sensitivity analysis was not performed for the opposite scenario, assuming that the calculation of time and distance savings made using Google Maps is, in itself, the minimum.

Table 5. Sensitivity analysis: 20% increase in costs. Main results (€).

	Concept	Telemedicine	Usual Care	Difference
Healthcare system costs	Primary care staff phone call	51,210		51,210
	Hospital staff	165,366	350,816	−185,451
User's costs	Patient: consultation time	50,221	247,565	−197,344
	Patient: travel time	1154	382,748	−381,594
	Travel cost (private car)	69,893	268,146	−198,253
	Total	337,844	1249,275	−911,431
	Total per patient	6.47	23,93	−17.46

4. Discussion

4.1. In Relation to the Study with 2016 Data

The study concludes that, in the given context, telemedicine is an unequivocally preferable option to usual care from an economic point of view. The strength of this diagnosis is similar to that derived from the analysis performed with 2016 data for the specific case of teledermatology, i.e., the result of including other specialties (teleulcers, teleophthalmology and teleaudiometries), lengthening the time period (by using the complete sample available) and adding the indirect cost approach of the caregiver results in savings per visit 35% above the base case studied by Vidal Alaball et al. with 2016 data [12] (Table 6). We note that once caregivers' opportunity costs are introduced, the most important differential corresponds precisely to the calculation of the cost in terms of the time of users. The similarity of results between the different types of costs reflects the robustness of the methodology used.

Table 6. Differential costs per visit. Comparison between studies.

Type of Costs		Previous Study [12] (€)	Baseline Scenario (€)	Previous Study [12] (% of total)	Baseline Scenario(% of total)
Healthcare system costs	Primary care staff	0.77	0.82	22.60	14.33
	Hospital staff	−3.42	−2.96		
User's costs	Time	−6.31	−9.64	77.40	85.67
	Travel cost	−2.76	−3.17		
Total		−11.71	−14.95	100	100

4.2. Sensitive Variables

The magnitude of the result is highly sensitive to the parameter corresponding to the opportunity cost (lost productivity) of the user and this has been calculated homogeneously among the different beneficiary profiles (minors, of working-age and retirees); although an eventual differential calculation by profile would not change the results, it would far better approximate the representative total of the savings. It should be borne in mind that in contexts with higher labor productivity of both professionals and users, the results of the analysis would be much more favorable to telemedicine.

With regard to the extrapolation of these conclusions and with the "travel time" factor, it is worth keeping in mind that the study was performed in a mostly rural and semirural setting. The average distance per journey may be higher than in urban settings, although it is not clear if the journey time would be higher (as moving within a city is much slower). Whatever the case, the results show that both factors (i.e., travel and time lost) are sufficient to reach the same conclusion, namely, that even if telemedicine did not save on travel costs (being "zero kilometer"), it would be cost-effective, and even if it did not save anything in terms of time (for the user and the healthcare system), it would also be cost-effective.

As to the assumption that patients travel by car, it is reasonable to assume that some of them use public transport. If we consider this possibility, telemedicine savings would be even higher, since in rural settings, where the frequency of public transport is very low, the potential savings in terms of travel costs (using public transport instead of private transport) would clearly be far outweighed by more travel time (with and without waiting time). In the context involved in the study, which was almost devoid of a railway network (except in the south of the city of Manresa), it is unlikely that the bus is faster than private transport.

4.3. Factors not Included in the Analysis

While it is true that this assessment includes the differential essential elements between the two analyzed models, it does not include objective or easily monetizable intangible factors such as the users' and professionals' satisfaction with the service or the improved management of cases in function of their clinical severity. This improvement in care management could reduce waiting lists to the access of GPs, one of the biggest problems in the Catalan healthcare system. In this context, telemedicine allows for better allocation of care time according to the complexity of the case. Future lines of research ought to quantify these factors, which are complementary but key in order to evaluate the service's effectiveness.

In addition, the type of analysis performed assumes that clinical effectiveness is equivalent. Although a time period which includes aspects strictly related to management seems sufficient to make a good diagnosis, as is the case, and despite the complexity of the information which would be needed, we ought to try to ensure the hypothesis of equivalence in health impact and add any significant and differential costs which go beyond and which can be calculated in a rigorous manner.

It needs to be borne in mind that as doctors are remunerated, their increased productivity does not imply a direct translation into the healthcare provider's income account; instead, the freer the practitioners, the fewer practitioners the healthcare provider will need to hire. In other words, savings might occur in the mid-term, as opposed to the short term.

It should also be considered that the increased ease with which referrals can be made might have incentivized GPs to use interconsultation as a second opinion tool to support the diagnosis of patients they would normally have treated. This might have increased the ratio of saved face-to-face visits.

Finally, it should be mentioned that the study also assumed that the differential cost of expenses such as cameras or clinical software is zero, since this was the case, but in the case of introducing this service from scratch in another context, these costs would have to be taken into account. In any case, the magnitude of the savings made by the service makes it unlikely that including them could significantly alter the results of the analysis.

5. Conclusions

The results show that telemedicine minimizes the costs of the two agents included in the analysis (i.e., the user and the healthcare system); from either perspective, telemedicine is better than usual care from an economic point of view. However, it was observed that from the € 14.95 saving per visit, approximately 85% benefits the patient, showing that this kind of intervention is especially convenient for the user, particularly for the time saving which it offers.

Author Contributions: Conceptualization, F.L.S. and J.V.-A.; methodology, F.L.S. and J.V.-A.; software, F.L.S.; validation, J.F.P. and X.G.G.; formal analysis, F.L.S.; investigation, F.L.S. and J.V.-A.; resources, F.L.S. and J.V.-A.; data curation, F.L.S.; writing—original draft preparation, F.L.S., C.A.M., J.V.-A.; writing—review and editing, F.L.S., C.A.M. and J.V.-A.; visualization, F.L.S., J.V.-A., J.F.P., X.G.G., J.M.P., F.G.C., C.A.M., A.G.-A.; supervision, F.G.C. and A.G.-A.; project administration, F.L.S.; funding acquisition, F.L.S. and J.V.-A. All authors have read and agreed to the published version of the manuscript.

Funding: This research received no external funding.

Acknowledgments: This study was conducted with the support of the Secretary of Universities and Research of the Department of Business and Knowledge at the Generalitat de Catalunya. We are also grateful to the staff at the Technical and Support Area of Gerència Territorial de la Catalunya Central for their help during data collection. The manuscript highly benefited from the comments of two anonymous reviewers.

Conflicts of Interest: The authors declare no conflict of interest.

References

1. Bashshur, R.; Shannon, G.; Krupinski, E. The taxonomy of telemedicine. *Telemed J. E Health* **2011**, *17*, 484–494. [CrossRef] [PubMed]
2. NICE. *Evidence Standards Framework for Digital Health Technologies*; NICE: London, UK, 2019.
3. WHO. *Guideline: Recommendations on Digital Interventions for Health System Strengthening*; World Health Organization: Geneva, Switzerland, 2019.
4. Kruse, C.S.; Soma, M.; Pulluri, D.; Nemali, N.T.; Brooks, M. The effectiveness of telemedicine in the management of chronic heart disease—A systematic review. *JRSM Open* **2017**, *8*, 2054270416681747. [CrossRef] [PubMed]

5. Delgoshaei, B.; Mobinizadeh, M.; Mojdekar, R.; Afzal, E.; Arabloo, J.; Mohamadi, E. Telemedicine: A systematic review of economic evaluations. *Med. J. Islam. Repub. Iran* **2017**, *31*, 113. [CrossRef] [PubMed]
6. Lee, J.Y.; Lee, S.W.H. Telemedicine cost-effectiveness for diabetes management: A systematic review. *Diabetes Technol. Ther.* **2018**, *20*, 492–500. [CrossRef] [PubMed]
7. Warren, R.; Carlisle, K.; Mihala, G.; Scuffham, P.A. Effects of telemonitoring on glycaemic control and healthcare costs in type 2 diabetes: A randomized controlled trial. *J. Telemed. Telecare* **2018**, *24*, 586–595. [CrossRef] [PubMed]
8. Lee, J.J.; English, J.C., 3rd. Teledermatology: A review and update. *Am. J. Clin. Dermatol.* **2018**, *19*, 253–260. [CrossRef] [PubMed]
9. Natafgi, N.; Shane, D.M.; Ullrich, F.; MacKinney, A.C.; Bell, A.; Ward, M.M. Using tele-emergency to avoid patient transfers in rural emergency departments: An assessment of costs and benefits. *J. Telemed. Telecare* **2018**, *24*, 193–201. [CrossRef] [PubMed]
10. Langabeer, J.R., 2nd; Champagne-Langabeer, T.; Alqusairi, D.; Kim, J.; Jackson, A.; Persse, D. Cost-benefit analysis of telehealth in pre-hospital care. *J. Telemed. Telecare* **2017**, *23*, 747–751. [CrossRef] [PubMed]
11. Vestergaard, A.S.; Hansen, L.; Sørensen, S.S.; Jensen, M.B.; Ehlers, L.H. Is telehealthcare for heart failure patients cost-effective? An economic evaluation alongside the Danish TeleCare North heart failure trial. *BMJ Open* **2020**, *10*, e031670. [CrossRef] [PubMed]
12. Vidal-Aballi, J.; Garcia Domingo, J.L.; Garcia Cuyàs, F.; Peña, J.M.; Matco, G.F.; Rosanas, J.D.; Valmaña, G.S. A cost savings analysis of asynchronous teledermatology compared to face-to-face dermatology in Catalonia. *BMC Health Serv. Res.* **2018**, *18*, 650. [CrossRef] [PubMed]
13. Vidal-Aballi, J.; Franch-Parella, J.; Seguí, F.L.; Cuyàs, F.G.; Peña, J.M. Impact of a Telemedicine Program on the Reduction in the Emission of Atmospheric Pollutants and Journeys by Road. *Int. J. Environ. Res. Public Health* **2019**, *16*, 4366. [CrossRef] [PubMed]
14. Vidal-Aballi, J.; Álamo-Junquera, D.; López-Aguilá, S.; García-Altés, A. Evaluation of the impact of teledermatology in decreasing the waiting list in the Bages region (2009–2012). *Aten. Primaria* **2015**, *47*, 320. [CrossRef] [PubMed]
15. Institut Català de la Salut. Llibre de Retribucions 2019. Available online: http://ics.gencat.cat/web/.content/documents/transparencia/personal/2019-Taules-retributives-estatutaris-gener-juny.pdf (accessed on 18 March 2020).
16. Unió Catalana d'Hospitals. Xè Conveni Col·Lectiu de Treball D'establiments Sanitaris D'hospitalització, Assistència, Consulta i Laboratoris D'anàlisis Clíniques. Available online: https://www.uch.cat/negociacio-collectiva-/convenis-collectius-del-sector-sanitari-100/xe-conveni-collectiu-de-treball-destabliments-sanitaris-dhospitalitzacio-assistencia-consulta-i-laboratoris-danalisis-cliniques.html (accessed on 18 March 2020).
17. Sistema d'Avaluació d'Inversions en Transport (SAIT). Available online: http://territori.gencat.cat/ca/03_infraestructures_i_mobilitat/carreteres/SAIT (accessed on 18 March 2020).

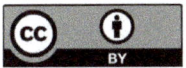

© 2020 by the authors. Licensee MDPI, Basel, Switzerland. This article is an open access article distributed under the terms and conditions of the Creative Commons Attribution (CC BY) license (http://creativecommons.org/licenses/by/4.0/).

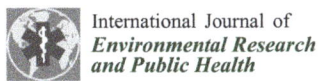

Article

Health Advertising on Short-Video Social Media: A Study on User Attitudes Based on the Extended Technology Acceptance Model

Jie Zhao [1,*] and Jianfei Wang [1,2]

1. School of Business, Anhui University, Hefei 230601, China; m17201037@stu.ahu.edu.cn
2. School of Management, Hefei University of Technology, Hefei 230602, China
* Correspondence: zhaojie@ahu.edu.cn

Received: 19 January 2020; Accepted: 24 February 2020; Published: 26 February 2020

Abstract: The rapid development of short-video social network platforms provides us with an opportunity to conduct health-related advertising and recommendation. However, so far, there are no empirical evidence on whether users are willing to accept health-related short-video advertisements. Here, acceptance refers to purchase intention, meaning that users will read short-video ads, share ads with others, or even open the product link embedded in ads to purchase the product. In this paper, we make the first attempt to model and quantify user acceptance of health-related short-video advertisements. Particularly, we propose a new research model that enhances the Technology Acceptance Model (TAM) with two new designs. First, we propose four new antecedents including social interaction, intrusiveness, informativeness, and relevance into the original TAM to reflect the features of short-video social networks. Second, we introduce two mediator variables including perceived usefulness and attitude so that we can better study how different factors affect user acceptance of health-related short-video ads. We perform a survey on the Internet and conduct an empirical analysis of the surveyed data. The results show that the four antecedents as well as the perceived ease of use have significant influences on perceived usefulness, attitude, and purchase intention. Further, perceived usefulness plays a valid mediating role in attitude and purchase intention. We also found that users' perceived ease of use on health-related short-video ads cannot significantly predict users' attitudes toward ads. This is a new finding in social media-oriented ads. Finally, we integrate the empirical findings and present reasonable suggestions for advertisers and marketers to promote health-related short-video ads.

Keywords: public health; short video; social network; social media; TAM

1. Introduction

Social media is one of the most promising tools in the digital advertising environment [1,2]. Since 2016, short video has become an important field for the expansion of social media such as Tik Tok, Facebook live, YouTube, Snapchat, Instagram, Douyin (Chinese), and Douyu (Chinese). These real-time interactive information platforms provide a free and easy-to-access online resource for live videos for anchors and viewers. For example, Figure 1 shows a typical short video (15 s by default) on the largest Chinese live-video platform Douyin (https://www.douyin.com/), where people can use self-generated videos to share with others something interesting, such as new products and nice places. In Figure 1, the user is introducing a new Swisse product from Australia. So far, short video has gradually developed into a popular social media channel. For example, a recent report showed that the number of short-video users in China had reached 422 million [3].

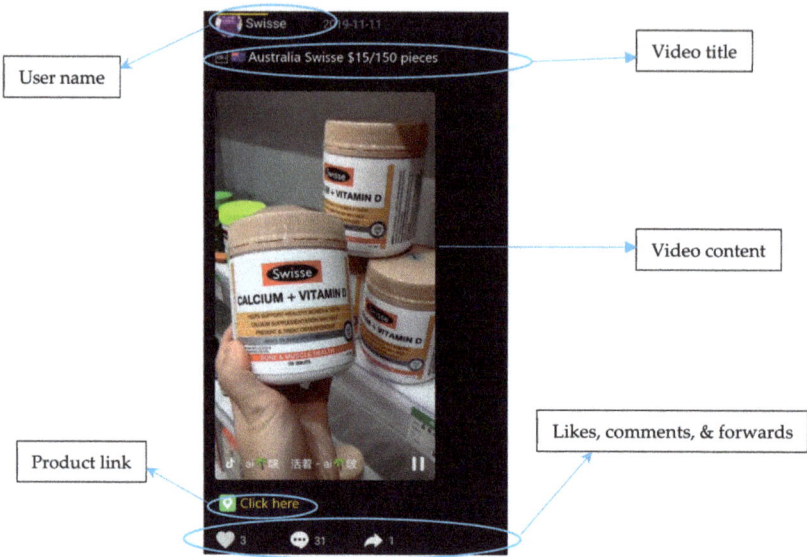

Figure 1. An example of health-related short videos on Douyin (http://www.douyin.com).

The rapid development of short-video platforms introduces new opportunities for health promotion, e.g., health-related advertising and recommendation. Compared with traditional social media, short-video platforms have little time delay and can support one-on-one as well as many-to-many social interaction by videos and the barrage (scrolling texts on the screen). For example, the largest Chinese live-video platform Douyin (https://www.douyin.com/) provides one-on-one video interaction that allows one user discusses some topics with another user through live video. At the same time, other users can watch the live video and interact with others via barrages, text reviews, emojis, and images. This new form of social interaction on short-video social network platforms has been demonstrated to be an effective way of advertising [4]. However, in health-related short-video platforms, an important issue is to know users' intentions of accepting health-related short-video advertisements.

Therefore, this study attempts to investigate whether and how short-video ads affect users' purchase intentions on health-related products. Particularly, we take the Technology Acceptance Model (TAM) as the base model and extend social interaction, intrusiveness, informativeness, and relevance as four new antecedents to the perceived usefulness of health-related short-video ads. Then, we set perceived usefulness and attitude as two mediate factors and validate their mediating effect in the model. Finally, we conduct an empirical analysis of questionnaire data from the Internet and short-video social network platforms based on the structural equation model. Briefly, following the research framework of the TAM model, we aim to study the following research questions:

RQ1: What are the key factors that affect the perceived usefulness of health-related short-video ads?
RQ2: How do the factors affect the perceived usefulness of health-related ads?
RQ3: How do perceived usefulness and perceived ease of use affect user attitudes and purchase intention on health-related short-video ads?
RQ4: What kind of relationship exists between user attitudes toward health-related short-video ads and users' purchase intention on health-related products?
RQ5: What is the mediating effect of perceived usefulness and user attitudes to users' purchase intention on health-related products?

In summary, we make the following contributions in this paper:

(1) We extend the Technology Acceptance Model (TAM) with new antecedents including social interaction, intrusiveness, informativeness, and relevance to analyze the users' response to health-related short-video ads. To the best of our knowledge, this is the first study that extends the TAM model to analyze user acceptance of health-related short-video ads.
(2) We conduct a survey on the Internet and short-video social network platforms and perform systematical data analysis over the surveyed data. The data analysis consists of many aspects, including measurement model evaluation, structural model evaluation, and mediating effect analysis. The results show that social interaction, intrusiveness, informativeness, relevance, and the TAM factors (perceived usefulness and perceived ease of use) have a significant influence on user acceptance of health-related short-video ads. Further, we find that users' perceived ease of use on health-related short-video ads cannot significantly predict users' attitudes toward ads. This is a new finding that is contrary to previous studies in social media-oriented ads.
(3) We integrate the empirical findings and present reasonable suggestions for advertisers and marketers to better develop health-related short-video ads.

The remainder of this paper is structured as follows. Section 2 describes the related work and the differences between previous studies and this paper. Section 3 presents the research model as well as the hypothesis propositions. Section 4 describes the data collection and measurements. Section 5 presents the results of data analysis. Section 6 discusses the research implications and suggestions. Finally, in Section 7, we conclude the entire paper.

2. Related Work

2.1. Short-Video Advertising

Digital advertising significantly influences users' attitudes and intentions to purchase [5]. There are many studies about the factors that influence the effectiveness of online advertising [6], video advertising [7], and social media advertising [2]. Although short-video ads are a promising form of online advertising, this ad form has not been adequately examined in the research. The core of short-video ads is "video + sociality", and it has become an important field for the expansion of social media. Therefore, we study our questions mainly based on the research of social media advertising. Some quote video studies, of course.

There have been some existing studies on informativeness and intrusiveness and how such concerns may influence users' attitudes toward advertising and product purchase intentions [8–16]. Generally, informativeness is defined as the information value provided by media like texts, images, or videos [11] and intrusiveness is defined as the degree to which people deem the presentation of information as contrary to their goals [14]. Both informativeness and intrusiveness have been regarded as key factors to predict the helpfulness of messages in the research of social networks. For example, Dehghani et al. [12] conducted an empirical study on YouTube ads and found that a high value of informativeness led to a high level of user acceptance of YouTube ads, meaning that informativeness is a positive factor affecting users' attitude toward YouTube ads. Meanwhile, they found intrusiveness is a negative factor, meaning that a high value of intrusiveness led to a low level of user acceptance of YouTube ads. Lee and Hong empirically investigated that informativeness has a potential contribution to a positive online behavior based on the theory of reasoned action and the social influence theory [13]. Jung found perceived ad relevance influences advertising effectiveness while it could increase privacy concerns, which ultimately raise ad avoidance in social media [16].

Relevance is another factor that may affect user acceptance of advertising. Relevance has been widely adopted in web search and online recommendation [17]. For instance, a web search engine can rank the searching results according to the relevance between the user query and the returned web pages. In the online recommendation in E-commerce, the relevance between the user profile and products is usually used to predict the items that may fit within the users' interests. Similarly, the relevance between a user's interest and short-video advertisements may also affect the user acceptance of short-video ads [18]. Therefore, we will also consider relevance as a construct in the research model of this study, which will be detailed in Section 3.

On the other hand, according to the social influence theory [19], a high level of social interactions can enhance the feelings of affection, trust, belongingness, and warmth. Currently, most people are engaged in short videos by mobile apps. The mobile short-video apps offer people real-time interaction with other ones. In addition, platforms like Douyin and Tik Tok allow users to interact with short videos. For example, users can click the product link and fill a form to deliver their purchase interest to vendors. Therefore, social interaction can be a key factor affecting user acceptance of short-video ads.

So far, short-video ads are still in the early developing stage. Existing work has paid little attention to how the new features of short videos impact users' attitudes toward purchase behavior. Based on previous experiences in social media ads, many researchers claimed that two aspects of information should be considered in the context of social media ads [20–22]. The first one, product information, focuses on informativeness, relevance, and intrusiveness of information [20]. The second one, personal interaction, refers to social interaction, which reflects the impact of social identity and group norms on community users' group intention of accepting advertising [21]. Windels et al. examined the differences between native advertisements and friend referrals on social networking sites. They found that social relationships did not always work [22]. In this paper, we consider these related studies as well as the features of short-video ads to design antecedents toward the perceived usefulness of users and the attitude to short-video ads. As a result, four antecedents including informativeness, relevance, intrusiveness, and social interaction are designed in our study.

2.2. Technology Adoption Model (TAM)

The Technology Acceptance Model (TAM) was developed to describe users' behavior to accept or reject the use of new technologies [23]. The TAM model defines two variables, namely perceived usefulness and perceived ease of use, to quantify user attitude to information technology, which in turn can be used to measure user acceptance of information technologies.

Although the TAM model is initially designed to explain and predict the behavior of individuals on the use of information systems, it has been used in many studies [24–26]. Previous studies have demonstrated the applicability of the TAM model to online advertising. For example, Demangeot and Broderick examined a modified technology acceptance model (TAM) that was developed to test the intention to use SMS advertising [27]. Based on the ability of TAM and short video including a wide variety of online media services and SNS, it is a reasonable choice to consider the TAM model to model and quantify user acceptance of short-video ads.

The TAM model has been widely adopted in many existing studies. In this paper, we also adopt the TAM model as the basic research model. There are two reasons. First, many studies in social media have applied the TAM model to analyze the acceptance factors of online advertising and social network advertising. The research scope of this paper, i.e., short video, has the characteristics of both online media and social networks; thus, it is a reasonable choice to select the TAM model. Second, the basic factors in the TAM model, namely perceived usefulness (PU) and perceptual ease of use (PEOU), are suitable to distinguish the usefulness of live advertising and the impact of live-video technologies.

On the other hand, differing from the traditional TAM model, we integrate social interaction, intrusiveness, informativeness, and relevance with TAM and propose to use perceived usefulness as the mediate factor, forming an augmented TAM model that is more suitable for studying the intact path of short-video ads. Even though research integrating these external variables with the TAM is limited, available empirical findings generally support the influence of these factors on perceptions about users' ad attributes and adoption intentions.

In addition to the TAM model, another widely used model for predicting user acceptance of short-video ads is the Unified Theory of Acceptance and Use of Technology (UTAUT) model [28], which was proposed to incorporate various models of human behavior theory. The UTAUT model was constructed by extracting three variables that affect users' behavioral intentions, one variable that influences action, and four moderators that mediate the effects of the process. Some of the variables had similar concepts with variables that construct the TAM model. One major difference between UTAUT and TAM was that UTAUT proposed four control variables (i.e., gender, age, experience, and voluntariness) to further enhance the predictive power of the model. Based on UTAUT, Venkatesh et al. incorporated three other constructs into UTAUT, namely hedonic motivation, price value, and habit, extending UTAUT into UTAUT 2 [29]. Compared to UTAUT, the extensions proposed in UTAUT2 produced a substantial improvement in the variance explained in behavioral intention. As a result, both UTAUT and UTAUT 2 have been actively used in predicting users' purchase behavior in many areas like healthcare systems [30] and social-network-based advertising [1]. However, as suggested by Venkatesh et al. [29], in order to increase the applicability of the original UTAUT as well as the UTAUT 2 model, other relevant factors are usually needed to be extended to meet the specific requirements of different applications, technologies, countries, etc.

In summary, both TAM and UTAUT are actively utilized in the research of user adoption of new technologies. Whether or not to use TAM or UTAUT mainly depends on the particular type of the application. In this paper, we select TAM rather than UTAUT as the basic model for analyzing user acceptance of health-related short-video ads for the following reasons. First, UTAUT is a behavioral model aiming to explain the behavior of people in the use of information systems [31], but in this study, the content of short-videos, as measured by the antecedents named informativeness, relevance, and intrusiveness in our model, is also an important factor. Second, the UTAUT model is more complex than TAM; thus, extending TAM is easier than extending UTAUT. Nevertheless, as Venkatesh et al. [29] and Dwivedi et al. [32] reported, most studies only employed a subset of the UTAUT model, and the moderators were typically removed. To this end, the TAM model can have similar predictive power as the UTAUT model without moderators. However, it is still worth investigating the extension of the UTAUT or UTAUT 2 model to predict the user adoption of health-related short-video ads in the future.

3. Research Model and Hypotheses

3.1. Research Model

In this paper, we first selected the main factors in the TAM model as basic independent variables, i.e., perceived usefulness (PU), perceived ease of use (PE), and ad attitudes (AT). Further, we introduced social interaction (SI), informativeness (IR), intrusiveness (IN), and relevance (RE) as new antecedents of perceived usefulness. The selection of the four factors (i.e., SI, IR, IN, RE) was mostly based on two aspects. First, previous studies in social media have shown that these factors are critical to the usefulness of social media advertising [2,12,16]. Second, these factors are suitable for short-video ads, as they reflect the information features of live video ads. Thus, it is reasonable to introduce them to the research model. As a result, the perceived usefulness (PU) in our research model became a mediator variable. The purchase intention (PI) was set to be the dependent variable. In the study of behavior intention, attitude has been commonly recognized as a variable that affects the willingness of behavior. Thus, we chose attitude as another mediator variable. On this basis, this paper put forward the research model of user responses to health-related short-video advertisements. Figure 2 shows the components of the proposed research model.

3.2. Research Hypothesis

According to the research model, there are three independent variables, namely perceived usefulness (PU), perceived ease of use (PE), and ad attitude (AT), and four antecedent variables, namely social interaction (SI), informativeness (IR), intrusiveness (IN), and relevance (RE). In addition, there are two mediator variables called perceived usefulness (PU) and ad attitude (AT). These variables are supposed to impact the dependent variable named purchase intention (PI).

To reveal the relationships among these factors, we propose hypotheses to the research questions presented earlier, as listed in Table 1. The right column in Table 1 shows the corresponding hypotheses that are proposed to answer the research question. In the following subsections, we will explain each hypothesis.

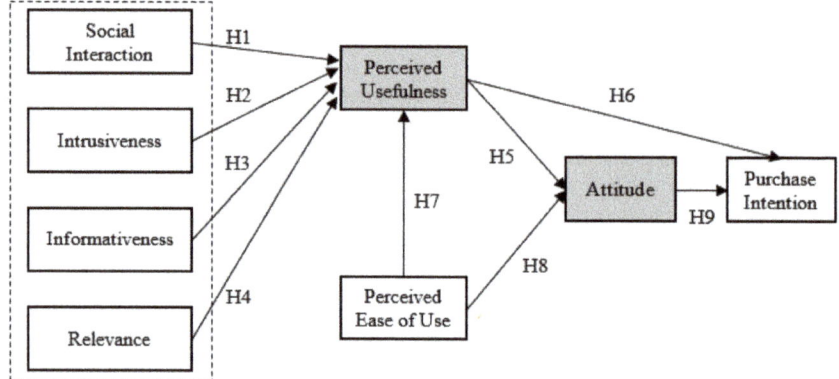

Figure 2. The research model extended from Technology Acceptance Model (TAM) [23] (each rectangle represents one variable. The mediator variables are shaded grey. Purchase intention is the dependent variable, and the remaining five are independent variables).

Table 1. Research questions and corresponding hypotheses.

Question Number	Research Question	Corresponding Hypotheses
RQ1	What are the key factors of short-video ads?	H1, H2, H3, H4
RQ2	How do the factors affect the perceived usefulness of health-related ads?	H1, H2, H3, H4
RQ3	How do perceived usefulness and perceived ease of use affect user attitudes and purchase intention on health-related short-video ads?	H5, H7, H8
RQ4	What kind of relationship exists between user attitudes toward health-related short-video ads and users' purchase intention on health-related products?	H9
RQ5	What is the mediating effect of perceived usefulness and user attitudes to users' purchase intention on health-related products?	H5, H6, H8, H9

Sociability has been defined as 'the extent to which the computer-mediated communication environment facilitates the emergence of social space by allowing social affordance [33]. Social interaction can mitigate users' perceptions of ad avoidance and enhance the effectiveness of ads [19]. Interactive online media are an increasingly preferred format for users and advertisers. Particularly, health-related short-video ads are more social than traditional social media advertising, whereby audiences can, in a timely manner, view, share, and post barrages on these ads with anchors and peer audiences. Given the massively real-time interactivity distinguishing live video from traditional social media, real-time interactivity may enhance the influence of social interactions or depress viewers' experience because of barrages filled with mobile screens. Therefore, we make the following hypothesis:

Hypothesis 1 (H1). *Social interaction of health-related short-video ads positively affects users' perceived usefulness (PU) of ads.*

Intrusiveness describes the extent to which the content is messy and irritating to users [34]. Intrusiveness in social media advertising will be negatively related to the perceived usefulness of ads [2,14,15]. When an inconsistent ad is posted with live videos, audiences may spend efforts on non-major tasks and cannot effectively deal with advertising information, resulting in the ineffectiveness of advertising. In addition, the small screen of a mobile phone may also make intrusiveness be a negative factor in live video ads. Moreover, intrusive ads may bring the negative emotion to users [35]. Hence, we make Hypothesis 2:

Hypothesis 2a (H2a). *The intrusiveness of health-related short-video ads negatively affects users' perceived usefulness (PU) of ads.*

Hypothesis 2b (H2b). *The intrusiveness of health-related short-video ads negatively affects users' perceived ease of use of ads.*

Informativeness represents the information that is helpful and resourceful [36]. It can inform users about product alternatives. Consumers tend to gain information more through unconditional, interpersonal information exchange [37]. Studies have found informativeness to be important in the formation of consumer attitudes to electronic commerce websites as well as to SNS advertising [10] and to social media advertising [13]. The informative content of a message positively influences the perceived value of online advertising [15]. Hence, we make Hypothesis 3:

Hypothesis 3 (H3). *Informativeness of health-related short-video ads positively affects users' perceived usefulness (PU) of ads.*

Relevance is used to capture users' general perception of similarity between short-video ads and live video content. According to the limited capacity model of attention [18], the total capacity allocated to process activities can be divided into the primary capacity for the most important task and the spare capacity for less important tasks. When an inconsistent ad is placed in the primary task field, audiences may reduce the likelihood of primary capability being allocated to processing the ad. Advertising relevance decreases ad skepticism and ad avoidance in e-mails, direct mails, telemarketing, and text messages [38]. Hence, we make Hypothesis 4:

Hypothesis 4 (H4). *The relevance of health-related short-video ads positively affects users' perceived usefulness (PU) of ads.*

Perceived usefulness (PU) refers to the degree to which individuals perceive the use of health-related short-video ads. If users think that short-video ads are useful, they are much likely to have a positive attitude on using them. Attracting and motivating short-video ads can also lead to purchase intention [2]. Hence, we make Hypotheses 5 and 6 as follows:

Hypothesis 5 (H5). *Users' perceived usefulness of health-related short-video ads positively affects their attitudes toward ads.*

Hypothesis 6 (H6). *Users' perceived usefulness of health-related short-video ads positively affects their purchase intentions.*

Perceived ease of use (PEOU) is defined as the mobile phone users' expectations about the effort required to use live video advertising messages. Short-video advertising requires some cognitive effort from users such as maneuvering through screens, reading the advertising, and making a quick evaluation of whether it is worthy (in terms of time or effort) to take further action. Therefore, the easier they perceive using short-video advertisements to be in general, the more likely they are to later engage in the action implied by the ad. Hence, we make Hypotheses 7 and 8:

Hypothesis 7 (H7). *Users' perceived ease of use of health-related short-video ads positively affects their perceived usefulness.*

Hypothesis 8 (H8). *Users' perceived ease of use of health-related short-video ads positively affects their attitudes toward ads.*

Attitude towards advertising is regarded as an important factor for advertising management because consumers' attitude can influence purchase intention [39]. Previous research has indicated that purchase intention is a critical indicator of advertising effectiveness and may be affected by indicators such as attitude towards ads [2,12,36]. For example, Lin and Kim found that the attitude towards ads affected brand awareness and purchase intentions [2]. Tran found that purchase intention was positively affected by ad attitude on Facebook [40]. Whether consumers prefer a product or an advertisement depends on the informativeness of the advertisement, i.e., whether the advertisement can provide the opportunity and convenient ways for purchase. Therefore, the informational nature of advertisement affects the consumer's purchase intention. Based on these observations, we make the following hypothesis:

Hypothesis 9 (H9). *Users' attitudes of health-related short-video ads positively affect their purchase intentions.*

Note that we only set up the Hypotheses H1–H4 to measure the impact of the four constructs on PU but not on PEOU. This is mainly because the constructs are all about the information offered by advertisements, but not about the operations or behavior of advertising. On the other hand, the perceived ease of use (PEOU) refers to the ease of operations that users perceive, i.e., PEOU is operation related. Thus, in this paper, we only focus on the impact of the constructs on PU.

4. Data Collection and Measurement

4.1. Data Collection

We mainly conducted questionnaires on users who have online shopping experiences due to mobile live ads, so that we could gain useful feedback from experienced users on short-video platforms. The data for this study were collected using an online survey in Douyu.com (a famous short-video platform in China) during January 2018, which lasted for three weeks. Three hundred and fifty questionnaires were sent to the viewers with anchors' help, and 289 questionnaires were received. Thirty-three questionnaires that contained inconsistent answers or incomplete information filling were removed from the data set.

Note that it is not possible to ask the Douyu platform to only present health-related short-video ads to the participants, because the platform does not offer the function of filtering health-related short-videos (actually, this could be a complicated task which needs effective algorithms). We offered the participants three weeks to return questionnaires, and all questions were restricted to health-related short-video ads (an example is given in Figure 1). Although we do not know what health-related videos the participants watched, we believe that the involved short-videos covers a wide range of health-related products. This is because the number of short videos on the Douyu platform is dramatically increasing day by day. In addition, different users have various interests, so the platform will recommend different short-video ads to each user.

Specifically, we asked three Douyu anchors for help, namely Prisoner, Valila, and Liu shaji, to distribute the questionnaires to their fans. The time span of the questionnaires was from January 3, 2018 to January 24, 2018. Consequently, we collected 256 valid questionnaires, which met the analytical requirements of the structural equation model.

In the data set, the proportions of males and females were 53.5% and 46.5%, respectively. There were 79.8% users that were under 30 years old. The duration of using live videos ranged from 0 to 2 years, and 58.6% of the users had experienced live videos for 1 to 2 years. Furthermore. 50.4% of the users were undergraduates and graduates (see Table 2). The attributes of the surveyed data were similar to those in the IResearch report (IResearch, The research report on the China mobile live video market, http://wreport.iresearch.cn/uploadfiles/reports/636161408839324949.pdf).

Table 2. Statistics of the surveyed users.

Measure	Frequency	Percentage (%)
Gender		
female	119	46.5
male	137	53.5
Age		
<30	204	79.8
≥30	52	20.2
Education		
Below bachelor's	79	30.9
Bachelor's	129	50.4
Master's	39	15.2
Ph.D.	9	3.5
Years of using short videos		
Less than 1 year	45	17.6
1–2 years	150	58.6
More than 2 years	61	23.8
Short video Usage		
Everyday	79	30.9
5–6 days per week	70	27.3
3–4 days per week	66	25.8
Once or twice a week	41	16

4.2. Measurement

The survey was designed using a multi-item approach. All variables were carried out by a five-point Likert-scale, ranging from strongly disagree (1) to strongly agree (5). Items were borrowed from previous literature and modified for the context of this study.

The questionnaire consisted of three parts:

(1) Sample Selection: Users who have online shopping experiences due to mobile live ads are considered as samples in this study.
(2) Sample Characteristics: This part mainly measures the sample statistical data of participants.
(3) Variable Questionnaire: This study included eight latent variables, including Social interaction (SI), Intrusiveness (IR), Informativeness (IN), Relevance (RE), Perceived Usefulness (PU), Perceived ease of use (PE), Ad attitudes (AT), and Purchase Intention (PI).

The whole items are shown in Table 3.

Table 3. Summary of measurement scales constructs (in the table, short video refers to health-related short videos).

Construct	Item	Source
Social Interaction	SI1: Short video ads provide me the opportunity to have lively, interesting, and engaging interaction with others SI2: In general, I think that short video ads strongly facilitate social interactions SI3: Overall, I am very satisfied with the social aspects of short video ads	Animesh et al.(2011) [41]; Fan et al.(2017) [19]
Intrusiveness	IR1: Short video ads are an insult to one's intelligence IR2: Short video ads are bothersome IR3: Short video ads are disappointing IR4: Short video ads are irritating	Chowdhury et al. (2010) [42]; Pintado et al. (2017) [15]
Informativeness	IN1: Short video ads are a good source of information on products IN2: Short video ads offer opportune information on products IN3: Short video ads are a good source of updated information	Chowdhury et al. (2010) [42]; Pintado et al. (2017) [15]
Relevance	RE1: The presentation style of short video ads is my favorite one RE2: The theme of advertising is very close to my interest RE3: The function of advertising fits well with my needs	Wang et al. (2013) [43]; Fan et al. (2017) [19]
Perceived Usefulness	PU1: Short video ads would enable me to purchase favorite products PU2: Short video ads would enable me to broaden my understanding of the product or service PU3: Short video ads provide valuable information for products	Ducoffe (1996) [8]; Lin & Kim (2016) [2]
Perceived Ease of Use	PE1: Learning how to participate in short video ads would be easy for me (viewing, clicking and commenting) PE2: Participating in short video ads takes less time and effort PE3: Short video ads can link products directly	Ducoffe (1996) [8]; Lin & Kim (2016) [2]
Ad Attitude	AT1: I like the sponsored advertisement section in short video AT2: I like pictures uploaded by ad sponsors on short videos AT3: I'll be positive about short video ads AT4: I like the style of short video ads	Taylor et al. (2011) [10]; Lin & Kim (2016) [2]
Purchase Intention	PI1: I will buy miscellaneous products shown on short video ads PI2: I intend to purchase products shown on short video ads PI3: I will recommend products shown on short videos to others	Lin & Kim (2016) [2]

5. Data Analysis and Results

The research model was tested using AMOS 21, a structural modeling technique that is well suited for estimating parameters and theoretical models. In Section 5.1, we use confirmatory factor analysis

(CFA) to validate the reliability and validity of the measurement model. In Section 5.2, we perform maximum likelihood estimation (MLE) and the bootstrapping method to examine the structural model. In Section 5.3, we measure the mediating effects of PU and AT in the research model. In Section 5.4, we summarize the conclusion of the research.

Before measuring the model, we examined whether common method bias was a concern in this study with two tests of common method variance (CMV) [44]. First, an exploratory factor analysis of all items extracted eight factors, which explained 73.72% of all the variance, with no single factor accounting for significant loadings (at the $p < 0.10$ level) for all items. Second, single method-factor approaches indicated that there was no significant difference among the method factors (ΔCMIN/DF = −0.032, ΔGFI = 0.009, ΔAGFI = 0.001, ΔIFI = 0.003, ΔRMSEA = −0.002). Thus, we concluded that CMV was not a concern in this data set.

5.1. Measurement Model Evaluation

The measurement model evaluation mainly included three parts, namely reliability analysis, convergent validity, and discriminant validity.

Reliability is usually examined by using internal consistency reliability and composite reliability. As shown in Table 4, the coefficient alpha for the eight variables scored in the range from 0.800 to 0.907 (more than 0.70 [45]). The composite reliability (CR) of all constructs was above 0.70 [46]. The reliability of the model was achieved.

Convergent validity is usually examined by using composite reliability (CR) and average variance extracted (AVE). As shown in Table 4, all items load significantly on their respective constructs and none of the loadings is below the cutoff value of 0.70. AVE of each variable was more than 0.50 [47]. Thus, convergent validity was achieved.

Discriminant validity is analyzed to examine whether a measurement is not a reflection of any other measurement or not. As shown in Table 5, the square root of AVE for each variable is greater than the other correlation coefficients. The discriminant validity of the model is achieved.

Table 4. Statistics of construct items.

Variable	Item	Factor Loading	Cronbach's α	CR	AVE	Mean	S. D.
Social Interaction	SI1	0.76	0.800	0.805	0.580	3.753	0.895
	SI2	0.70					
	SI3	0.82					
Intrusiveness	IR1	0.78	0.889	0.899	0.691	3.787	0.886
	IR2	0.84					
	IR3	0.89					
	IR4	0.81					
Informativeness	IN1	0.84	0.886	0.884	0.717	2.354	0.974
	IN2	0.85					
	IN3	0.85					
Relevance	RE1	0.84	0.907	0.909	0.769	3.777	0.946
	RE2	0.90					
	RE3	0.89					
Perceived Usefulness	PU1	0.77	0.828	0.824	0.609	3.583	0.990
	PU2	0.76					
	PU3	0.81					

Table 4. Cont.

Variable	Item	Factor Loading	Cronbach's α	CR	AVE	Mean	S. D.
Perceived Ease of use	PR1	0.85	0.898	0.898	0.746	3.900	0.926
	PR2	0.90					
	PR3	0.84					
Ad Attitude	AT1	0.77	0.862	0.867	0.621	3.768	1.002
	AT2	0.81					
	AT3	0.80					
	AT4	0.77					
Purchase Intention	PI1	0.86	0.892	0.893	0.735	3.620	1.145
	PI2	0.90					
	PI3	0.81					

Table 5. Correlations between constructs (AVE and squared correlations).

	1	2	3	4	5	6	7	8
1 Social Interaction	0.762							
2 Intrusiveness	−0.122	0.831						
3 Informativeness	0.116	−0.237	0.847					
4 Relevance	0.329	−0.248	0.253	0.78				
5 Perceived Ease of Use	0.003	0.241	−0.23	0.163	0.864			
6 Perceived Usefulness	0.224	−0.114	0.101	0.293	−0.021	0.877		
7 Ad Attitude	0.194	−0.127	0.131	0.6	0.174	0.171	0.788	
8 Purchase Intention	0.113	−0.08	0.082	0.344	0.073	0.1	0.353	0.857

Note: The numbers in the diagonal row are square roots of the average variance extracted.

5.2. Structural Model Evaluation

The research model was tested by using AMOS 23, and a bootstrapping resampling procedure (2000 samples) was used to ensure the solidity.

The resulting indices indicated a good model fit ($x2/df$ = 1.318; GFI = 0.903; RMSEA = 0.035; NFI = 0.909; CFI = 0.976; TLI = 0.972; RMR = 0.071; SRMR = 0.058).

Figure 3 shows that social interaction (SI), informativeness (IN), and relevance (RE) of health-related short-video ads were significant and positive predictors of perceive usefulness of ads (β = 0.23, p < 0.01; β = 0.22, p < 0.01; β = 0.20, p < 0.01). These findings support H1, H3, and H4, respectively, and this supports previous studies [12,19]. Similarly, intrusiveness (IR) of health-related short-video ads was a significant and negative predictor of the perceive usefulness of ads (β = −0.21, p < 0.01), and H2 is validated. This is consistent with previous research [2,15]. These four factors (SI, IR, IN, and RE) explained 29% of the variance in the perceived usefulness of health-related short-video ads. Additionally, comparing these four coefficients, we found social interaction was more important to users' perceived usefulness of ads. Users' perceived usefulness of health-related short-video ads positively affected their attitudes toward ads (β = 0.59, p < 0.001) and purchase intention (β = 0.21, p < 0.05); these results validate H5 and H6. Users' perceived ease of use of health-related short-video ads was a significant and positive predictor of perceived usefulness of ads (β = 0.27, p < 0.001), and H7 is validated. However, users' perceived ease of use of health-related short-video ads could not significantly predict users' attitudes toward ads. H8 is not validated and this is not consistent with Lin and Kim' research, as they found users' perceived ease of use of social media ads significantly predict users' attitudes [2]. This enlightens us that perceived ease of use may not be an important factor in health-related short-video ads. Therefore, only users' perceived usefulness of ads explained 37% of the variance in attitudes toward ads. Finally, users' attitudes of health-related short-video ads were found to positively predict their purchase intentions ($\beta = 0.23$, $p < 0.05$), and H9 is validated. Users' perceived usefulness of ads and attitudes toward ads accounted for 33% of the variance in purchase intentions.

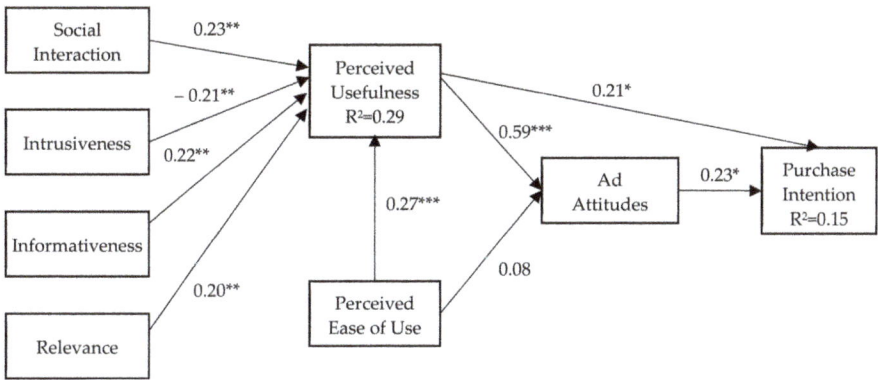

Note: *** $p < 0.001$, ** $p < 0.01$, * $p < 0.05$; R^2 is the coefficient of determination.

Figure 3. Results of structural model evaluation.

5.3. Mediating Effects Analysis

Mediation analyses were tested using the Preacher and Hayes' bootstrapping (2000 bootstrap samples) analysis with the PROCESS macro [48]. We focused on two mediate variables (perceived usefulness and ad attitudes) to find the impact path of user responses to health-related short-video advertisements because users' perceived ease of use of health-related short-video ads cannot significantly predict users' attitudes toward ads. The results are shown in Table 6.

The mediating path (Social Interaction→PU→AT) tested the specific indirect effect of social interaction of ads on ad attitudes through perceived usefulness of ads. As both the upper and lower limits of the confidence interval (CI) were above zero (0.014, 0.166), this indirect effect can be interpreted as significantly positive. Similarly, the direct effect of the perceived usefulness of ads can be interpreted as significantly positive. Hence, the perceived usefulness of ads served as a partial mediating variable between social interaction and ad attitudes. That means those who perceived the sociality of health-related short-video ads believed that the ad was more useful, and this increased usefulness enhances the viewers' positive attitudes toward the ad.

The mediating path (Intrusiveness→PU→AT) tested the specific indirect effect of intrusiveness of ads on ad attitudes through perceived usefulness of ads. As both the upper and lower limits of the confidence interval (CI) were above zero (−0.134, −0.018), this indirect effect can be interpreted as significantly positive. The perceived usefulness of ads served as a partial mediating variable between intrusiveness and ad attitudes. That means those who perceived intrusiveness of health-related short-video ads believed that the ad was less useful, and this decreased usefulness enhances the viewers' negative attitudes toward the ad.

Table 6. Mediating effects analysis.

Path	Effect	Bootstrapping (2000 Bootstrap Samples)				Result
		Bias-Corrected 95% CI		Percentile 95% CI		
		Lower	Upper	Lower	Upper	
Social Interaction→PU→AT	total	0.104	0.418	0.095	0.407	Partial mediation
	direct	0.024	0.348	0.014	0.33	
	indirect	0.014	0.166	0.013	0.162	
Intrusiveness→PU→AT	total	−0.355	−0.088	−0.355	−0.087	Partial mediation
	direct	−0.285	−0.02	−0.282	−0.018	
	indirect	−0.134	−0.018	−0.133	−0.017	
Informativeness→PU→AT	total	0.118	0.367	0.113	0.358	Partial mediation
	direct	0.025	0.308	0.018	0.299	
	indirect	0.011	0.164	0.01	0.162	
Relevance→PU→AT	total	0.079	0.366	0.071	0.36	Failed
	direct	0.017	0.32	0.008	0.313	
	indirect	−0.003	0.159	−0.01	0.147	
Perceived Ease of Use →PU→AT	total	0.129	0.467	0.123	0.459	Partial mediation
	direct	0.051	0.378	0.035	0.363	
	indirect	0.024	0.188	0.02	0.184	
Social Interaction→PU→PI	total	−0.081	0.287	−0.082	0.287	Failed
	direct	−0.164	0.21	−0.163	0.21	
	indirect	0.015	0.199	0.009	0.176	
Intrusiveness→PU→PI	total	−0.272	0.072	−0.273	0.068	Failed
	direct	−0.22	0.133	−0.221	0.133	
	indirect	−0.144	−0.012	−0.14	−0.011	
Informativeness→PU→PI	total	−0.138	0.189	−0.126	0.197	Failed
	direct	−0.2	0.135	−0.193	0.143	
	indirect	0.01	0.161	0.006	0.155	
Relevance→PU→PI	total	0.013	0.353	0.013	0.354	Failed
	direct	−0.059	0.3	−0.05	0.308	
	indirect	−0.001	0.161	−0.01	0.141	
Perceived Ease of Use→PU→PI	total	0.099	0.479	0.085	0.466	Partial mediation
	direct	0.009	0.383	0.002	0.378	
	indirect	0.018	0.195	0.014	0.185	
Perceived Usefulness→AT→PI	total	0.216	0.615	0.218	0.618	Full mediation
	direct	−0.007	0.511	−0.015	0.507	
	indirect	0.026	0.368	0.024	0.358	

The mediating path (Informativeness→PU→AT) tested the specific indirect effect of informativeness of ads on ad attitudes through perceived usefulness of ads. Perceived usefulness of ads served as a partial mediating variable between informativeness and ad attitudes (CI: 0.011, 0.164). That means those who perceived informativeness of health-related short-video ads believed that the ad was more useful, and this increased usefulness enhances the viewers' positive attitudes toward the ad.

The mediating path (PEOU→PU→AT) tested the specific indirect effect of perceived ease of use of ads on ad attitudes through perceived usefulness of ads. Perceived usefulness of ads served as a partial mediating variable between perceived ease of use and ad attitudes (CI: 0.024, 0.188). That means those who perceived ease of use of health-related short-video ads believed that the ad was more useful, and this increased usefulness enhances the viewers' positive attitudes toward the ad.

Similarly, the perceived usefulness of ads served as a partial mediating variable between perceived ease of use and purchase intentions (CI: 0.018, 0.195). That means those who perceived ease of use of health-related short-video ads believed that the ad was more useful, and this increased usefulness enhances the viewers' purchase intentions.

Finally, the mediating path (PU→AT→PI) tested the specific indirect effect of perceived usefulness of ads on purchase intention through ad attitudes. The indirect effect was significant (CI: 0.026, 0.368) while the direct effect was not significant (CI: −0.007, 0.511). Hence, ad attitudes served as a full mediating variable between perceived usefulness and purchase intention. That means users' attitude toward health-related short-video ads was a key path to the effectiveness of ads.

In summary, there were four impact paths of user responses to health-related short-video advertisements. First, social interaction had an indirect effect on purchase intentions through perceived usefulness and ad attitudes in serial (SI→PU→AT→PI). Second, intrusiveness had an indirect effect on purchase intentions through perceived usefulness and ad attitudes in serial (IR→PU→AT→PI). Third, informativeness had an indirect effect on purchase intentions through perceived usefulness and ad attitudes in serial (IN→PU→AT→PI). Fourth, perceived ease of use had an indirect effect on purchase intentions through perceived usefulness and ad attitudes in serial (PE→PU→AT→PI).

5.4. Summary of Hypothesis Validation

By combing the results described in Section 5.1–Section 5.3, we present the summary of the hypothesis validation in Table 7.

Table 7. Summary of hypotheses validation.

Number	Hypothesis	Validation Result
H1	Social interaction of health-related short video ads positively affects users' perceived usefulness (PU) of ads.	Established
H2	Intrusiveness of health-related short video ads negatively affects users' perceived usefulness (PU) of ads.	Established
H3	Informativeness of health-related short video ads positively affects users' perceived usefulness (PU) of ads.	Established
H4	Relevance of health-related short video ads positively affects users' perceived usefulness (PU) of ads.	Established
H5	Users' perceived usefulness of health-related short video ads positively affects their attitudes toward ads.	Established
H6	Users' perceived usefulness of health-related short video ads positively affects their purchase intentions.	Established
H7	Users' perceived ease of use of health-related short video ads positively affects their perceived usefulness.	Established
H8	Users' perceived ease of use of health-related short video ads positively affects their attitudes toward ads.	Not established
H9	Users' attitudes of health-related short video ads positively affect their purchase intentions.	Established

The validation-result column in Table 7 shows the final validation results of each hypothesis, from which we can see that H1-H4 are well established. These hypotheses correspond with the research questions RQ1 and RQ2 presented in Table 1. This implies that five qualities (social interaction, intrusiveness, informativeness, relevance, and perceived ease of use) of health-related short-video ads help enhance the perceived usefulness of ads. Among all the factors, according to different coefficients, social interaction of health-related short-video ads made a more valuable contribution to advertising usefulness. Thus, advertisers and marketers should not only focus on social interaction, intrusiveness, informativeness, relevance, and the perceived ease of use of health-related short-video ads, but also pay more attention to social interaction.

Regarding hypotheses H5, H7, and H8, which aim to answer RQ3, only the perceived usefulness of health-related short-video ads helped produce positive user attitudes. H9 answers RQ4, finding that positive user attitudes significantly promotef purchase intentions. Combined with the analysis of the mediating effects in Section 5.3, we found four impact paths of user responses to health-related short-video advertisements (SI→PU→AT→PI; IR→PU→AT→PI; IN→PU→AT→PI; PE→PU→AT→PI). This answers RQ5. Thus, advertisers and marketers may maximize resource utilization through the impact paths.

6. Discussions

6.1. Research Implications

(1) The study of this paper is based on the background of online ads in the health-related short video, which has become an important field for the expansion of social media and a part of people's daily life. Due to the value of short-video ads, it is necessary to explore user responses to short-video advertisements. We propose a research model based on the integration of the TAM model, social interaction, intrusiveness, informativeness, and relevance. This model augments the application of the widely used TAM model and offers referential values for other related researches. In addition, we present empirical results on user acceptance of participating in health-related short-video ads. These results can provide new research insights for advancing health-related short-video advertisements, e.g., a socially interactive mechanism for mobile ads.

(2) This paper studies users' purchase intention towards health-related short-video ads and is valuable for advertisers and marketers to realize the importance of developing health-related short-video advertisements. With the rapid development of technologies and social entertainment, users' attitudes toward online ads may have changed a lot. Short video has been a promising tool for seeking business opportunities and establishing brand expression, and advertisers need to keep reforming their advertising strategy to meet user needs.

(3) According to the empirical study conducted in this paper, the five factors (social interaction, intrusiveness, informativeness, relevance, and perceived ease of use) defined in the research model are helpful to enhance the perceived usefulness of health-related short-video ads, which can in turn affect user acceptance of health-related short-video ads. The results indicated that social interaction, informativeness, and relevance of advertisements are all positive factors, while intrusiveness is a negative factor, meaning that the increasing of intrusiveness will lower the user acceptance of health-related short-video ads. These results are consistent to what were revealed by previous studies [12,15,19]. Furthermore, compared with other factors, social interaction showed a higher impact to the perceived usefulness of short-video ads. This is a new finding of the study. While advertisers should be mindful of multiple aspects of ads, including intrusiveness, informativeness, relevance, and perceived ease of use, they should largely focus their efforts on the social interactions that stem from these ads.

(4) We also find that users' perceived ease of use of health-related short-video ads cannot significantly predict users' attitudes toward short-video ads. This does not support Lin and Kim' research conclusions [2], i.e., users' perceived ease of use of social media ads significantly predict users' attitudes toward ads. To this end, the perceived ease of use may not be an important factor in health-related short-video ads.

(5) We find four impact paths of user responses to health-related short-video advertisements (SI→PU→AT→PI; IR→PU→AT→PI; IN→PU→AT→PI; PE→PU→AT→PI) by mediating effects analysis. Thus, advertisers and marketers can maximize resource utilization through the impact paths and promote the effectiveness of health-related short-video ads.

6.2. Suggestions

The empirical analysis of this study can offer some useful hints for advertisers to advance short-video ads. Below, we present some suggestions for advertisers and marketers to better develop health-related short-video ads:

(1) Consider various factors when promoting short-video ads.

The results of this study show that the five factors (social interaction, intrusiveness, informativeness, relevance, and perceived ease of use) defined in the model can all positively affect the perceived usefulness of short-video ads. Thus, we suggest that advertisers should consider all five factors rather than focusing on one or some specific factors. For example, if advertisers neglect the 'relevance' factor, they might issue short-video ads in which the video content is irrelevant to the topic of the ads.

(2) Emphasize the social interactions of short-video ads.

Our study shows that social interaction is more influential to the perceived usefulness of short-video ads compared with other factors. Thus, we suggest advertisers to pay more attention to the social interactions of short-video ads, which is a shortcoming of current short-video ads. As shown in Figure 1, current short-video ads provide few ways for social interaction. They are much like an introduction of a product, which neglect the use of social interaction. However, the results of this study show that social interaction is a key construct for enhance user acceptance of short-video ads. Therefore, we strongly suggest advertisers to design social-interaction tools in short-video ads. For example, they can embed a voting button in a video by using new technologies like HTML5 to let video viewers submit their choices.

(3) Focus on users' perceived usefulness of short-video ads.

Through the mediating factor analysis, we found that users' perceived usefulness of short-video ads plays an important role in the impact path from the influential factors to users' purchase intention. Therefore, enhancing users' perceived usefulness of short-video ads is the key point of improving the effectiveness of short-video ads. On the one hand, advertisers should improve the quality of short-video ads, e.g., by increasing the informativeness and relevance of ads, or by providing new kinds of social interactions to attract users' attention. On the other hand, advertisers should avoid issuing any false advertisements, which are much harmful to consumers' confidence on products. Once users find that the short-video ads issued by an advertiser are over-claimed or false, the fast spreading of word-of-mouth on social network platforms will do considerable harm to the reputation of the advertiser.

(4) Advance ads on short-video social network platforms.

Short videos provide a free, real-time, and easy-to-access online way for enterprises to deliver ads to potential users. Recently, the number of the users on short-video social network platforms has shown a dramatical increasing trend, because live videos provide more attractive presentation than conventional textual web pages or tweets. Thus, it is important for enterprises to develop their short-video-based advertising systems and departments to advance ads on short-video social network platforms. Accordingly, the live short video as a new style of advertising could be utilized as a new tool to enhance the market competitiveness of enterprises.

7. Conclusions and Future Work

In this paper, we analyze the major factors that influence user responses to health-related short-video advertisements. Particularly, we made three contributions. First, we extended the Technology Acceptance Model (TAM) with new antecedents including social interaction (SI), intrusiveness (IR), informativeness (IN), and relevance (RE) to analyze the users' response to health-related short-video ads. We also introduced two mediate factors, i.e., perceived usefulness (PU) and ad attitude (AT), to reflect the influence of independent variables on the dependent variable named purchase intention (PI). To the best of our knowledge, this is the first study that extends the TAM model to analyze user acceptance of health-related short-video ads. Second, we conducted a survey on the Internet and short-video social network platforms and performed systematical data analysis over the surveyed data. The data analysis consisted of many aspects, including measurement model evaluation, structural model evaluation, and mediating effect analysis. The results showed that social interaction, intrusiveness, informativeness, relevance, and the TAM factors (perceived usefulness and perceived ease of use) had a significant influence on user acceptance of health-related short-video ads. Further, we found that users' perceived ease of use on health-related short-video ads could not significantly predict users' attitudes toward ads. This is a new finding that is contrary to previous studies in social media-oriented ads. Third, we presented reasonable suggestions for advertisers and marketers to better develop health-related short-video ads.

This study is beneficial for advertisers to realize the importance of understanding the effectiveness of health-related short-video ads. Base on the empirical results of this study, we gained some new findings, some of which are contrary to existing research. These findings are helpful to reveal the major factors that influence users' ad attitudes and intentions to purchase and to quantify the impacts of these factors on them. The suggestions made based on the empirical results of this study can provide some management ideas for advertisers and academia to develop health-related short-video ads.

Some limitations of this study can be summarized as follows. First, although hundreds of valid questionnaires are theoretically enough to conduct data analysis, in this big data era, this number is relatively small to draw reliable and robust conclusions. Second, the results of this study have shown that the four antecedents, as well as the perceived ease of use, have significant influences on perceived usefulness, attitude, and purchase intention towards mobile live ads. However, the inherent theoretical basis has not been revealed yet. Third, the survey in this study has some limitations. Currently, we are only able to survey people on a Chinese short-video platform. The model, as well as the results, may not extend to people in other countries or on other platforms. In addition, as the respondents in the survey mainly cover young people (79.8% of them were under 30 years old), the results may not suit those advertisements that target old people.

Thus, in the future, there are some research issues that are worth further investigating. First, a further study on secondary data collected from some crowdsourcing platforms like Amazon Mechanical Turk [49] could be better to analyze user acceptance of advertising and marketing on short-video platforms. Second, because users' decision-making behavior could be impacted by other factors, future work can be focused on other possible factors, such as users' educational background and online experiences. Finally, in addition to the TAM model, it is also worth studying other research models within the big data and online community context [50].

Author Contributions: J.Z.: Conceptualization, project administration, supervision, and writing—original draft, J.W.: Data curation, formal analysis, investigation, and software. All authors have read and agreed to the published version of the manuscript.

Funding: This paper is partially supported by the National Science Foundation of China (No. 71273010).

Acknowledgments: We would like to thank the editors and anonymous reviewers for their suggestions and comments to improve the quality of the paper.

Conflicts of Interest: The authors declare no conflict of interest.

References

1. Alalwan, A. Investigating the impact of social media advertising features on customer purchase intention. *Int. J. Inf. Manag.* **2018**, *42*, 65–77. [CrossRef]
2. Lin, C.; Kim, T. Predicting user response to sponsored advertising on social media via the technology acceptance model. *Comput. Hum. Behav.* **2016**, *64*, 710–718. [CrossRef]
3. China Internet Network Information Center (CNNIC). The forty-first China statistical report on the development of the Internet. Available online: www.cnnic.net.cn/hlwfzyj/hlwxzbg/hlwtjbg/201801/P020180131509544165973.pdf (accessed on 3 January 2020).
4. Wang, X.; Tian, Y.; Lan, R.; Yang, W.; Zhang, X. Beyond the Watching: Understanding Viewer Interactions in Crowdsourced Live Video Broadcasting Services. *IEEE Trans. Circuits Syst. Video Technol.* **2019**, *29*, 3454–3468. [CrossRef]
5. Hamouda, M. Understanding social media advertising effect on consumers' responses: An empirical investigation of tourism advertising on Facebook. *J. Enterprise Inf. Management.* **2018**, *31*, 426–445. [CrossRef]
6. Krämer, J.; Schnurr, D.; Wohlfarth, M. Winners, losers, and Facebook: The role of social logins in the online advertising ecosystem. *Manag. Sci.* **2019**, *65*, 1678–1699. [CrossRef]
7. Zhang, H.; Cao, X.; Ho, J.; Chow, T. Object-level video advertising: An optimization framework. *IEEE Trans. Ind. Inform.* **2017**, *13*, 520–531. [CrossRef]
8. Ducoffe, R. Advertising value and advertising on the web. *J. Advert. Res.* **1996**, *36*, 21.
9. Khalis, A.; Mikami, A. Talking face-to-Facebook: Associations between online social interactions and offline relationships. *Comput. Hum. Behav.* **2018**, *89*, 88–97. [CrossRef]
10. Taylor, D.; Lewin, J.; Strutton, D. Friends, fans, and followers: Do ads work on social networks? How gender and age shape receptivity. *J. Advert. Res.* **2011**, *51*, 258–275. [CrossRef]
11. Sun, X.; Han, M.; Feng, J. Helpfulness of online reviews: Examining review informativeness and classification thresholds by search products and experience products. *Decis. Support Syst.* **2019**, *124*, 113099. [CrossRef]
12. Dehghani, M.; Niaki, M.K.; Ramezani, I.; Sali, R. Evaluating the influence of YouTube advertising for attraction of young customers. *Comput. Hum. Behav.* **2016**, *59*, 165–172. [CrossRef]
13. Lee, J.; Hong, I.B. Predicting positive user responses to social media advertising: The roles of emotional appeal, informativeness, and creativity. *Int. J. Inf. Manag.* **2016**, *36*, 360–373. [CrossRef]
14. Stafford, M.; Faber, R. *Advertising, Promotion, and New Media*; Taylor & Francis Group: New York, NY, USA, 2015.
15. Pintado, T.; Sanchez, J.; Carcelén, S.; Alameda, D. The effects of digital media advertising content on message acceptance or rejection: Brand trust as a moderating factor. *J. Internet Commer.* **2017**, *16*, 364–384. [CrossRef]
16. Jung, A. The influence of perceived ad relevance on social media advertising: An empirical examination of a mediating role of privacy concern. *Comput. Hum. Behav.* **2017**, *70*, 303–309. [CrossRef]
17. Panniello, U.; Hill, S.; Gorgoglione, M. The impact of profit incentives on the relevance of online recommendations. *Electron. Commer. Res. Appl.* **2016**, *20*, 87–104. [CrossRef]
18. Kahneman, D. *Attention and Effort. Prentice-Hall Series in Experimental Psychology*; Prentice-Hall: Englewood Cliffs, NJ, USA, 1973.
19. Fan, S.; Lu, Y. Sumeetgupta, Social media in-feed advertising: The impacts of consistency and sociability on ad avoidance. *Proc. PACIS* **2017**. Article No. 190.
20. Mao, E.; Zhang, J. What affects users to click on display ads on social media? The roles of message values, involvement, and security. *J. Inf. Priv. Secur.* **2017**, *13*, 84–96. [CrossRef]
21. Zeng, F.; Huang, L.; Dou, W. Social factors in user perceptions and responses to advertising in online social networking communities. *J. Interact. Advert.* **2009**, *10*, 1–13. [CrossRef]
22. Windels, K.; Heo, J.; Jeong, Y.; Porter, L.; Jung, A.; Wang, R. My friend likes this brand: Do ads with social context attract more attention on social networking sites? *Comput. Hum. Behav.* **2018**, *84*, 420–429. [CrossRef]
23. Davis, F. Perceived usefulness, perceived ease of use and user acceptance of information technology. *Mis. Q.* **1989**, *13*, 319–340. [CrossRef]
24. Zhao, J.; Zhu, C.; Peng, Z.; Xu, X.; Liu, Y. User willingness toward knowledge sharing in social networks. *Sustainability* **2018**, *10*, 4680. [CrossRef]
25. Marakarkandy, B.; Yajnik, N.; Dasgupta, C. Enabling internet banking adoption: An empirical examination with an augmented technology acceptance model (TAM). *J. Enterp. Inf. Manag.* **2017**, *30*, 263–294. [CrossRef]

26. Zhao, J.; Fang, S.; Jin, P. Modeling and quantifying user acceptance of personalized business modes based on TAM, trust and attitude. *Sustainability* **2018**, *10*, 356. [CrossRef]
27. Demangeot, C.; Broderick, A.J. Consumer perceptions of online shopping environments: A gestalt approach. *Psychol. Mark.* **2010**, *27*, 117–140. [CrossRef]
28. Venkatesh, V.; Morris, M.; Davis, G.; Davis, F. User acceptance of information technology: Toward a unified view. *Mis. Q.* **2003**, *27*, 425–478. [CrossRef]
29. Venkatesh, V.; Thong, J.; Xu, X. Consumer acceptance and use of information: Extending the unified theory of acceptance and use of technology. *Mis. Q.* **2012**, *36*, 157–178. [CrossRef]
30. Kim, S.; Lee, K.; Hwang, H.; Yoo, S. Analysis of the factors influencing healthcare professionals' adoption of mobile electronic medical record (EMR) using the unified theory of acceptance and use of technology (UTAUT) in a tertiary hospital. *BMC Med Inform. Decis. Mak.* **2016**, *16*, 12. [CrossRef]
31. Im, I.; Hong, S. Kang, An international comparison of technology adoption: Testing the UTAUT model. *Inf. Manag.* **2011**, *48*, 1–8. [CrossRef]
32. Dwivedi, Y.; Rana, N.; Jeyaraj, A.; Clement, M.; Williams, M. Re-examining the unified theory of acceptance and use of technology (UTAUT): Towards a revised theoretical model. *Inf. Syst. Front.* **2019**, *21*, 719–734. [CrossRef]
33. Kreijns, K.; Kirschner, P.A.; Jochems, W.; van Buuren, H. Measuring perceived sociability of computer-supported collaborative learning environments. *Comput. Educ.* **2007**, *49*, 176–192. [CrossRef]
34. McCoy, S.; Everard, A.; Galletta, D.; Moody, G. Here we go again! The impact of website ad repetition on recall, intrusiveness, attitudes, and site revisit intentions. *Inf. Manag.* **2017**, *54*, 14–24. [CrossRef]
35. Hühn, A.; Khan, V.; Ketelaar, P.; Jonathan, V.; Konig, R.; Rozendaal, E.; Batalas, N.; Markopoulos, P. Does location congruence matter? A field study on the effects of location-based advertising on perceived ad intrusiveness, relevance & value. *Comput. Hum. Behav.* **2017**, *73*, 659–668.
36. Du, B.; Wang, Z.; Zhang, L.; Zhang, L.; Liu, W.; Shen, J.; Tao, D. Exploring representativeness and informativeness for active learning. *IEEE Trans. Cybern.* **2017**, *47*, 14–26. [CrossRef]
37. de Mooij, M.; Hofstede, G. The Hofstede model: Applications to global branding and advertising strategy and research. *Int. J. Advert.* **2010**, *29*, 85–110. [CrossRef]
38. Nie, H.; Yang, Y.; Zeng, D. Keyword generation for sponsored search advertising: Balancing coverage and relevance. *IEEE Intell. Syst.* **2019**, *34*, 14–24. [CrossRef]
39. Can, L.; Kaya, N. Social networking sites addiction and the effect of attitude towards social network advertising. *Procedia-Soc. Behav. Sci.* **2016**, *235*, 484–492. [CrossRef]
40. Tran, T. Personalized ads on Facebook: An effective marketing tool for online marketers. *J. Retail. Consum. Serv.* **2017**, *39*, 230–242. [CrossRef]
41. Animesh, A.; Pinsonneault, A.; Yang, S.; Oh, W. An odyssey into virtual worlds: Exploring the impacts of technological and spatial environments on intention to purchase virtual products. *Mis. Q.* **2011**, *35*, 789–810. [CrossRef]
42. Chowdhury, H.; Parvin, N.; Weitenberner, C.; Becker, M. Consumer attitude toward mobile advertising in an emerging market: An empirical study. *Int. J. Mob. Mark.* **2006**, *1*, 1–12.
43. Wang, N.; Shen, X.; Sun, Y. Transition of electronic word-of-mouth services from web to mobile context: A trust transfer perspective. *Decis. Support Syst.* **2013**, *54*, 1394–1403. [CrossRef]
44. Podsakoff, P.; MacKenzie, S.; Lee, J.; Podsakoff, N. Common method biases in behavioral research: A critical review of the literature and recommended remedies. *J. Appl. Psychol.* **2003**, *88*, 879. [CrossRef]
45. Nunnally, J.; Bernstein, I. Psychometric Theory (3rd Ed.). McGrawHill, New York, USA, 1994.
46. Hair, J.; Black, C.; Babin, J.; Anderson, R.; Tatham, R. *Multivariate Data Analysis*, 5th version; Prentice-Hall: Upper Saddle River, NJ, USA, 1998.
47. Fornell, C.; Larcker, D. Evaluating structural equation models with unobservable variables and measurement error. *J. Mark. Res.* **1981**, *18*, 39–50. [CrossRef]
48. Preacher, K.; Hayes, A. Asymptotic and resampling strategies for assessing and comparing indirect effects in multiple mediator models. *Behav. Res. Methods* **2008**, *40*, 879–891. [CrossRef]
49. Amazon Mechanical Turk. Available online: https://www.mturk.com (accessed on 3 January 2020).

50. Zhao, J.; Wang, J.; Fang, S.; Jin, P. Towards sustainable development of online communities in the big data era: A study of the causes and possible consequence of voting on user reviews. *Sustainability* **2018**, *10*, 3156. [CrossRef]

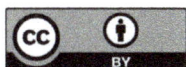

© 2020 by the authors. Licensee MDPI, Basel, Switzerland. This article is an open access article distributed under the terms and conditions of the Creative Commons Attribution (CC BY) license (http://creativecommons.org/licenses/by/4.0/).

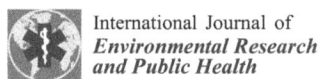

Article

Teleconsultations between Patients and Healthcare Professionals in Primary Care in Catalonia: The Evaluation of Text Classification Algorithms Using Supervised Machine Learning

Francesc López Seguí [1,2], Ricardo Ander Egg Aguilar [3], Gabriel de Maeztu [4], Anna García-Altés [5], Francesc García Cuyàs [6], Sandra Walsh [7], Marta Sagarra Castro [8] and Josep Vidal-Alaball [9,10,*]

1. TIC Salut Social—Ministry of Health, 08028 Barcelona, Spain; flopez@ticsalutsocial.cat
2. CRES&CEXS—Pompeu Fabra University, 08003 Barcelona, Spain
3. Faculty of Medicine, Barcelona University, 08036 Barcelona, Spain; ricardo.anderegg@gmail.com
4. IOMED Medical Solutions, 08041 Barcelona, Spain; gabriel.maeztu@iomed.es
5. Agency for Healthcare Quality and Evaluation of Catalonia (AQuAS), Catalan Ministry of Health, 08005 Barcelona, Spain; agarciaaltes@gencat.cat
6. Sant Joan de Déu Hospital, Catalan Ministry of Health, 08950 Barcelona, Spain; 31557fgc@gmail.com
7. Institut de Biologia Evolutiva (UPF-CSIC), Pompeu Fabra University, 08003 Barcelona, Spain; sandra.walsh34@gmail.com
8. Centre d'Atenció Primària Capellades, Gerència Territorial de la Catalunya Central, Institut Català de la Salut, 08786 Sant Fruitós de Bages, Spain; msagarra.cc.ics@gencat.cat
9. Health Promotion in Rural Areas Research Group, Gerència Territorial de la Catalunya Central, Institut Català de la Salut, 08272 Sant Fruitós de Bages, Spain
10. Unitat de Suport a la Recerca de la Catalunya Central, Fundació Institut Universitari per a la recerca a l'Atenció Primària de Salut Jordi Gol i Gurina, 08272 Sant Fruitós de Bages, Spain
* Correspondence: jvidal.cc.ics@gencat.cat

Received: 15 December 2019; Accepted: 7 February 2020; Published: 9 February 2020

Abstract: *Background*: The primary care service in Catalonia has operated an asynchronous teleconsulting service between GPs and patients since 2015 (eConsulta), which has generated some 500,000 messages. New developments in big data analysis tools, particularly those involving natural language, can be used to accurately and systematically evaluate the impact of the service. *Objective*: The study was intended to assess the predictive potential of eConsulta messages through different combinations of vector representation of text and machine learning algorithms and to evaluate their performance. *Methodology*: Twenty machine learning algorithms (based on five types of algorithms and four text representation techniques) were trained using a sample of 3559 messages (169,102 words) corresponding to 2268 teleconsultations (1.57 messages per teleconsultation) in order to predict the three variables of interest (avoiding the need for a face-to-face visit, increased demand and type of use of the teleconsultation). The performance of the various combinations was measured in terms of precision, sensitivity, F-value and the ROC curve. *Results*: The best-trained algorithms are generally effective, proving themselves to be more robust when approximating the two binary variables "avoiding the need of a face-to-face visit" and "increased demand" (precision = 0.98 and 0.97, respectively) rather than the variable "type of query" (precision = 0.48). *Conclusion*: To the best of our knowledge, this study is the first to investigate a machine learning strategy for text classification using primary care teleconsultation datasets. The study illustrates the possible capacities of text analysis using artificial intelligence. The development of a robust text classification tool could be feasible by validating it with more data, making it potentially more useful for decision support for health professionals.

Keywords: machine learning; teleconsultation; primary care; remote consultation; classification

1. Introduction

eConsulta is an asynchronous teleconsultation service between patients and GPs as part of the electronic health records of the public primary healthcare system of Catalonia. In operation since the end of 2015, this secure messaging service was designed to complement face-to-face consultations with primary healthcare teams (PHT). It was gradually implemented up until 2017, when the service became available to every PHT; currently, all of them have used this tool at least once.

An earlier study analysed the reasons why patients sought a consultation, which resulted in a patient–doctor interaction, as well as the subjective perception of the GP if they avoided a face-to-face visit or if it led to a consultation which otherwise would not have occurred, by means of a retrospective review of text messages relating to each case [1]. The results show there was a broad consensus among GPs that eConsulta has the potential to resolve patient queries (avoiding the need for a face-to-face visit in 88% of cases) for every type of consultation. In addition, GPs declared that ease of access led to an increase in demand (queries which otherwise would not have been made) in 28% of cases. Therefore, the possibility of eConsulta replacing a conventional appointment stands at between 88% and 63% (88% × (1 − 28%)). The most common use of e-consultation was for the management of test results (35%), clinical enquiries (16%) and the management of repeat prescriptions (12%).

Technology offers new possibilities for policy evaluation in conjunction with the aforementioned classical approaches. Artificial intelligence tools are already widely used in the field of healthcare in areas such as the prediction and management of depression, voice recognition for people with speech impediments, the detection of changes in the biopsychosocial status of patients with multiple morbidities, stress control, the treatment of phantom limb pain, smoking cessation, personalized nutrition by prediction of glycaemic response, to try to detect signs of depression and in particular for reading medical images [2–6]. The generation of data implies a huge potential for the impact assessment of these interventions with new analytical tools.

The classification of texts in the medical field has also been used to conduct a review of influenza detection and prediction through social networking sites [7–9] and in the analysis of texts from internet forums [10,11]. More specifically, in the framework of teleconsultations, a US-based study used machine learning to annotate 3000 secure message threads involving patients with diabetes and clinical teams according to whether they contained patient-reported hypoglycaemia incidents [12]. As far as the authors are aware, no study has looked into the development of a text classification algorithm in the context of teleconsultations between patients and primary care physicians.

The present study aims to evaluate specific text classification algorithms for eConsulta messages and to validate their predictive potential. The algorithms have been trained using a vector representation of text from the body of the message and the three variable annotations that primary healthcare professionals in Central Catalonia used in a previous study: avoiding the need for a face-to-face visit, increased demand and type of use of the teleconsultation [1]. Our study represents an exhaustive exploratory analysis of text classification algorithms of teleconsultation messages between GPs and patients that can provide useful information for future research and a potential use for decision support in healthcare.

2. Methodology

2.1. Data Acquisition

The teleconsultations that had previously been classified that were used as the basis for training the algorithm are those which were acquired in the study by a previous study (López) (Table 1). They are part of the health records of the *Gerència Territorial de la Catalunya Central* of the *Institut Català de la Salut* covering the period from when the tool was first used until the date of its extraction for analysis purposes (8 April 2016 to 18 August 2018). Message deidentification was performed by substituting all possible names contained in the Statistical Institute of Catalonia database [13] with a common token and removing all other personal attributes. The classification method used for the conversations is described and justified by López et al. 2019: Every healthcare professional who received an eConsulta labelled it according to whether, in their opinion, it avoided the need for a face-to-face consultation, led to an increased demand and by type of teleconsultation (Appendix A.1). These results of this annotation, with the corresponding messages, were used to train the text classification model using the three variables previously mentioned (Table 2).

Table 1. Data recorded by the teleconsulting system.

Conversation Title	Conversation ID	Message ID	From	To	Message	Files Attached?
Travelling to Australia	C1	M1	Mr. John Patient	Ms. Jane Doctor	Dear doctor, I'm travelling to Australia on 15 December. Do I need to have any vaccinations? Many thanks	No
		M2	Ms. Jane Doctor	Mr. John Patient	Hi, vaccination is required for travel to Australia	No

Table 2. Annotation by the GP.

Conversation ID	Face-to-Face Visit Avoided?	Increased Demand?	Type of Visit
C1	Yes	No	6 (Vaccinations)

Most of the data were received with a tabular arrangement, and the texts and their labels were in different files that were merged according to the Conversation ID. The data cleaning was a multi-step process. Regarding the text: First, all the tokens of anonymized names were changed to a standard name of the country "Juan". The title was merged with the body of the message, adding the token "xxti" before the title and "tixx" after the title; that way we would not lose the information that this was the title. The texts were all converted to lowercase, and we extracted the length (in words and in characters) of every message to use as extra independent variables. As additional variables, the day of the month and time of the day were extracted from the date of the message.

2.2. Vector Representation of Text in eConsulta Messages

The emails needed to be represented in some way in order to use them as input for the models. A common practice in machine learning is the vector representation of words. These vectors capture hidden information about the language, such as word analogies and semantics, and improve the performance of text classifiers.

Four techniques have been used to generate the vector representation of texts. The Bag of Words (BoW) approach counts the number of times pairs of words appear in each document. The document is represented as a vector of a finite vocabulary. The Term Frequency–Inverse Document Frequency (TF–IDF) method assigns paired words a weight depending on the number of times they appear in a particular document (the Term Frequency), while discounting its frequency in other documents (Inverse Document Frequency): The more documents a word appears in, the less valuable that word is as a signal to differentiate any given document. Word2Vec is a two-layered neuronal network that trains and processes text. Its input is a corpus of text and its output is a set of vectors for the words in the corpus, with words represented by numbers. The initial vector assigned to a word cannot be used to accurately predict its context, meaning its components must be adjusted (trained) through the contexts in which they are found. In this way, repeating the process for each word, word vectors with similar contexts end up in nearby vector spaces. Fasttext [14] is used to obtain word2vec vectors. Finally, the objective of Doc2vec is to create a numerical representation of a document, regardless of its length. This approach represents each document by a dense vector, which learns to predict the words in the document [15]. In all cases, before carrying out the vectorization of the texts, these were first tokenized and any stop-words eliminated (those which are taken to have no meaning in their own right, such as articles, pronouns or prepositions).

In each instance, the vectors were enriched by supplementing them with similar texts in Catalan and Spanish [16]. The external data used to enrich the corpus were models of interactions extracted from online databases with colloquial language similar to that used in eConsulta. Where augmented BOW, TF-IDF and Word2Vec were used, word and character length and word density were also used as predictor variables.

2.3. Training and Testing AI Algorithms

The task addressed in this study is a multiclass classification with respect to the type of visit and two binary classifications for the other two variables (avoiding visit and increased demand). For each text vector representation algorithm five different algorithms were implemented: Random Forest, Gradient Boosting (lightGBM), Fasttext, Multinomial Naive Bayes and Naive Bayes Complement [17]. Bayesian text classifiers are the most standard algorithms in this setting. A convolutional neural network was also used using the augmented Word2vec vectors. We tested the performance of the algorithms through a stratified 10-fold cross-validation: During 10 iterations/trainings, 9 divisions served as learning and 1 as a test.

The coefficients of interest to evaluate the goodness of the algorithms were precision (the fraction of relevant instances between the retrieved instances/proportion of correct predictions of the total of all predicted cases) and sensitivity (the number of correct classifications for the positive class "true positive"). It was decided not to use the "accuracy" coefficient since it is a metric that, given an unbalanced dataset like the one under investigation, can result in a very high score in spite of the fact that the classifier works poorly, since it assesses the number of total hits without taking into account whether most of the data is of the same class. The F value is used to determine a weighted single value of accuracy and completeness. The diagnostic value is assessed by means of the ROC curve. The goodness-of-fit of all the coefficients is represented as a value between 0 and 1.

Python 3.7 and the following libraries were used for the algorithm training: numpy [18], matplotlib [19], seaborn [20], altair [21], scikit-learn [22], pandas [23], gensim [24], nltk [25], fasttext [14], pytorch [26] and lightGBM [27]. The majority of the code was carried out on Jupyter Notebooks [28].

2.4. Ethical Considerations

The study was approved by the Ethical Committee for Clinical Research at the Foundation University Institute for Primary Health Care Research Jordi Gol and Gurina, registration number P19/096-P, and carried out in accordance with the Declaration of Helsinki [29].

3. Results

In order to assess the predictive potential of eConsulta messages regarding the three variables of interest, we first aimed to identify the best combination of algorithms. A total of 3559 messages (169,102 words) corresponding to 2268 teleconsultations (1.57 messages per teleconsultation) were analysed in a framework of 20 different combinations of vector representation of text and machine learning algorithms (Table 3). We assessed the performance of the combinations of algorithms though a stratified 10-fold cross-validation analysis. Figure 1 shows the performance of the most stable algorithm (best metrics, in general) according to the predictor variable.

Table 3. Text representations and algorithms used.

Text Representations	Algorithms
BoW	Random Forest
TF–IDF	Gradient Boosting (lightGBM)
Word2Vec	Fasttext
Doc2Vec	Multinomial Naive Bayes
	Complement Naive Bayes

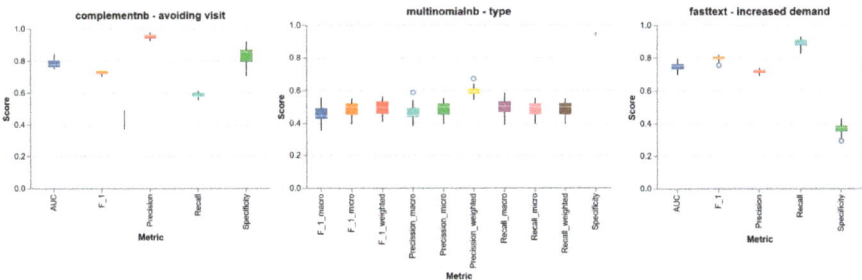

Figure 1. Performance metrics of algorithms.

Specific combinations of algorithms per variable generally perform very well. Table 4 shows the evaluation metrics (mean + standard deviation of the 10 iterations) of the combination of algorithm and numerical representation of the text which has a better performance for each target variable. For all of the cases, the vectors obtained directly from the original texts have been more useful than those enriched with external texts. Table 4 shows that algorithms are generally effective, showing they are better when approximating the two binary variables (avoiding the need for a face-to-face visit, increased demand) than the variable "type of query". Thus, eConsulta's classifiers have a promising and robust predictive value, especially for binary variables.

Table 4. Results of the best algorithm/text representation combination, according to the variable to be approximated. Average (SD) of the 10 iterations.

Variable	Precision	Recall	F1	Roc_AUC
Avoiding the need of a face-to-face visit	Random Forest TF-IDF 0.98 (0.026)	FastText Word2Vec 0.99 (0.005)	FastText Word2Vec 0.92 (0.004)	ComplementNB TF-IDF 0.79 (0.032)
Increased demand	Random Forest TF-IDF 0.97 (0.057)	FastText Word2Vec 0.89 (0.029)	FastText Word2Vec 0.79 (0.018)	FastText Word2Vec 0.75 (0.031)
Type of use of the teleconsultation (micro averaged score)	MultinomialNB BOW 0.48 (0.049)	MultinomialNB BOW 0.48 (0.049)	MultinomialNB BOW 0.48 (0.049)	

As a whole, the results illustrate eConsulta's algorithm classifiers potential predictive value and provide a valuable insight into the implementation of AI methodologies for healthcare teleconsultation.

4. Discussion

Limitations

Several limitations apply to this study and the results must be understood in light of these shortcomings. First, our classifier is restricted to one dataset and the training set was relatively small. Although the study used all the available information, more data is needed to generalize the model and avoid overfitting.

The amount of data with which the algorithms were tested is especially relevant in the case of trying to calculate the variable "type of message", since the number of types which contain the classification [13], meaning the quantity of messages of each with which the classification algorithm has been trained, is minimal, thus diminishing its predictive capacity. This may have had implications to our approach and subsequent results. What is required is not only more messages, they must also contain as much information as possible. Validating the algorithm requires a replication of the proposed methodology with a larger data set, together with the analysis of subgroups. Likewise, the goodness of fit of the results may be caused by overfitting: The model explains this set of data well, but could show weaknesses when generalizing to others, limiting its potential for extrapolation. Because of that, this study includes exhaustive detail of the methodology used in order that it can be replicated.

Second, an error analysis was not conducted. This analysis might have helped us to understand why certain posts where misclassified or classified correctly.

Using complex mathematical models makes it difficult to explain why some work better than others. The vectors would need to be evaluated at a lower level in order to have a better idea as to which characteristics redirect the model towards one decision or another. This analysis is of interest for future applications of these techniques on a larger scale or for applications related to medical practice.

5. Conclusions

In Catalonia, the number of conversations and messages now stand at approximately 370,000 and 500,000, respectively. Applying a classification algorithm like the one proposed here would help us understand the nature of the conversations and their impact in real time. Future research should evaluate the use of automation (to send a diagnostic test, generate an alert or "thank you" and close the case) as a tool for decision support for healthcare professionals to improve the management of clinical cases and to save GPs time. Natural Language Processing approaches should further analyse the content of the teleconsultations and proactively offer clinicians agile resources to deal with the cases.

This article has shown that the implementation of an algorithm for the prediction of factors such as a reduction in the number of face-to-face visits, induced demand or type of consultation is technically feasible and potentially useful in the context of service planning, management of the demand and evaluation. This study presents a combination of algorithms based on machine learning and a more efficient representation of vectors for this type of data. This study is an initial exploration into the potential of teleconsultation and the promising use of artificial intelligence for the evaluation of digital health interventions.

Author Contributions: Conceptualization, F.L.S., J.V.-A.; methodology, R.A.E.A., G.d.M.; software, R.A.E.A., G.d.M., S.W.; validation, F.L.S., R.A.E.A., G.d.M., A.G.-A., F.G.C., S.W., M.S.C., J.V.-A.; formal analysis, F.L.S., R.A.E.A., J.V.-A.; investigation, F.L.S., R.A.E.A., G.d.M., S.W., J.V.-A.; resources, F.L.S., J.V.-A.; data curation, R.A.E.A.; writing—original draft preparation, F.L.S., J.V.-A.; writing—review and editing, F.L.S., R.A.E.A., G.d.M., A.G.-A., F.G.C., S.W., J.V.-A.; visualization, F.L.S., A.G.-A., F.G.C., S.W., M.S.C., J.V.-A.; supervision, F.L.S., A.G.-A., F.G.C., M.S.C., J.V.-A.; project administration, F.L.S.; funding acquisition, F.L.S. All authors have read and agreed to the published version of the manuscript.

Acknowledgments: This study was conducted with the support of the Secretary of Universities and Research of the Department of Business and Knowledge at the *Generalitat de Catalunya*. We would like to thank the staff at the Technical and Support Area of *Gerència Territorial de la Catalunya Central* for their assistance during the data collection phase.

Conflicts of Interest: The authors declare no conflict of interest.

Abbreviations

GP	General Practitioner
BOW	Bag of Words
TF-IDF	Term Frequency—Inverse Document Frequency
ROC	Receiver Operating Characteristics

Appendix A

Reasons for using eConsulta

Appendix A.1 Administrative

1   Management of test results

    ◦   The patient provides the results of tests carried out in an external centre in order that they are recorded in their medical history.

- The GP provides the results of tests with normal results.
- The GP deals with questions related to tests requested by the patient.
- The GP requests tests after conducting a follow-up teleconsultation.

2. Temporary disability management

- The patient communicates changes to their health related to an upcoming temporary disability.
- The GP tracks the progress of a temporary disability in conjunction with face-to-face visits.

3. Management of visits/referrals

- The patient has an enquiry which the GP thinks ought to be dealt with by a specialist and refers them. They can also report incidents resulting from any referrals made.
- The GP resolves incidents relating to the timing of visits.
- The GP cancels visits from other clinicians in cases in which the problem has been resolved following completion of the e-consultation.
- Validation of appointments with other specialists where the citizen needs more information about the motivation of the appointment.

4. Request for a clinical report/sick-note

- The patient asks for a report/sick-note while consulting their medical history.
- The GP asks the patient for more information in order to prepare the report.

5. Repeat prescriptions

- The patient asks for their prescription to be updated if it has been modified by an external specialist, either because they do not use it or because it has expired.
- The GP warns the patient that their prescription is about to expire and updates it.
- The GP cancels an unnecessary prescription following an e-consultation.

6. Vaccinations

- Updates of immunization schedules and general enquiries regarding vaccinations.
- Questions concerning vaccinations for travel overseas.

7. Other administrative issues: Any administrative procedure which can be resolved without being physically present.

Appendix A.2 Medical

8. Medical enquiries: The patient has a question about their health that can be resolved without a physical examination. They can also attach photographs to accompany the description.
9. Issues regarding medicines: the patient asks a question about a prescription.
10. Questions regarding anticoagulants and dosage.

Appendix A.3 Others

11. Messages sent in error: The patient made a mistake.
12. Other.
13. Test messages.

References

1. López Seguí, F.; Vidal Alaball, J.; Sagarra Castro, M.; García Altés, A.; García Cuyàs, F. Does teleconsultation reduce face to face visits? Evidence from the Catalan public primary care system. *JMIR Prepr.* **2019**. [CrossRef]
2. Triantafyllidis, A.K.; Tsanas, A. Applications of Machine Learning in Real-Life Digital Health Interventions: Review of the Literature. *JMIR* **2019**, *21*, e12286. [CrossRef] [PubMed]
3. Luo, W.; Phung, D.; Tran, T.; Gupta, S.; Rana, S.; Karmakar, C.; Shilton, A.; Yearwood, J.; Dimitrova, N.; Ho, T.B.; et al. Guidelines for Developing and Reporting Machine Learning Predictive Models in Biomedical Research: A Multidisciplinary View. *JMIR* **2016**, *18*, e323. [CrossRef] [PubMed]
4. Li, Z.; Keel, S.; Liu, C.; He, Y.; Meng, W.; Scheetz, J.; Lee, P.Y.; Shaw, J.; Ting, D.; Wong, T.Y.; et al. An Automated Grading System for Detection of Vision-Threatening Referable Diabetic Retinopathy on the Basis of Color Fundus Photographs. *Diabetes Care.* **2018**, *41*, 1–8. [CrossRef] [PubMed]

5. Gulshan, V.; Peng, L.; Coram, M. Development and validation of a deep learning algorithm for detection of diabetic retinopathy in retinal fundus photographs. *JAMA* **2016**, *316*, 2402–2410. [CrossRef] [PubMed]
6. Vidal-Alaball, J.; Dídac Royo, F.; Zapata, M.A.; Gomez, F.M.; Fernandez, O.S. Artificial Intelligence for the Detection of Diabetic Retinopathy in Primary Care: Protocol for Algorithm Development. *JMIR Res. Protoc.* **2019**, *8*, e12539. [CrossRef] [PubMed]
7. Alessa, A.; Faezipour, M. Preliminary Flu Outbreak Prediction Using Twitter Posts Classification and Linear Regression with Historical Centers for Disease Control and Prevention Reports: Prediction Framework Study. *JMIR Public Health Surveill.* **2019**, *5*, e12383. [CrossRef] [PubMed]
8. Xu, S.; Markson, C.; Costello, K.L.; Xing, C.Y.; Demissie, K.; Llanos, A.A. Leveraging Social Media to Promote Public Health Knowledge: Example of Cancer Awareness via Twitter. *JMIR Public Health Surveill.* **2016**, *2*, e17. [CrossRef] [PubMed]
9. Doan, S.; Ritchart, A.; Perry, N.; Chaparro, J.D.; Conway, M. How Do You #relax When You're #stressed? A Content Analysis and Infodemiology Study of Stress-Related Tweets. *JMIR Public Health Surveill.* **2017**, *3*, e35. [PubMed]
10. McRoy, S.; Rastegar-Mojarad, M.; Wang, Y.; Ruddy, K.J.; Haddad, T.C.; Liu, H. Assessing Unmet Information Needs of Breast Cancer Survivors: Exploratory Study of Online Health Forums Using Text Classification and Retrieval. *JMIR Cancer* **2018**, *4*, e10. [CrossRef] [PubMed]
11. Bobicev, V.; Sokolova, M.; El Emam, K.; Jafer, Y.; Dewar, B.; Jonker, E.; Matwin, S. Can Anonymous Posters on Medical Forums be Reidentified? *JMIR* **2013**, *15*, e215. [CrossRef] [PubMed]
12. Chen, J.; Lalor, J.; Liu, W.; Druhl, E.; Granillo, E.; Vimalananda, V.G.; Yu, H. Detecting Hypoglycemia Incidents Reported in Patients' Secure Messages: Using Cost-Sensitive Learning and Oversampling to Reduce Data Imbalance. *JMIR* **2019**, *21*, e11990. [CrossRef] [PubMed]
13. IDESCAT. Noms de la Població. Available online: http://www.idescat.cat/noms/ (accessed on 24 September 2019).
14. Bojanowski, P.; Grave, E.; Jouilin, A.; Mikolov, T. Enriching word vectors with subword information. *Trans. Assoc. Comput. Linguist.* **2017**, *5*, 135–146. [CrossRef]
15. Le, Q.; Tomas, M. Distributed representations of sentences and documents. In Proceedings of the International Conference on Machine Learning, Beijing, China, 21–26 June 2014.
16. Ljubesic, N.; Toral, A. caWaC-A web corpus of Catalan and its application to language modeling and machine translation. *LREC* **2014**, *L14-1647*, 1728–1732.
17. Rennie, J.D.; Shih, L.; Teevan, J.; Karger, D.R. Tackling the poor assumptions of naive bayes text classifiers. In Proceedings of the 20th International Conference on Machine Learning (ICML-03), Washington, DC, USA, 21–24 August 2003.
18. Van Der Walt, S.; Chris Colbert, S.; Varoquaux, G. The NumPy array: A structure for efficient numerical computation. *Comput. Sci. Eng.* **2011**, *13*, 22. [CrossRef]
19. Hunter, J.D. Matplotlib: A 2D Graphics Environment. *Comput. Sci. Eng.* **2007**, *9*, 9–95. [CrossRef]
20. mwaskom/seaborn: v0. 9.0. Available online: https://zenodo.org/record/1313201 (accessed on 30 January 2020).
21. Altair. Available online: https://altair-viz.github.io/index.html (accessed on 8 February 2020).
22. Pedregosa, F.; Grisel, O.; Blondel, M.; Prettenhofer, P.; Weiss, R.; Dubourg, V.; Vanderplas, J.; Passos, A.; Cournapeau, D. Scikit-learn: Machine Learning in Python. *JMLR* **2011**, *12*, 2825–2830.
23. McKinney, W. Data structures for statistical computing in python. In Proceedings of the 9th Python in Science Conference, Austin, TX, USA, 9–15 July 2010; Volume 445.
24. Rehurek, R.; Sojka, P. Software framework for topic modelling with large corpora. In Proceedings of the LREC 2010 Workshop on New Challenges for NLP Frameworks, Valetta, Malta, 22 May 2010.
25. Bird, S.; Loper, E.; Klein, E. *Natural Language Processing with Python*; O'Reilly Media Inc.: Newton, MA, USA, 2009.
26. Paszke, A. Automatic differentiation in pytorch. In Proceedings of the 31st Conference on Neural Information Processing Systems (NIPS 2017), Long Beach, CA, USA, 4–9 December 2017.
27. Ke, G.; Meng, Q.; Finley, T.; Wang, T.; Chen, W.; Ma, W.; Ye, Q.; Liu, T. Lightgbm: A highly efficient gradient boosting decision tree. In Proceedings of the 31st Conference on Neural Information Processing Systems (NIPS 2017), Long Beach, CA, USA, 4–9 December 2017.

28. Kluyver, T.; Ragan-Kelley, B.; Pérez, F.; Granger, B.; Bussonnier, M.; Frederic, J.; Kelley, K.; Hamrick, J.; Grout, J.; Corlay, S.; et al. Jupyter Notebooks-a publishing format for reproducible computational workflows. *ELPUB* **2016**. [CrossRef]
29. World Medical Association. World Medical Association Declaration of Helsinki. Ethical Principles for Medical Research Involving Human Subjects Helsinki. 2013. Available online: https://www.wma.net/what-we-do/medical-ethics/declaration-of-helsinki/ (accessed on 27 January 2020).

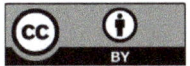

© 2020 by the authors. Licensee MDPI, Basel, Switzerland. This article is an open access article distributed under the terms and conditions of the Creative Commons Attribution (CC BY) license (http://creativecommons.org/licenses/by/4.0/).

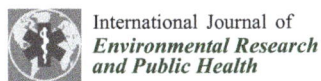

International Journal of
Environmental Research and Public Health

Article

Impact of a Telemedicine Program on the Reduction in the Emission of Atmospheric Pollutants and Journeys by Road

Josep Vidal-Alaball [1,2,*], Jordi Franch-Parella [3,*], Francesc Lopez Seguí [4,5], Francesc Garcia Cuyàs [6] and Jacobo Mendioroz Peña [1,2]

1. Health Promotion in Rural Areas Research Group, Institut Català de la Salut, 08272 Sant Fruitós de Bages, Spain; jmendioroz.cc.ics@gencat.cat
2. Unitat de Suport a la Recerca de la Catalunya Central, Fundació Institut Universitari per a la Recerca a l'Atenció Primària de Salut Jordi Gol i Gurina, 08007 Barcelona, Spain
3. Faculty of Social Sciences, Universitat de Vic-Universitat Central de Catalunya, 08242 Manresa, Spain
4. TIC Salut Social-Ministry of Health, 08005 Barcelona, Spain; flopez@ticsalutsocial.cat
5. CRES&CEXS-Pompeu Fabra University, 08005 Barcelona, Spain
6. Sant Joan de Déu Hospital, Catalan Ministry of Health, 08950 Barcelona, Spain; 31557fgc@gmail.com
* Correspondence: jvidal.cc.ics@gencat.cat (J.V.-A.); jfranch@umanresa.cat (J.F.-P.)

Received: 3 October 2019; Accepted: 6 November 2019; Published: 8 November 2019

Abstract: This retrospective study evaluates the effect of a telemedicine program developed in the central Catalan region in lowering the environmental footprint by reducing the emission of atmospheric pollutants, thanks to a reduction in the number of hospital visits involving journeys by road. Between January 2018 and June 2019, a total of 12,322 referrals were made to telemedicine services in the primary care centers, avoiding a total of 9034 face-to-face visits. In total, the distance saved was 192,682 km, with a total travel time saving of 3779 h and a total fuel reduction of 11,754 L with an associated cost of €15,664. This represents an average reduction of 3248.3 g of carbon dioxide, 4.05 g of carbon monoxide, 4.86 g of nitric oxide and 3.2 g of sulphur dioxide. This study confirms that telemedicine reduces the environmental impact of atmospheric pollutants emitted by vehicles by reducing the number of journeys made for face-to-face visits, and thus contributing to environmental sustainability.

Keywords: telemedicine; carbon dioxide; air pollutants; vehicle emissions; primary care

1. Introduction

The distance travelled and time spent by patients when visiting a doctor may limit patients' access to medical care. Fortunately, telemedicine overcomes geographical barriers to healthcare, which is particularly beneficial for patients in rural communities or in places where there is a shortage of doctors or a shortage of health services [1–4].

In the central Catalan region, the Bages, Moianès and Berguedà counties have developed several telemedicine programs: the most consolidated is Teledermatology while the most innovative are Teleulcers, Teleeyelids and Teleaudiometries. Teledermatology is a service that has provided a speedy service to thousands of users, thus avoiding numerous unnecessary hospital visits [5], and representing a saving of €11.4 per face-to-face visit avoided [6]. Meanwhile, Teleulcers it is a more specialized service that, with less patient volume, has managed to improve the quality of care for people with chronic ulcers [7]. Teleeyelids and Teleaudiometries, which are in the process of being evaluated, are the most recent telemedicine programs introduced in the region.

The first three telemedicine programs all operate in the same way; the primary care physician or a nurse takes a photograph of the injury or injuries and attaches it to the patient's electronic health record together with their clinical notes. The use of the patient's electronic health record ensures the images are handled securely, since they do not need to be sent by email or uploaded to an external server. Hospital specialists can access the patient's electronic health record, review the images and suggest treatment or an action plan. The primary care physician or nurse can review the instructions and telephone the patient to give them the results of the consultation. This can usually all be done in less than 5–7 working days. If the specialist has any doubts, they can ask the primary care professional to book the patient for a face-to-face consultation.

The teleaudiometry program is similar to other telemedicine programs, but it does not involve taking photographs. Patients are instead referred to a primary care center where an audiometry test is performed. This is uploaded to the patient's electronic health record, together with specific clinical information. The patient's otorhinolaryngologist accesses the electronic health record, reviews the audiometry test and suggests an action plan. The primary care physician reviews the instructions and telephones the patient to give them the results of the consultation as with the other programs.

Numerous studies provide evidence showing the benefits of telemedicine from the point of view of both the patient and the health system [8]. Recently some studies have analyzed the environmental impact of the savings offered by telemedicine programs due to the fact that the patient does not need to make a journey to their health center [9–12]. In the current climate of growing interest in reducing the environmental footprint of health care activities [13,14], this study evaluates the effect of a telemedicine program in lowering a procedure's environmental footprint by reducing the emission of atmospheric pollutants due to a reduction in the number of hospital visits involving journeys by road.

2. Materials and Methods

The cases that were studied came from the existing telemedicine program, which includes Teledermatology, Teleulcers, Teleeyelids and Teleaudiometries in the Institut Català de la Salut's primary health centers and tertiary referral hospitals in the Bages, Berguedà and Moianès counties; the Sant Joan de Déu Hospital (Althaia Foundation) in Manresa and the Hospital Comarcal Sant Bernabé de Berga, located in Central Catalonia. Patients from primary care centers in the Bages and Moianès counties are referred to the Hospital Sant Joan de Déu de Manresa, while patients in Berguedà are referred to the Hospital Comarcal Sant Bernabé de Berga (Figure 1). The analysis was conducted from January 2018 to June 2019.

This retrospective study uses administrative data and evaluates the impact of telemedicine services on reducing the distance travelled and the associated savings in terms of time and money, as well as the reduction in atmospheric pollutants. The savings in the distance travelled are calculated in terms of the round trip from the primary care center to the hospital.

The reduction in the emission of atmospheric pollutants and greenhouse gases is calculated by multiplying the kilometers that are not travelled by emissions per kilometer. The savings made are calculated as the difference between the cost of travelling to the referral hospital and the cost of travelling to the nearest primary care center. Finally, the time saved through the use of telemedicine is defined as the total round-trip from the primary care center to the referral hospital. Google Maps was used to calculate both the distances travelled and the time saved on the trip via the existing road network. The "fastest route with the usual traffic" search option was used to make the calculations, and involved an equal number of diesel and petrol cars. The emission of atmospheric pollutants per km is shown in Table 1.

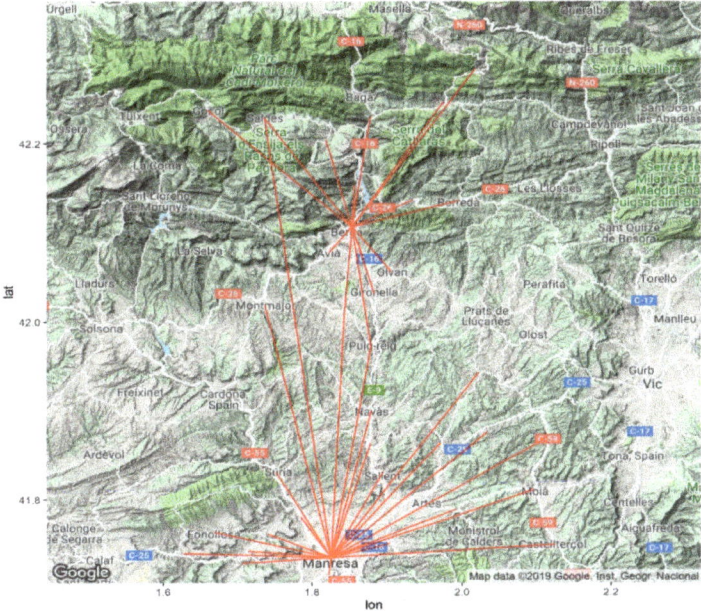

Figure 1. Map showing the primary care centers and their associated referral hospitals in Manresa and Berga.

Table 1. Emission of pollutants per km. Source: Mobility and emissions. Extra-urban cycle (gasoline and diesel fuel). Available at: http://mobilitat.gencat.cat/ca/detalls/Article/mobilitat_emissions (Date of access: 20 September 2019).

Pollutant	Formula	Emissions per km (g)
Carbon dioxide	CO_2	152.5
Carbon monoxide	CO	0.19
Nitric Oxide	NO_x	0.228
Sulphur dioxide	SO_2	0.15

The telemedicine service was considered to have replaced a face-to-face consultation when no face-to-face visit occurred in relation to the same type of specialist in the three months following the telemedicine consultation. Microsoft Excel and R 3.6.1 were used for data processing and quantitative analysis.

3. Results

As noted in Table 2, between January 2018 and June 2019, a total of 12,322 referrals were made to telemedicine services in the primary care centers which are within the catchment areas of the 2 referral hospitals, avoiding a total of 9034 face-to-face visits. The remaining 3288 telemedicine consultations were referred to a specialist for a face-to-face consultation. Thus, the percentage of face-to-face visits prevented through the use of telemedicine was 73.3%. The most widely used telemedicine service was Teledermatology, with 9352 cases and a reduction in face-to-face visits of 69.66%, followed by Teleaudiometries (2465 cases and a 86.10% reduction in visits), Teleeyelids (350 cases and a 74.6% reduction in visits) and Teleulcers (155 cases and 87.8% reduction in visits).

Table 2. Face-to-face visits and visits prevented through telemedicine.

	Teledermatology	Teleaudiometries	Teleeyelids	Teleulcers	Total
Origin of Visits	9352	2465	350	155	12,322
V. Referred	2837	343	89	19	3288
V. Prevented	6515	2122	261	136	9034
% V. Prevented	69.66%	86.10%	74.6%	87.8%	73.3%

Table 3 shows the distance of saved visits due to the telemedicine program and time and travel cost savings in terms of unused fuel. The average distance of a round trip between a primary care center and the referral hospital was 21.3 km, with an average travel time savings of 25 min. In total, the distance saved was 192,682 km, with a total travel time savings of 3779 h and a total fuel reduction of 11,754 L with an associated cost of €15,664.

Table 3. Reduction in journeys by distance, time, fuel and cost. Cost of fuel available at: https://www.dieselgasolina.com (Accessed on: 17 September 2019).

Kms	
Average journey saved in km (return)	21.3 km
Total journeys saved (return)	192,682 km
Time	
Average journey saved in minutes (return)	25 min
Total journeys saved in hours (return)	3779 h
Total reduction in petrol consumption	11,754 L
Cost of fuel saved	15,664 euros

A breakdown of the reduction in the emissions of pollutants is shown in Table 4. Total reduction in pollutants is 29.384 tonnes of carbon dioxide, 36.61 kg of carbon monoxide, 43.93 kg of nitric oxide and 28.9 kg of sulphur dioxide. This represents an average reduction of 3248.3 g of carbon dioxide, 4.05 g of carbon monoxide, 4.86 g of nitric oxide and 3.2 g of sulphur dioxide.

Table 4. Reduction in the emissions of pollutant gases.

Carbon Dioxide	
Average (return) journey	3248.3 g
Total journeys	29.384 t
Carbon monoxide	
Average journey	4.05 g
Total journeys	36.61 kg
Nitric oxide	
Average journey	4.86 g
Total journeys	43.93 kg
Sulphur dioxide	
Average journey	3.2 g
Total journeys	28.9 kg

4. Discussion

In this study, the results of a fully functioning and fully developed telemedicine program comprising four different services, Teledermatology, Teleulcers, Teleeyelids and Teleaudiometries, have been analyzed in terms of journeys to hospitals prevented, time saved, reductions in fuel consumption and reductions in the emission of pollutant and greenhouse gases. The rural and dispersed nature of the area involved increases the effectiveness of telemedicine. The three counties featured in the study have a total population of 228,622, with 66.65% living in rural areas, with an urban area defined as having a population greater than 20,000. From the patient's point of view, they avoid an unnecessary journey to hospital, save on the journey time and reduce their fuel consumption while receiving the same standard of care. From the environmental point of view, there is a reduction in the emission of pollutants and greenhouse gases.

The results are consistent with those from 2016 [6], involving the same geographical area, and relating specifically to the Teledermatology service. Of a total of 5606 consultations, 80.3% were dealt with telematically, while the remaining 19.7% were referred to a specialist for a face-to-face consultation. In 2016, Teledermatology reduced journeys by a total of 99,368 km. This represented 1928 h of travel time saved. CO_2 emissions were reduced by 15.2 tonnes. The study included a cost-saving analysis that concluded that using teledermatology instead of face-to-face dermatology consultations could save up to €11.4 per patient visited. Other studies also suggest that the reduction in visits as a result of telemedicine services and the consequent reduction of pollutant emissions is significant [15,16]. A recent study conducted by the vascular surgery division of the Henry Ford hospital in Detroit between October 2015 and November 2017 [17] analyzed the impact of telemedicine on 87 patients. The results showed that the average reduction in pollutants per consultation was 1118 g of carbon dioxide, 294 g of carbon monoxide, 21.6 g of nitric oxide and 32.3 g of other volatile organic compounds. The average distance saved on a round trip was 50.2 km, with an average duration of 39 min. The total reduction in fuel consumption was 734 L with an associated cost of $622. This includes $2.50 for parking. Another study by the University of Kansas Medical Center, involving 132 patients and a total of 257 consultations shows an average saving per journey of $86.13 [18], while in another study by the University of Kentucky, the distance and time saved per visit as a result of telemedicine was 102 km and 66.8 min, respectively [19].

The present study has certain limitations. A prospective analysis would be able to obtain more detailed and individualized information, including data related to the loss of working hours and salary, the degree of driving-related stress, waiting time and additional costs such as parking. None of these costs are included in the current study. In addition, this study does not take into account factors that increase the cost of telemedicine such as the use of platforms or the need for equipment connected to the internet.

For the purposes of the study, the type of transport used has been taken to be a private vehicle with average emissions. The use of public transport or emissions that deviate from the average (whether due to lower emissions through the use of hybrid or electric cars, or higher emissions through the use of outdated and obsolete cars) have not been taken into account. However, public transport is not always easily available in rural areas.

Future studies ought to look at the monetary value of the pollutants which were not emitted, because telemedicine, in addition to saving on direct costs, can contribute to environmental sustainability.

5. Conclusions

This study confirms that telemedicine reduces the environmental impact of atmospheric pollutants emitted by vehicles by reducing the number of journeys made for face-to-face visits to see a specialist. The distance saved results in time saved and reductions in fuel and pollutants. Further studies ought to include more information on alternative face-to-face models, wasted working hours and the associated impact on earnings, as well as a cost-effectiveness analysis of face-to-face visits compared to telemedicine. The expansion of telemedicine programs ought to be considered an option as part of a global strategy to reduce the emission of atmospheric pollutants.

Author Contributions: Conceptualization, J.V.-A.; Data curation, J.V.-A. and F.L.S.; Formal analysis, J.V.-A., J.F.-P. and F.L.S.; Investigation, J.F.-P. and F.G.C.; Methodology, J.V.-A. and J.F.-P.; Resources, J.M.P.; Software, F.L.S.; Supervision, J.V.-A., F.G.C. and J.M.P.; Validation, J.F.-P., F.G.C. and J.M.P.; Visualization, J.F.-P. and F.L.S.; Writing–original draft, J.V.-A., J.F.-P., F.L.S., F.G.C. and J.M.P.; Writing–review & editing, J.V.-A., J.F.-P. and F.L.S.

Funding: This research received no external funding.

Acknowledgments: A big thank you to the staff at the Technical and Support Area of Gerència Territorial de la Catalunya Central for their help during the data collection phase. This study was conducted with the support of the Secretary of Universities and Research of the Department of Business and Knowledge at the Generalitat de Catalunya.

Conflicts of Interest: The authors declare no conflict of interest.

References

1. Bradford, N.K.; Caffery, L.; Smith, A. Telehealth services in rural and remote Australia: A systematic review of models of care and factors. *Rural Remote Health* **2016**, *16*, 3808. [PubMed]
2. Saleh, N.; Abdel Hay, R.; Hegazy, R.; Hussein, M.; Gomaa, D. Can teledermatology be a useful diagnostic tool in dermatology practice in remote areas? An Egyptian experience with 600 patients. *J. Telemed. Telecare* **2016**, *23*, 233–238. [CrossRef] [PubMed]
3. Vidal-Aballí, J.; Mendioroz Peña, J.; Sauch Valmaña, G. Rural-urban differences in the pattern of referrals to an asynchronous teledermatology service. *Int. Arch. Med.* **2018**, *11*, 1–5. [CrossRef]
4. Jetty, A.; Moore, M.A.; Coffman, M.; Petterson, S.; Bazemore, A. Rural Family Physicians Are Twice as Likely to Use Telehealth as Urban Family Physicians. *Telemed. e-Health* **2018**, *24*, 268–276. [CrossRef] [PubMed]
5. Vidal-Aballí, J.; Álamo-Junquera, D.; López-Aguilá, S.; García-Altés, A. Evaluación del impacto de la teledermatología en la disminución de la lista de espera en la comarca del Bages (2009-2012). *Aten. Primaria* **2014**, *47*, 9–10.
6. Vidal-Aballí, J.; Garcia Domingo, J.L.; Garcia Cuyàs, F.; Mendioroz Peña, J.; Flores Mateo, G.; Deniel Rosanas, J.; Sauch Valmaña, G. A cost savings analysis of asynchronous teledermatology compared to face-to-face dermatology in Catalonia. *BMC Health Serv. Res.* **2018**, *18*, 650. [CrossRef] [PubMed]
7. Navarro, A.; Badrenas, A.; Vidal-Aballí, J.; Boix, C. Teleúlceres, una alternativa assistencial amb més d'un any d'experiència. *Ann. Med.* **2014**, *97*, 159–162.
8. Ekeland, A.G.; Bowes, A.; Flottorp, S. Effectiveness of telemedicine: A systematic review of reviews. *Int. J. Med. Inform.* **2010**, *79*, 736–771. [CrossRef] [PubMed]
9. Oliveira, T.C.; Barlow, J.; Gonçalves, L.; Bayer, S. Teleconsultations reduce greenhouse gas emissions. *J. Health Serv. Res. Policy* **2013**, *18*, 209–214. [CrossRef] [PubMed]
10. Smith, A.C.; Kimble, R.M.; O'Brien, A.; Mill, J.; Wootton, R. A telepaediatric burns service and the potential travel savings for families living in regional Australia. *J. Telemed. Telecare* **2007**, *13*, 76–79. [CrossRef]
11. Audebert, H.J.; Meyer, T.; Klostermann, F. Potentials of telemedicine for green health care. *Front. Neurol.* **2010**, *1*, 10. [CrossRef] [PubMed]
12. Holmner, Å.; Ebi, K.L.; Lazuardi, L.; Nilsson, M. Carbon footprint of telemedicine solutions—Unexplored opportunity for reducing carbon emissions in the health sector. *PLoS ONE* **2014**, *9*, e105040. [CrossRef] [PubMed]
13. Sherman, J.D.; MacNeill, A.; Thiel, C. Reducing Pollution from the Health Care Industry. *JAMA* **2019**, *322*, 1043–1044. [CrossRef] [PubMed]
14. Yellowlees, P.M.; Chorba, K.; Burke Parish, M.; Wynn-Jones, H.; Nafiz, N. Telemedicine can make healthcare greener. *Telemed. e-Health* **2010**, *16*, 229–232. [CrossRef] [PubMed]
15. Whetten, J.; Montoya, J.; Yonas, H. ACCESS to Better Health and Clear Skies: Telemedicine and Greenhouse Gas Reduction. *Telemed. e-Health* **2019**, *25*, 960–965. [CrossRef] [PubMed]
16. Wootton, R.; Bahaadinbeigy, K.; Hailey, D. Estimating travel reduction associated with the use of telemedicine by patients and healthcare professionals: Proposal for quantitative synthesis in a systematic review. *BMC Health Serv. Res.* **2011**, *11*, 185. [CrossRef] [PubMed]

17. Paquette, S.; Lin, J.C. Outpatient telemedicine program in vascular surgery reduces patient travel time, cost, and environmental pollutant emissions. *Ann. Vasc. Surg.* **2019**, *59*, 167–172. [CrossRef] [PubMed]
18. Spaulding, R.; Belz, N.; DeLurgio, S.; Williams, A.R. Cost savings of telemedicine utilization for child psychiatry in a rural Kansas community. *Telemed. J. E Health* **2010**, *16*, 867–871. [CrossRef] [PubMed]
19. Soares, N.S.; Johnson, A.O.; Patidar, N. Geomapping telehealth access to developmental behavioral pediatrics. *Telemed. J. E Health* **2013**, *19*, 585–590. [CrossRef] [PubMed]

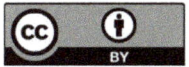

© 2019 by the authors. Licensee MDPI, Basel, Switzerland. This article is an open access article distributed under the terms and conditions of the Creative Commons Attribution (CC BY) license (http://creativecommons.org/licenses/by/4.0/).

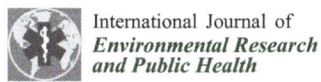

Article

Social Media, Thin-Ideal, Body Dissatisfaction and Disordered Eating Attitudes: An Exploratory Analysis

Pilar Aparicio-Martinez [1,2,3,*], Alberto-Jesus Perea-Moreno [4], María Pilar Martinez-Jimenez [4], María Dolores Redel-Macías [5], Claudia Pagliari [6] and Manuel Vaquero-Abellan [3]

1. Departamento de Enfermería, Universidad de Córdoba, Campus de Menéndez Pidal, 1470 Córdoba, Spain
2. Usher Institute of Population Health Sciences and Informatics, University of Edinburgh, Edinburgh EH8 9YL, UK
3. Grupo Investigación epidemiológica en Atención primaria (GC-12) del Instituto Maimónides de Investigación Biomédica de Córdoba (IMIBIC), Hospital Universitario Reina Sofía, 14071 Córdoba, Spain; mvaquero@uco.es
4. Departamento de Física Aplicada, Universidad de Córdoba, ceiA3, Campus de Rabanales, 14071 Córdoba, Spain; aperea@uco.es (A.-J.P.-M.); fa1majip@uco.es (M.P.M.-J.)
5. Departamento Ingeniería Rural, Ed Leonardo da Vinci, Campus de Rabanales, Universidad de Córdoba, Campus de Excelencia Internacional Agroalimentario, ceiA3, 1470 Cordoba, Spain; mdredel@uco.es
6. eHealth Research Group, Usher Institute of Population Health Sciences and Informatics, University of Edinburgh, Edinburgh EH8 9YL, UK; claudia.pagliari@ed.ac.uk
* Correspondence: n32apmap@uco.es; Tel.: +34-67-972-7823

Received: 25 September 2019; Accepted: 26 October 2019; Published: 29 October 2019

Abstract: Disordered eating attitudes are rapidly increasing, especially among young women in their twenties. These disordered behaviours result from the interaction of several factors, including beauty ideals. A significant factor is social media, by which the unrealistic beauty ideals are popularized and may lead to these behaviours. The objectives of this study were, first, to determine the relationship between disordered eating behaviours among female university students and sociocultural factors, such as the use of social network sites, beauty ideals, body satisfaction, body image and the body image desired to achieve and, second, to determine whether there is a sensitive relationship between disordered eating attitudes, addiction to social networks, and testosterone levels as a biological factor. The data (N = 168) was obtained using validated surveys (EAT-26, BSQ, CIPE-a, SNSA) and indirect measures of prenatal testosterone. The data was analysed using chi-square, Student's t-test, correlation tests and logistic regression tests. The results showed that disordered eating attitudes were linked to self-esteem ($p < 0.001$), body image ($p < 0.001$), body desired to achieve ($p < 0.001$), the use of social media ($p < 0.001$) and prenatal testosterone ($p < 0.01$). The findings presented in this study suggest a relationship between body image, body concerns, body dissatisfaction, and disordered eating attitudes among college women.

Keywords: social media; disordered eating behaviours; body image; female; university students

1. Introduction

Mental health problems have increased, especially among young people, over the last decade [1]. The most common mental problems are behavioural, emotional, and hyperkinetic disorders. Among these illnesses, disordered eating behaviours are rapidly increasing in a short time, especially among young women [2,3]. These disordered attitudes are defined as afflictions in which people suffer severe disruption in their eating behaviours, thoughts and emotions. The people who suffer from these complaints are usually preoccupied with food and weight. In this sense, disordered eating is used to describe a range of irregular eating behaviours that may or may not warrant a diagnosis of a specific disordered eating attitude [4].

These disorders usually occur in women in their twenties or during adolescence [3]. People who suffer these disorders usually present altered attitudes, behaviours, weight perception and physical appearance [5]. Moreover, disordered eating behaviours or attitudes are defined as unhealthy or maladaptive eating behaviours, such as restricting or binging and/or purging [6]. These behaviours are not categorized as an eating disorder, though they are considered a phase of diagnosed eating disorders [7].

The concern from health care systems is based on the fact that these severe mental disorders usually puts in danger the well-being and health of the people who suffer them [5]. One-third of the women in the world have suffered from these mental problems at some point in their life [6]. If they are inadequately treated, they may develop severe clinical disorders [8]. Moreover, around 1% of the people with these disordered eating attitudes struggle with unhealthy and emotional problems through all their lives [6].

Out of the population with disordered eating attitudes, 16% of them present overeating, 20% purged by vomiting, and 61% food restraining [9]. These frequencies changed as people aged, with food restriction being more common in older women and vomiting during adolescence [10]. Moreover, recent data have discussed the increase of how the minimum age of the people with disorders is around 12 years of age and decreasing. Meanwhile, the prevalence of disordered eating attitudes appears to increase as young adults or adolescents grow older [10].

Although these diseases have a crucial psychobiological component, social and cultural factors have a significant influence. Among these factors, advertising has been described as an internalizing or normalizing means to spread unrealistic beauty ideals. Therefore, a higher incidence of these diseases is presented in advanced and modern societies and people with the best living conditions, mostly caused by the popularization of thin and muscular ideals [11–13].

Several biological factors have been linked to disordered eating attitudes, with up to 50% of disordered eating being described as familiarly transmitted [5,14]. Researchers have also suggested that neurotransmitters in the brain are involved in disordered eating attitudes and, therefore, eating disorders [15,16]. Additionally, the hormones have been linked as factors to puberty, body perception and body concerns [17,18]. Testosterone is included among those hormones highly studied, with blood samples providing a more precise method of examination. Nevertheless, different researchers pointed out the possibility of using indirect markers to avoid taking biological samples and creating risks for the participants. In this sense, most studies have linked testosterone and estrogenic levels via the 2D:4D digital ratio as an indirect indicator [19], which heavily dictates attractiveness [17]. This ratio, which is based on the difference in length of the phalanges of the hands (2D:4D ratio) having a lower ratio as an indicator of the existence of a higher level of testosterone, is used for the determination of intrauterine testosterone levels during gestation [20]. This ratio has reflected the relationship with self-perception, body image, body dissatisfaction, and disordered eating behaviours [20,21]. Based on these studies, the hormone levels, and the indirect marker, might appear to have essential roles in disordered eating attitudes [22]. Nevertheless, other authors have described how biological or genetic factors are essential, but may not determine, these disordered eating attitudes [23].

Other factors, such as ethical or familiar factors, contribute to the development of this disordered eating behaviours [24]. In this sense, previous studies have established that the probability of developing a disordered eating attitude or a diagnosis of eating disorders is higher if the mother had a disordered eating or self-esteem problems [25,26]. Moreover, ethnicity has been linked to the perception of beauty ideals, self-esteem and body perception [27,28].

Another critical factor is the media by which beauty ideals have been promoted. The media plays a vital role in formulating what is attractive in society, increasing the thin beauty ideal among females being unattainable [29,30]. These ideals confirmed the way young people perceived themselves and, therefore, how they value themselves [10,31]. This contradiction between what society portrays as a role model and the real body that many young women have has resulted in body concerns. Body concerns usually maintain over time and increase body dissatisfaction. This body dissatisfaction emerges because of the distortion on the body image, its perception and, therefore, body concern [32,33]. This dissatisfaction also plays an essential role in disordered eating attitudes since it provokes emotional and psychological distress [34].

In this sense, the theory of social comparison and numerous studies have studied the relationship between body dissatisfaction and disordered eating attitudes to better understand the causes of these illnesses. These previous works showed that real comparisons with other people leads to a distortion of body image and may favour disorderly feeding [11,29,35]. Additionally, Fredrickson and Roberts (1997) suggested that sexualization and self-objectification promoted via media should be considered as a risk factor for disordered eating attitudes [36–38]. Based on previous and recent studies it seems that the role of the media in disordered eating attitudes is noteworthy [1,11,39].

This paper presents a research study in which these objectives have been pursued: first, to determine the relationship between disordered eating attitudes in female university students and sociocultural factors, such as the use of social network sites, beauty ideals, body satisfaction, the body image and the body image desired to achieve. Second, to determine whether there is a sensitive relationship between disordered eating attitudes, addiction to social networks, and other biological factors, such as testosterone levels.

2. Background

College-aged women may be at particular risk for body dissatisfaction and disordered eating practices due to the unhealthy weight gain that often occurs during this life stage [3,31]. The promotion of beauty ideals in the media disseminates disordered eating [40,41], drive for thinness and body dissatisfaction among female college students [42]. Furthermore, the growth of social networking sites (SNS), such as Facebook or Instagram, has also increased the exposure to thin and fit ideals [2,43,44]. The social media are more used than any other media as a mean of communication. These internet-based sites pulled the users to create personal profiles and share, view, comment and 'like' peer-generated content [20].

Importantly, young people, almost 90% of them (ages 18–29), reported being active users and being continuously exposed to different content and images in this medium [14,45]. Among the most active users of these media stands out the influencers. These new media role models have a significant impact in the last tendencies, the news and the trends that young people are following [46]. In this sense, researchers have also pointed out how social media and influencers may have the key to decrease body dissatisfaction and body concerns. Nevertheless, substantial studies have shown that economic interests are linked with the promotion of dieting in social media, or even surgery [47].

The last publications concluded that the most dangerous social media was Instagram, followed by Facebook and Twitter. These conclusions were based on the instant satisfaction of reviewing and having peer views in the images posted by the users [48]. Especially on Instagram, the message is accommodated according to the image uploaded [47].

These studies concluded that the influence of the advertising and the promotion of the thin and muscular ideals might more be connected with the perception that young people has regarding body, dieting and social media [49]. Additionally, the objectification suggests that the media's sexual objectification of women modifies their body appearance. Due to this, it could be concluded that self-perception slowly shapes attractiveness resulting in a modification in the body-image, body dissatisfaction and disordered eating attitude. That being said, the proposed hypotheses are as follows:

Hypothesis 1 (H1). *Among young women, self-image will be linked to body dissatisfaction, the thin-ideal and the desire to change one's body shape.*

Hypothesis 2 (H2). *The level of body dissatisfaction among female college students will be high and be linked to self-esteem.*

Hypothesis 3 (H3). *The young women's eating behaviours will be linked to the degree of body dissatisfaction and the frequency of using social media.*

Hypothesis 4 (H4). *The young women's body image and body description will be slightly connected to prenatal testosterone levels.*

3. Methodology

3.1. Design and Sample

In the first phase, a cross-sectional study was carried out focused on female college students, aged from 18 to 25 years. The sample was recruited to participate in an in-person survey from April to May 2018 from the University of Cordoba. The selection of the sample was based on non-probability convenience sampling. This method of sampling was selected based on the accessibility of the students and previous scheduling with the professors.

The final sample was constituted by 168 subjects, from biological, education, informatics and nursing degrees who agreed to participate in the study voluntarily. The initial sample was 224, though the final sample was 168 after applying the exclusion terms. The mean age of the sample was 20 ± 0.76.

3.2. Measures

All the surveys used in the study are validated in different languages, including Spanish. Moreover, these surveys are used globally among health professionals and researchers in the health field [50].

The demographic and anthropometric data were not included in this study since the objective focused on the socio-cultural and individual factors. In this sense, the perception of young people was focused on social media, self-appearance, specific social network sites and distorted eating behaviours.

The EAT-26 with the reduced version of 26 items, was used to assess the frequency of disordered eating attitudes [51,52]. This test measures the low, medium and high risk of having a disordered eating attitude. Moreover, three different disordered eating behaviours can be reflected depending on the answers to each item. In this sense, these three subscales are dieting (focused on questions 1, 6, 7, 10, 11, 12, 14, 16, 17, 22, 23, 24, 26), bulimia and food preoccupation (focused on questions 3, 4, 9, 18, 21, 25) and food oral control (2, 5, 8, 13, 15, 8, 20). Total scores were calculated by taking the sum of the 26 items, based on the value from 0 to 3, where higher scores, over 20 points, indicated higher levels of disordered eating behaviours. This validated survey based on screening disorder eating attitudes when the score is over 20 points [52]. Nevertheless, this survey does not provide a definite diagnosis of eating disorders; therefore, a clinical evaluation is needed. This evaluation can be carried out via individual interviews.

The body satisfaction questionnaire (BSQ) [53], whose Spanish adaptation was completed by Raich [54], was used. The stereotypes perception survey from the University of Granada was also used [55].

The questions referring to body image included illustrations of women's bodies. These illustrations comprise seven body images that vary from underweight to obese, numbered from 1 to 7. Additionally, a specific section focused on body satisfaction, examining their satisfaction on a scale from 1 to 7, with lower scores relating to higher levels of body dissatisfaction. In this section, one of the questions examined the steps each young person would take to attain a body type that corresponded to the ideal.

The body image concerns were observed by using the BSQ, a self-report instrument evaluating weight and shape preoccupations [54]. Sample items include: "Have you been so worried about your shape that you have felt you ought to diet?"; "Have you noticed the shape of others and felt that your shape compared unfavourably?" The questions were answered on a six-point Likert scale (1 = never, five = always).

The Appearance Evaluation (AE) subscale of the Multidimensional Body-Self Relations Questionnaire-Appearance Scales (MBSRQ) was used to measure self-perception and stereotypes [56]. Participants rate the extent to which they agree with seven statements (e.g., "Most people would consider me good-looking") on a five-point scale (1 = disagree, 5 = agree) with lower scores indicating lower self-perception and stereotypes.

Finally, self-esteem was evaluated by the Rosenberg survey (CIPE-a) composed of ten questions, which provided us with high, medium or low levels of self-esteem. The questions were given a scale on a four-point scale (1 = disagree, 4 = agree), with lower scores indicating lower self-esteem [57].

On the other hand, the survey that focused on social networks had preliminary yes/no items about having social network accounts on Twitter, Facebook, Instagram, YouTube or Snapchat. Participants indicated how often they access/check their respective accounts daily on a five-point scale: hardly ever, sometimes, usually, all most all the time and always. Additionally, the participants' daily use (hours per day in social networks and highly visual social media, i.e., Instagram, Snapchat), number of accounts and importance given to these was rated on a 1 (strongly disagree) to 5 (strongly agree) scale.

Meanwhile, addiction to social networks was evaluated by a validated survey called the Social Networks Addiction Questionnaire (SNSA) [50]. The survey is based on the DSM-IV-TR [27], a diagnostic instrument that does not recognize psychological addictions as disorders but as a prior stage that can lead to addiction. The survey is formed by 24 items applying a five-point rating system (from 0 to 4), taking into account the frequency from "never" to "always" [56].

The study has focused on the indirect determination of intrauterine testosterone levels during the gestation, determined experimentally from the difference in length of the phalanges of the hands (2D:4D ratio). This measure was selected to determine the possible relation with sociocultural factors indirectly. The selection of this method was based on reducing the risks, vulnerability and protecting biological or genetic material from the participants. When the ratio is higher, i.e., the difference between the second and fourth finger, lower levels of testosterone are implied [21]. 2D:4D is an indicator of testosterone and oestrogen levels [58], which heavily dictate attractiveness [17]. Therefore, this digit ratio may be related to self-perception, body image, body dissatisfaction and disordered eating attitudes.

3.3. Instruments

The instruments used to obtain the image of the hands were a Canon Camera EOS700D (produced by Canon Inc., which is a Japanese company founded in Ota, Tokyo) and a Manfrotto Compact Advance tripod (produced by Manfrotto, which is an Italian company founded in, produced and distributed form the USA). Additionally, free access software GeoGebra (https://www.geogebra.org), which is a free access software founded in Austria and later updated and mass produced in USA, was used to analyse the indirect marker of testosterone levels (2D:4D ratio).

3.4. Procedure

Participants approved a participant information statement, consent form and questionnaires, followed by the approval of the Research Ethics Committee of Public Health System in Cordoba (Ethical Approval number 273, reference 3773).

The participants were undergraduate students with health, education, life and engineering studies. The recruitment took place in different classrooms of the University, the objective of the study, ethical indications, risks for the participants and voluntary participation in the study being previously explained. During the recruitment a teacher and a researcher were present in the classroom the entire time.

The inclusion of the participants was based on an initial survey, which was provided previously in the same classroom. In this survey, the students were asked about the previous diagnosis of conduct or emotional disorders, addiction to technologies, abuse of substances and having a social network account. Those students that had a previous diagnosis of conduct, emotional disorders, or addiction were eliminated from the sample and were not given the survey of the study. Those students that did not have an account on any social network were also excluded from the study (Figure 1).

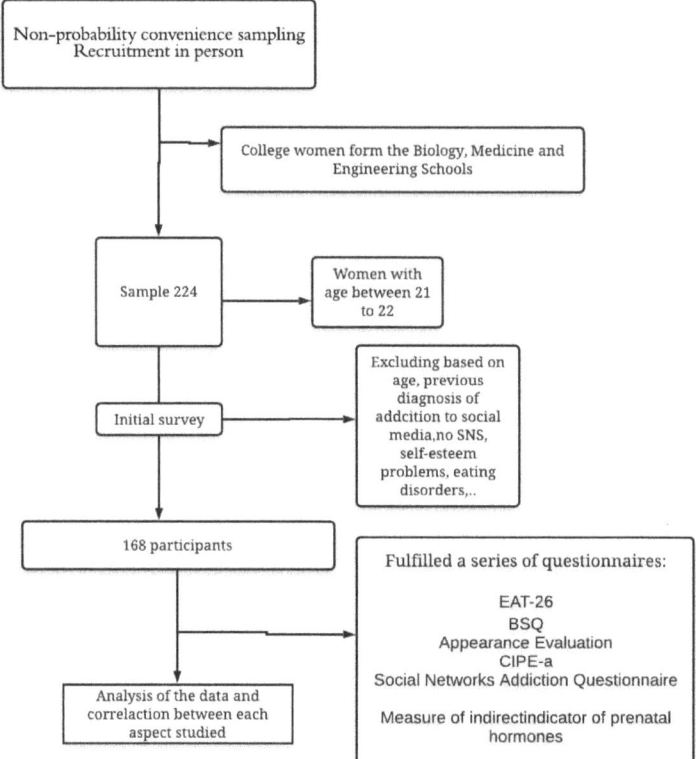

Figure 1. Flow chart of the recruitment and selection of the sample.

3.5. Statistical Analysis

Mean and standard deviation (SD) were calculated for the quantitative variables and frequencies in the case of qualitative variables. Firstly, we studied the normalization of the data using the Kolmogorov-Smirnov test ($p < 0.05$). Moreover, Cronbach's alpha test was used for determining the consistency among the scales and subscales and, especially, the SNS test showed acceptable value (0.77) and the EAT-26 (0.83) was excellent. In order to assess the first objective, the χ^2 test was used for the qualitative variables, such as gender and body image, and the Student's *t*-test was applied to compare quantitative variables, such as the EAT-26 score and age. Additionally, correlational analyses were used to examine relations between all variables.

Moreover, the second set of analyses examined the impact of the relationship between disordered eating attitudes and the rest the factors measured. For this purpose, the crude and adjusted odds ratio (OR) values were calculated for the logistic regression. In the end, the ROC (receiver operating characteristic) curves and the validity indices were used for the diagnostic accuracy of disordered eating attitudes having body dissatisfaction and social networks addiction.

4. Results

First Phase

The initial analysis of the data showed that women ($N = 168$) had a range of age between 21 and 22, 96.7% of them being Caucasian ethnicity. Moreover, the body image that they had was in range between 3 and 4, which may imply a normal weight. The perception that they had of themselves was fatter (3.56 ± 1.2) when compared to the desired body image (2.99 ± 0.83) (Table 1). Additionally, the most common description of body satisfaction showed low and medium-high levels of body satisfaction (48.7%). In this sense, the difference among the group with lower and higher levels of body satisfaction was related to the body image given by the women ($\chi^2 = 113.64$, $p < 0.001$).

Table 1. Mean, standard deviation and confidence intervals.

Factors Studied in Women	Mean (SD)	CI 95%
Self-image	3.56 (1.2)	3.38–3.75
Disordered eating	18.34 (10.7)	16.70–19.97
Self-description	3.99 (0.98)	3.84–4.14
Body satisfaction	4.32 (1.48)	4.1–4.54
Desired body image	2.99 (0.83)	2.86–3.12
Method of change	1.98 (0.82)	1.76–2.01
Zone to change	3.37 (1.95)	3.08–3.67
Self-perception	2.76 (0.89)	2.62–2.89
Stereotypes	2.59 (0.75)	2.48–2.71
Self-esteem	31.10 (4.7)	30.3–31.8
SNS addiction	14.69 (10.37)	13.11–16.26
Use of social media	3.13 (0.72)	3.02–3.24
Frequency of connections	3.46 (0.92)	4.32–3.6
Duration of the connections	3.2 (1.17)	3.02–3.38
Importance of social media	2.8 (0.87)	2.67–2.94

Moreover, the results from the data showed that almost 93% of the women desired to change at least three zones of their body using at least two different methods (1.98 ± 0.82). The methods most used were physical activity (92%), diet (48%), surgery (24%) and beauty or alimentary products (23%). Among the zones to be modified by a surgical procedure 68% of the women indicated breast implants.

The analysis of the results from the EAT-26 test showed that most of the women had a medium probability of having disordered eating attitudes (18.34 ± 10.7). Figure 2 reflects the frequency of the scores from the EAT-26 related to body satisfaction.

The figure displays a higher frequency of scores over 20 points in disordered eating behaviours in the lower points of the body satisfaction scale. This figure implies that there were more values over 20 points when women suffered higher levels of body dissatisfaction. Additionally, the analysis between the score in the disordered eating behaviour test and level of body satisfaction showed significant differences among individuals with low and high levels of body satisfaction and scores over 20 points in the EAT-26 ($\chi^2 = 375.34$, $p < 0.001$). Moreover, a more in-depth analysis of the data, based on women with more than 20 points in the EAT-26, 48 out of 168 women showed that 40.81% had food oral control, 38.77% presented bulimia and food preoccupation and 20.5% dieting.

Further study of the data was carried out in order to address the possible correlations between the body image that women perceived of themselves and the other variables analysed. In Table 2, the correlations between the body image and the different variables have shown significant value with numerous factors, including disordered eating attitudes, self-esteem, desired body image or number of methods. These correlations were positive for a fatter body image in higher scores in the EAT-26 and more methods used to modify the body image and the current body image. Moreover, negative correlations were found for a curvier description that the women gave about their body and higher desires for a thinner body image, higher body dissatisfaction and lower levels of self-esteem.

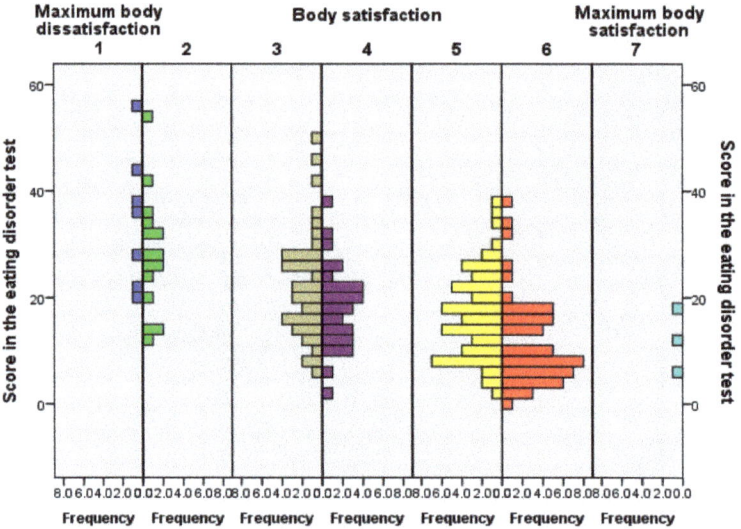

Figure 2. Results from the EAT-26 related to body satisfaction.

Table 2. Correlations with body image that women perceived of themselves.

Factors Studied in Women	Correlation	p-Value
Disordered eating attitudes	0.29	<0.001
Self-description	0.72	<0.001
Body satisfaction	−0.39	<0.001
Desired image	−0.46	<0.001
Method of change	0.22	<0.01
Self-perception	−0.38	<0.001
Stereotypes	0.38	<0.001
Self-esteem	−0.34	<0.001
2D:4D ratio	0.17	<0.05

Another variable that determines a "fatter" body image is the level of prenatal testosterone, measured by the 2D:4D ratio. This result displayed a positive relationship implying that a higher 2D:4D ratio, lower levels of intrauterine testosterone, may lead to a fatter body image.

On the other hand, Table 3 exposed the analysis of correlations between the score obtained in EAT-26 for disordered eating attitudes and the other factors analysed. This test displayed a negative correlation between having a higher score in the test and having lower levels of body satisfaction, self-esteem, the desired of having a thinner body image and worse perception of their own body.

Moreover, the positive correlations were obtained for numerous factors studied. The most highlighting positive correlations were reflected for a higher score in the SNS addiction test, a fatter body image and a higher difference in the 2D:4D ratio. These results implied that a higher 2D:4D ratio or fatter body image may lead to a higher score in the EAT-26.

The logistic regression model was used to define a disordered eating behaviour related to having lower levels of body satisfaction, the desired to achieve a thinner body image, lower levels of self-esteem, higher score in the SNS addiction test, higher duration of connection to this media and higher difference between the second and fourth finger (Table 4).

Table 3. Correlations with having higher scores in the disordered eating attitudes test.

Factors Studied in Women	Correlation	p-Value
Body Image	0.32	<0.001
Self-description	0.34	<0.001
Body satisfaction	−0.64	<0.001
Method of change	0.37	<0.01
Self-perception	−0.38	<0.001
Stereotypes	0.57	<0.001
Desired image	−0.19	<0.05
Zone to change	0.35	<0.001
Self-esteem	−0.49	<0.001
Addiction to SNS	0.18	<0.05
2D:4D ratio	0.41	<0.001

Table 4. Logistic regression for disordered eating attitudes.

Factors Studied in Women	Non-Adjusted				Adjusted	
	ED (Yes)	ED (No)	OR	CI	OR	CI
Body Dissatisfaction	3.35 (1.48)	4.73 (0.21)	0.49	0.38–0.64	0.54	0.33–0.87
Desired image	2.76 (0.14)	3.19 (0.07)	0.56	0.37–0.83	0.24	0.11–0.52
Stereotypes	3.15 (0.69)	2.35 (0.98)	5.17	2.95–9.06	2.56	1.16–0.65
Self-esteem	2.80 (0.53)	3.26 (0.39)	0.10	0.043–0.24	0.15	0.04–0.63
Addiction to SNS	0.96 (0.11)	0.68 (0.57)	1.71	0.56–0.74	0.48	0.23–1.01
Duration of the connections	3.43 (0.17)	3.03 (0.09)	1.32	1.4–1.76	1.68	1.05–2.69
Testosterone levels (2D:4D ratio)	1.20 (0.79)	0.6 (0.79)	2.49	1.62–3.62	3.13	1.60–6.12

From the analysis based on levels of self-esteem and social networks, the results showed that most women have high levels of self-esteem (31.1 ± 4.7) and low levels of addictive behaviour to social network sites (14.69 ± 10.37). Furthermore, the results of the social network sites presented a high dispersion of the results. In this sense, the confidence intervals (95%) were focused on medium levels regarding addictive behaviour to SNS (13.11–16.26).

Based on this, the correlations for the score in the SNS addition test were studied. The results indicated positive significance for the number of methods used to change their body image (<0.001), higher desired of a thinner body ($p < 0.001$), lower levels of self-esteem ($p < 0.001$), greater number of social media accounts ($p < 0.001$), longer duration of the connections ($p < 0.001$) and the importance given to the social networks ($p < 0.001$). Nevertheless, the difference between the second and fourth phalange (2D:4D ratio) showed no significance with scores in the social network addiction test.

Finally, based on the results from the logistic regression, a probabilistic model was obtained. This model could diagnose 42.9% of the population with disordered eating attitudes (R^2 Cox and Snell 0.429) by knowing if the person had scored high in the SNS addiction test, body image, body dissatisfaction and high desire of having a thinner body. The specificity (90.3), sensibility (68.9) and valid index (84.6) results were optimal. Finally, the curve of the model was analysed (Figure 3) obtaining an acceptable probabilistic high risk of a disordered eating attitudes (area = 0.94, $p < 0.001$, CI 0.88–0.97).

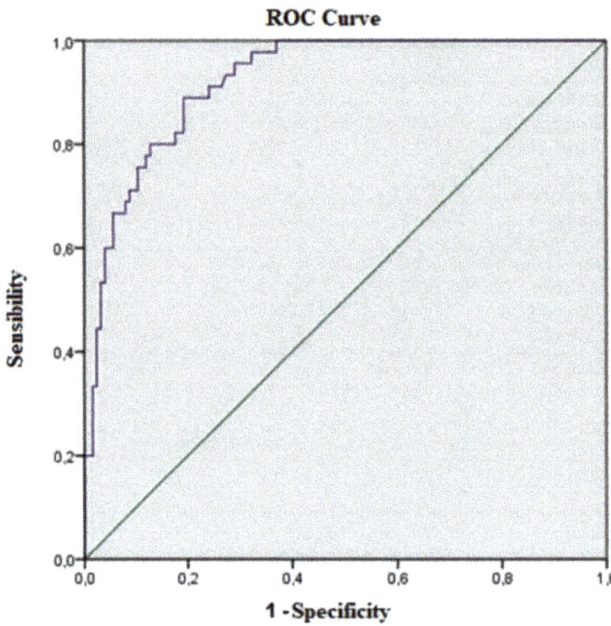

Figure 3. ROC curve from the logistic model for disordered eating.

5. Discussion

This study has reflected how different factors, such as the level of self-esteem (Table 1), might play a significant role in disordered eating behaviours. Among these factors the body image that women perceived over themselves stood out as a significant element. In this sense, according to previous researchers, body image is multidimensional, being made of perceptual, behavioural and cognitive-affective domains created by the individual [46]. This perception is dependent on a variety of elements, including social media and beauty ideals. In the case of social media, the results from this study showed a relationship between the body image, body ideals and the use of social media (Tables 2 and 3). Furthermore, previous publications explained that the desire to achieve the beauty ideal emerges as the internalization of the portrayed image exposed by the media [59,60]. Homan (2010) discussed how, among female college students, two principal beauty ideals coexist: the athletic-ideal and thin-ideal [61]. The internalization of the athletic-ideal predicts compulsive exercise [61–63]. Meanwhile, the thin-ideal internalization predicts food restriction and body dissatisfaction, both leading to disordered eating attitudes and possible origins for eating disorders [64–66]. These results confirm the association obtained between the desire of having a thinner body image and the use of the media since this media is the primary source to promote such ideals (Table 3).

The issue resides on the fact that the thin-ideal produces a worse body image with a tendency toward frustration based on a fatter body image than desired. This concern among young women results in making different choices to obtain the desired image, such as surgery [67,68]. In this sense, the results from this paper also showed a high frequency of women determined to undergo plastic surgery to improve their image, being focused on breast surgery.

Notwithstanding, internalization of the fit-ideal has been studied as a predictor of the use of social media content related to health and fitness [69,70]. In this case, the fit ideal or athletic ideal may become a replacement for the other ideals, leading to healthier behaviour [71].

The results (Table 2) have established that body dissatisfaction might be a potential agent in body image and desire to change this body image. These publications also accord with our earlier observations, which showed that levels of body dissatisfaction were associated with the desire of changing the body image in order to achieve a thinner body, especially using dieting [72]. Based on this, the results appear to match with previous works about how body dissatisfaction and body concerns in young women and teenagers may be related to disordered eating attitudes [27,73].

Another significant outcome was the link between body concerns, body dissatisfaction and levels of self-esteem (Table 2). These data are in accord with recent investigations which connected body dissatisfaction and self-esteem to mental illness and the role of emotional distress in behavioural disorders [48].

Another study found that body dissatisfaction and disordered eating attitudes could be related to a high level of intrauterine testosterone, measured by the 2D:4D ratio. The prenatal masculinization has been established as a potential intermediate phenotype for the development of these disorders in their offspring [74]. Following these studies, the results obtained in this paper seem to initially match such conclusions (Table 3) [75]. These results are partially consistent with the existing literature relating to dieting, alimentary products, such as supplements, negative affect, body dissatisfaction and the tendency to thinness [71]. Nevertheless, the results obtained regarding the hormonal levels may be related to the environmental conditions during the pregnancy more than the individual level of hormones [76].

The results of the study (Table 4) have shown how social network sites might play an important role in disordered eating attitudes. In the study carried out by Cohen et al. (2018), the influence of the social networks was determined by the content and the selfies that the users upload to them more than by the assiduity of the connections [20]. This is partially contradictory to the present results in which the addiction to SNS and the duration of the connections were linked to weight loss and unhealthy dieting. These results match with previous studies in the sociocultural factors, not included among biological measures [77,78]. Withstanding, it is important to note that the regression model obtained in this study have shown the probable role of factors, such as the degree of body satisfaction, self-esteem, use of SNS and other measures, such as the 2D:4D ratio, related to disordered eating behaviours.

Additionally, SNS addiction, which has been related to other mental disorders [79], has shown correlation with stereotypes, self-esteem, method of change, thinner body image and the desired part of the body to change. In this sense, prior investigations proved the addiction to social media as cause–effect of disordered behaviours [80,81].

The present study raises the possibility that disordered eating attitudes in women might be conditioned by the influence of the ideals of beauty imposed by the social environment and to a lesser extent by the exposure to intrauterine levels of testosterone extracted from the 2D:4D ratio of the phalanges. It is possible, therefore, that disordered eating attitudes are multidimensional disorders produced by the media, hormones, and factors related to body concerns. Although this study has focused on Spanish college students, the results (Table 2 and Figure 2) seem to match with previous works conducted in Caucasian women [82,83]. These studies seem to distant themselves from publications focused on Latina or African American young women or adolescents [84,85]. Nevertheless, it is possible, therefore, that because the study was carried out in Spanish college students, the results might not match university women from other countries.

Nevertheless, as with all research, the current findings need to be considered in light of possible limitations of the study. Therefore, biases and possibly incorrect data may have been included, and causal inferences cannot be drawn. Additionally, as with the majority of the body image literature, the current participants were university students, based on the sample and size of the sample caution is recommended in not generalizing these results to other samples or different samples. Nevertheless, these results seem to provide essential data regarding social media, disordered eating and the perception of the young people about themselves. Another limitation present in this study is the lack of inclusion of further cultural factors, such as the mother–child relationship, and anthropometric data, such as BMI.

All being said, the results from this manuscript and the comparison with previous works suggest how the initial hypothesis has been entirely or partially confirmed, showing how disordered eating behaviours are complex eating attitudes.

6. Conclusions

This paper has argued the relationship between body image, body concerns, body dissatisfaction, and disordered eating behaviours present in college women from the south of Spain. This study has identified that women reported moderate levels of body dissatisfaction and body concerns, which were consistently and strongly associated with disordered eating attitudes. In this sense, this work has established high levels of body dissatisfaction, and the link with the desire to achieve a thinner body image. Additionally, the study has shown how body dissatisfaction and desire to achieve the thin-ideal appear to be universal among college women.

Additionally, one of the more significant findings to emerge from this study was that the thin-ideal seems to be widespread in social media. This ideal can promote unhealthy measures, such as dieting, increase body dissatisfaction and disordered eating attitudes. In this sense, the desire to change the body image and taking unhealthy measures was common, given the proliferation of the use of the social network sites where images and content encourage women to aspire to unrealistic and unattainable body ideals. In this sense, the study associated body dissatisfaction, body concerns, and general mental well-being, demonstrating that interventions to improve body perception and satisfaction are essential. Additionally, this research found that higher levels of prenatal testosterone might decrease the probability of having a disordered eating attitude among women. That said, the current study suggests a connection between disordered eating attitudes, negative impacts of exposure to thin-ideal content, addiction to social media and intrauterine testosterone levels.

Concerning practical implications, researchers have asserted that increasing body appreciation may be easier than attempting to decrease body dissatisfaction and for those disordered eating attitudes. Furthermore, the findings regarding the negative impact of exposure to social media related to women's body satisfaction and body appreciation are notable. Despite the limitations present in this manuscript, the findings may help us to understand body concerns focused on the impact of exposure to social media.

In the end, future investigations should continue exploring differences in the levels of body dissatisfaction and disordered eating, including the differences between various ethnic groups. Given the findings regarding differences between those with higher and lower score in EAT-26, the role of social media may be essential in levels of body dissatisfaction and disordered eating attitudes within specific gender/age groups. Longitudinal research is needed to determine the direction of the association between the frequency of connections to social media and body dissatisfaction/disordered eating behaviours. Researchers may also consider culturally-relevant factors that may differentially influence such behaviours.

Author Contributions: Conceptualization: P.A.-M. and M.V.A.; methodology: P.A.-M. and M.P.M.-J.; validation: A.-J.P.-M.; formal analysis: P.A.-M. and A.-J.P.-M.; investigation: P.A.-M. and A.-J.P.-M.; resources: M.P.M.-J. and A.-J.P.-M.; data curation: M.D.R.-M.; writing—original draft preparation: P.A.-M., M.P.M.-J. and A.-J.P.-M.; writing—review and editing: M.V.A. and C.P.; visualization: C.P.; supervision: M.D.R.-M., C.P. and M.V.A.; project administration: M.V.A. and M.P.M.-J.; funding acquisition: M.V.A.

Funding: UCO Social Innova Project Galileo IV from the institution of OTRI of the University of Cordoba, Spain and the funding provided from "IDEP/Escuela de Doctorado" of the University of Cordoba.

Acknowledgments: We would also like to thank of UCO Social Innova Project Galileo IV from the institution of OTRI of the University of Cordoba, Spain and the funding provided from "IDEP/Escuela de Doctorado" of the University of Cordoba to one of the authors. The content is the responsibility of the authors and does not necessarily represent the official views of the OTRI.

Conflicts of Interest: The authors declare no conflict of interest.

References

1. Dowds, J. What do young people think about eating disorders and prevention programmes? Implications for partnerships between health, education and informal youth agencies. *JPMH* **2010**, *9*, 30–41. [CrossRef]
2. Fardouly, J.; Vartanian, L.R. Negative comparisons about one's appearance mediate the relationship between Facebook usage and body image concerns. *Body Image* **2015**, *12*, 82–88. [CrossRef]
3. Bailey, A.P.; Parker, A.G.; Colautti, L.A.; Hart, L.M.; Liu, P.; Hetrick, S.E. Mapping the evidence for the prevention and treatment of eating disorders in young people. *J. Eat. Disord.* **2014**, *2*, 5. [CrossRef]
4. Telch, C.F.; Pratt, E.M.; Niego, S.H. Obese women with binge eating disorder define the term binge. *Int. J. Eat. Disord.* **1997**, *24*, 313–317. [CrossRef]
5. Plateau, C.R.; Brookes, F.A.; Pugh, M. Guided recovery: An interpretative phenomenological analysis of service users' experiences of guided self-help for bulimic and binge eating disorders. *Cogn. Behav. Pract.* **2018**, *25*, 310–318. [CrossRef]
6. Reba-Harrelson, L.; von Holle, A.; Hamer, R.M.; Swann, R.; Reyes, M.L.; Bulik, C.M. Patterns and prevalence of disordered eating and weight control behaviors in women ages 25–45. *Eat. Weight Disord.* **2009**, *14*, e190–e198. [CrossRef] [PubMed]
7. Croll, J.; Neumarksztainer, D.; Story, M.; Ireland, M. Prevalence and risk and protective factors related to disordered eating behaviors among adolescents: Relationship to gender and ethnicity. *J. Adolesc. Health* **2002**, *31*, 166–175. [CrossRef]
8. Baranowksi, M.J.; Jorga, J.; Djordjevic, I.; Marinkovic, J.; Hetherington, M.M. Evaluation of adolescent body satisfaction and associated eating disorder pathology in two communities. *Eur. Eat. Disord. Rev.* **2003**, *11*, 478–495. [CrossRef]
9. Harris, J.K.; Duncan, A.; Men, V.; Shevick, N.; Krauss, M.J.; Cavazos-Rehg, P.A. Messengers and messages for tweets that used #thinspo and #fitspo hashtags in 2016. *Prev. Chronic Dis.* **2018**, *15*. [CrossRef]
10. Garousi, S.; Garrusi, B.; Baneshi, M.R.; Sharifi, Z. Weight management behaviors in a sample of Iranian adolescent girls. *Eat. Weight Disord.* **2016**, *21*, 435–444. [CrossRef]
11. Kraak, V.I.; Story, M. Influence of food companies' brand mascots and entertainment companies' cartoon media characters on children's diet and health: A systematic review and research needs. *Obes. Rev.* **2015**, *16*, 107–126. [CrossRef] [PubMed]
12. Otero, M.C.; Fernández, M.L.; Castro, Y.R. Influencia de la imagen corporal y la autoestima en la experiencia sexual de estudiantes universitarias sin trastornos alimentarios. *Int. J. Clin. Health Psychol.* **2004**, *4*, 357–370.
13. Calado, M.; Lameiras, M.; Sepulveda, A.R.; Rodríguez, Y.; Carrera, M.V. The mass media exposure and disordered eating behaviours in Spanish secondary students. *Eur. Eat. Disord. Rev.* **2010**, *18*, 417–427. [CrossRef]
14. Rodgers, R.F.; Faure, K.; Chabrol, H. Gender differences in parental influences on adolescent body dissatisfaction and disordered eating. *Sex. Roles* **2009**, *61*, 837–849. [CrossRef]
15. Walsh, B.T.; Devlin, M.J. Eating disorders: Progress and problems. *Science* **1998**, *280*, 1387–1390. [CrossRef] [PubMed]
16. Muris, P.; Meesters, C.; van de Blom, W.; Mayer, B. Biological, psychological, and sociocultural correlates of body change strategies and eating problems in adolescent boys and girls. *Eat. Behav.* **2005**, *6*, 11–22. [CrossRef]
17. Wade, T.J.; Shanley, A.; Imm, M. Second to fourth digit ratios and individual differences in women's self-perceived attractiveness, self-esteem, and body-esteem. *Personal. Individ. Differ.* **2004**, *37*, 799–804. [CrossRef]
18. Guo, S.-W.; Reed, D.R. The genetics of phenylthiocarbamide perception. *Ann. Hum. Biol.* **2012**, *38*, 111–142.
19. Manning, J.; Barley, L.; Walton, J.; Lewis-Jones, D.; Trivers, R.; Singh, D.; Thornhill, R.; Rohde, P.; Bereczkei, T.; Henzi, P.; et al. The 2nd: 4th digit ratio, sexual dimorphism, population differences, and reproductive success: Evidence for sexually antagonistic genes? *Evol. Hum. Behav.* **2000**, *21*, 163–183. [CrossRef]
20. Eichler, A.; Heinrich, H.; Moll, G.H.; Beckmann, M.W.; Goecke, T.W.; Fasching, P.A.; Muschler, M.-R.; Bouna-Pyrrou, P.; Lenz, B.; Kornhuber, J. Digit ratio (2D:4D) and behavioral symptoms in primary-school aged boys. *Early Hum. Dev.* **2018**, *119*, 1–7. [CrossRef]
21. Barut, C.; Tan, U.; Dogan, A. Association of height and weight with second to fourth digit ratio (2D:4D) and sex differences. *Percept. Mot. Skills* **2008**, *106*, 627–632. [CrossRef] [PubMed]

22. Jeevanandam, S.; Muthu, P.K. 2D:4D ratio and its implications in medicine. *J. Clin. Diagn. Res.* **2016**, *10*, CM01–CM03. [CrossRef] [PubMed]
23. Breithaupt, L.; Rallis, B.; Mehlenbeck, R.; Kleiman, E. Rumination and self-control interact to predict bulimic symptomatology in college students. *Eat. Behav.* **2016**, *22*, 1–4. [CrossRef] [PubMed]
24. Wood, N.A.R.; Petrie, T.A. Body dissatisfaction, ethnic identity, and disordered eating among African American women. *J. Couns. Psychol.* **2010**, *57*, 141–153. [CrossRef] [PubMed]
25. Loeb, K.L.; Hirsch, A.M.; Greif, R.; Hildebrandt, T.B. Family-based treatment of a 17-year-old twin presenting with emerging anorexia nervosa: A case study using the "Maudsley method". *J. Clin. Child Adolesc. Psychol.* **2009**, *38*, 176–183. [CrossRef]
26. Bourke-Taylor, H.M.; Jane, F.; Peat, J. Healthy mothers healthy families workshop intervention: A preliminary investigation of healthy lifestyle changes for mothers of a child with a disability. *J. Autism Dev. Disord.* **2019**, *49*, 935–949. [CrossRef]
27. Schaefer, L.M.; Burke, N.L.; Calogero, R.M.; Menzel, J.E.; Krawczyk, R.; Thompson, J.K. Self-objectification, body shame, and disordered eating: Testing a core mediational model of objectification theory among White, Black, and Hispanic women. *Body Image* **2018**, *24*, 5–12. [CrossRef]
28. Howard, L.M.; Heron, K.E.; MacIntyre, R.I.; Myers, T.A.; Everhart, R.S. Is use of social networking sites associated with young women's body dissatisfaction and disordered eating? A look at Black–White racial differences. *Body Image* **2017**, *23*, 109–113. [CrossRef]
29. Festinger, L. A theory of social comparison processes. *Hum. Relat.* **1954**, *7*, 117–140. [CrossRef]
30. Powell, E.; Wang-Hall, J.; Bannister, J.A.; Colera, E.; Lopez, F.G. Attachment security and social comparisons as predictors of Pinterest users' body image concerns. *Comput. Hum. Behav.* **2018**, *83*, 221–229. [CrossRef]
31. Neumark-Sztainer, D.; Wall, M.; Larson, N.I.; Eisenberg, M.E.; Loth, K. Dieting and disordered eating behaviors from adolescence to young adulthood: Findings from a 10-year longitudinal study. *J. Am. Diet. Assoc.* **2011**, *111*, 1004–1011. [CrossRef] [PubMed]
32. Caradas, A.A.; Lambert, E.V.; Charlton, K.E. An ethnic comparison of eating attitudes and associated body image concerns in adolescent South African schoolgirls. *J. Hum. Nutr. Diet.* **2001**, *14*, 111–120. [CrossRef] [PubMed]
33. Cohen, R.; Newton-John, T.; Slater, A. The relationship between Facebook and Instagram appearance-focused activities and body image concerns in young women. *Body Image* **2017**, *23*, 183–187. [CrossRef] [PubMed]
34. Hoare, E.; Marx, W.; Firth, J.; McLeod, S.; Jacka, F.; Chrousos, G.P.; Manios, Y.; Moschonis, G. Lifestyle behavioural risk factors and emotional functioning among schoolchildren: The Healthy Growth Study. *Eur. Psychiatry* **2019**, *61*, 79–84. [CrossRef]
35. Perez, M.; Ohrt, T.K.; Bruening, A.B. The effects of different recruitment and incentive strategies for body acceptance programs on college women. *Eat. Disord.* **2016**, *24*, 383–392. [CrossRef]
36. Moradi, B.; Huang, Y.-P. Objectification theory and psychology of women: A decade of advances and future directions. *Psychol. Women Q.* **2008**, *32*, 377–398. [CrossRef]
37. McKinley, N.M.; Hyde, J.S. The objectified body conciousness scale development and validation. *Psychol. Women Q.* **1996**, *20*, 181–215. [CrossRef]
38. Fredrickson, B.L.; Roberts, T.-A. Objectification theory: Toward understanding women's lived experiences and mental health risks. *Psychol. Women Q.* **1997**, *21*, 173–206. [CrossRef]
39. Groesz, L.M.; Levine, M.P.; Murnen, S.K. The effect of experimental presentation of thin media images on body satisfaction: A meta-analytic review. *Int. J. Eat. Disord.* **2002**, *31*, 1–16. [CrossRef]
40. Wyssen, A.; Coelho, J.S.; Wilhelm, P.; Zimmermann, G.; Munsch, S. Thought-shape fusion in young healthy females appears after vivid imagination of thin ideals. *J. Behav. Ther. Exp. Psychiatry* **2016**, *52*, 75–82. [CrossRef]
41. Brooks, K.R.; Mond, J.M.; Stevenson, R.J.; Stephen, I.D. Body image distortion and exposure to extreme body types: Contingent adaptation and cross adaptation for self and other. *Front. Neurosci.* **2016**, *10*, 334. [CrossRef] [PubMed]
42. Juarascio, A.S.; Shoaib, A.; Timko, C.A. Pro-eating disorder communities on social networking sites: A content analysis. *Eat. Disord.* **2010**, *18*, 393–407. [CrossRef] [PubMed]
43. Cohen, R.; Newton-John, T.; Slater, A. 'Selfie'-objectification: The role of selfies in self-objectification and disordered eating in young women. *Comput. Hum. Behav.* **2018**, *79*, 68–74. [CrossRef]

44. Hummel, A.C.; Smith, A.R. Ask and you shall receive: Desire and receipt of feedback via Facebook predicts disordered eating concerns: Facebook disordered eating. *Int. J. Eat. Disord.* **2015**, *48*, 436–442. [CrossRef] [PubMed]
45. van den Eijnden, R.J.J.M.; Lemmens, J.S.; Valkenburg, P.M. The social media disorder scale. *Comput. Hum. Behav.* **2016**, *61*, 478–487. [CrossRef]
46. Quick, V.M.; Byrd-Bredbenner, C. Disordered eating, socio-cultural media influencers, body image, and psychological factors among a racially/ethnically diverse population of college women. *Eat. Behav.* **2014**, *15*, 37–41. [CrossRef]
47. Instagram clamps down on diet and cosmetic surgery posts. *BBC News Technology*. 19 September 2019. Available online: https://www.bbc.com/news/technology-49746065 (accessed on 25 September 2019).
48. Chae, J. Virtual makeover: Selfie-taking and social media use increase selfie-editing frequency through social comparison. *Comput. Hum. Behav.* **2017**, *66*, 370–376. [CrossRef]
49. O'Donnell, N.H.; Willoughby, J.F. Photo-sharing social media for eHealth: Analysing perceived message effectiveness of sexual health information on Instagram. *J. Vis. Commun. Med.* **2017**, *40*, 149–159. [CrossRef]
50. Pichot, P.; Aliño, J.J.L.; Miyar, M.V. *Manual Diagnóstico y Estadístico de los Trastornos Mentales: DSM-IV*; Masson: Barcelona, Spain, 2001; ISBN 978-84-458-0297-7.
51. Garfinkel, P.E.; Newman, A. The eating attitudes test: Twenty-five years later. *Eat. Weight Disord.* **2001**, *6*, 1–21. [CrossRef]
52. Cooper, P.J.; Taylor, M.J.; Cooper, Z.; Fairburn, C.G. The development and validation of the body shape questionnaire. *Int. J. Eat. Disord.* **1987**, *6*, 485–494. [CrossRef]
53. Cash, T.F. Body image: Past, present, and future. *Body Image* **2004**, *1*, 1–5. [CrossRef]
54. Raich, R.M.; Mora, M.; Soler, A.; Avila, C.; Clos, I.; Zapater, L. Adaptación de un instrumento de evaluación de la insatisfacción corporal. *Clin. Salud* **1996**, *7*, 51–66.
55. Godoy, D. Imagen Corporal. Available online: https://test.ugr.es/limesurvey/index.php?sid=22944andlang=es (accessed on 7 June 2018).
56. Mayaute, M.E.; Blas, E.S. Construcción Y validación del cuestionario de adicción a redes sociales (ars). *Liberabit Rev. Peru. Psicol.* **2014**, *20*, 73–91.
57. Petersen, W. Society and the adolescent self-image. Morris Rosenberg. *Science* **1965**, *148*, 804. [CrossRef]
58. Romero-Martínez, A.; Moya-Albiol, L. Prenatal testosterone of progenitors could be involved in the etiology of both anorexia nervosa and autism spectrum disorders of their offspring. *Am. J. Hum. Biol.* **2014**, *26*, 863–866. [CrossRef]
59. Carrotte, E.R.; Prichard, I.; Lim, M.S.C. "Fitspiration" on social media: A content analysis of gendered images. *J. Med. Internet Res.* **2017**, *19*, e95. [CrossRef]
60. de Vries, D.A.; Vossen, H.G.M. Social media and body dissatisfaction: investigating the attenuating role of positive parent–adolescent relationships. *J. Youth Adolesc.* **2019**, *48*, 527–536. [CrossRef]
61. Homan, K. Athletic-ideal and thin-ideal internalization as prospective predictors of body dissatisfaction, dieting, and compulsive exercise. *Body Image* **2010**, *7*, 240–245. [CrossRef]
62. Kantanista, A.; Glapa, A.; Banio, A.; Firek, W.; Ingarden, A.; Malchrowicz-Mośko, E.; Markiewicz, P.; Płoszaj, K.; Ingarden, M.; Maćkowiak, Z. Body image of highly trained female athletes engaged in different types of sport. *Biomed. Res. Int.* **2018**, *2018*, 6835751. [CrossRef]
63. de Bruin, A.P.; Oudejans, R.R.D. Athletes' body talk: The role of contextual body image in eating disorders as seen through the eyes of elite women athletes. *J. Clin. Sport Psychol.* **2018**, *12*, 675–698. [CrossRef]
64. Hawkins, N.; Richards, P.S.; Granley, H.M.; Stein, D.M. The impact of exposure to the thin-ideal media image on women. *Eat. Disord.* **2004**, *12*, 35–50. [CrossRef] [PubMed]
65. Harrison, K. The body electric: Thin-ideal media and eating disorders in adolescents. *J. Commun.* **2000**, *50*, 119–143. [CrossRef]
66. Alberga, A.S. Fitspiration and thinspiration: A comparison across three social networking sites. *J. Eat. Disord.* **2018**, *6*, 39. [CrossRef]
67. Larson, K.; Gosain, A. Cosmetic surgery in the adolescent patient. *Plast. Reconstr. Surg.* **2012**, *129*, 135e–141e. [CrossRef]
68. Ching, B.H.-H.; Xu, J.T. Understanding cosmetic surgery consideration in Chinese adolescent girls: Contributions of materialism and sexual objectification. *Body Image* **2019**, *28*, 6–15. [CrossRef]

69. Holland, G.; Tiggemann, M. A systematic review of the impact of the use of social networking sites on body image and disordered eating outcomes. *Int. J. Eat. Disord.* **2016**, *17*, 100–110. [CrossRef]
70. Slater, A.; Varsani, N.; Diedrichs, P.C. #fitspo or #loveyourself? The impact of fitspiration and self-compassion Instagram images on women's body image, self-compassion, and mood. *Body Image* **2017**, *22*, 87–96.
71. Uhlmann, L.R.; Donovan, C.L.; Zimmer-Gembeck, M.J.; Bell, H.S.; Ramme, R.A. The fit beauty ideal: A healthy alternative to thinness or a wolf in sheep's clothing? *Body Image* **2018**, *25*, 23–30. [CrossRef]
72. Barker, E.T.; Bornstein, M.H. Global self-esteem, appearance satisfaction, and self-reported dieting in early adolescence. *J. Early Adolesc.* **2010**, *30*, 205–224. [CrossRef]
73. Griffiths, S.; Murray, S.B.; Krug, I.; McLean, S.A. The contribution of social media to body dissatisfaction, eating disorder symptoms, and anabolic steroid use among sexual minority men. *Cyberpsychol. Behav. Soc. Netw.* **2018**, *21*, 149–156. [CrossRef] [PubMed]
74. Quinton, S.J.; Smith, A.R.; Joiner, T. The 2nd to 4th digit ratio (2D:4D) and eating disorder diagnosis in women. *Personal. Individ. Differ.* **2011**, *51*, 402–405. [CrossRef] [PubMed]
75. Uban, K.A.; Herting, M.M.; Wozniak, J.R.; Sowell, E.R. Sex differences in associations between white matter microstructure and gonadal hormones in children and adolescents with prenatal alcohol exposure. *Psychoneuroendocrino* **2017**, *83*, 111–121. [CrossRef] [PubMed]
76. Seo, D.; Ray, S. Habit and addiction in the use of social networking sites: Their nature, antecedents, and consequences. *Comput. Hum. Behav.* **2019**, *99*, 109–125. [CrossRef]
77. Sumter, S.R.; Cingel, D.P.; Antonis, D. "To be able to change, you have to take risks #fitspo": Exploring correlates of fitspirational social media use among young women. *Telemat. Inform.* **2018**, *35*, 1166–1175.
78. Moessner, M.; Feldhege, J.; Wolf, M.; Bauer, S. Analyzing big data in social media: Text and network analyses of an eating disorder forum. *Int. J. Eat. Disord.* **2018**, *51*, 656–667. [CrossRef]
79. Pantic, I. Online social networking and mental health. *Cyberpsychol. Behav. Soc. Netw.* **2014**, *17*, 652–657. [CrossRef]
80. Abbasi, I.; Drouin, M. Neuroticism and Facebook addiction: How social media can affect mood? *Am. J. Fam. Ther.* **2019**, *47*, 199–215. [CrossRef]
81. Köse, Ö.B.; Doğan, A. The Relationship between Social Media Addiction and Self-Esteem among Turkish University Students. *Addicta Turk. J. Addict.* **2019**, *6*, 175–190. [CrossRef]
82. Sladek, M.R.; Salk, R.H.; Engeln, R. Negative body talk measures for Asian, Latina(o), and White women and men: Measurement equivalence and associations with ethnic-racial identity. *Body Image* **2018**, *25*, 66–77. [CrossRef]
83. Ceballos, N.; Czyzewska, M. Body Image in Hispanic/Latino vs. European American Adolescents: Implications for treatment and prevention of obesity in underserved populations. *J. Health Care Poor Underserved* **2010**, *21*, 823–838. [CrossRef] [PubMed]
84. Gordon, K.H.; Castro, Y.; Sitnikov, L.; Holm-Denoma, J.M. Cultural body shape ideals and eating disorder symptoms among White, Latina, and Black college women. *Cult. Divers. Ethn. Minority Psychol.* **2010**, *16*, 135–143. [CrossRef] [PubMed]
85. Stokes, D.M. Brown beauty: Body image, Latinas, and the media. *Body Image* **2016**, *16*, 8.

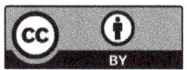

© 2019 by the authors. Licensee MDPI, Basel, Switzerland. This article is an open access article distributed under the terms and conditions of the Creative Commons Attribution (CC BY) license (http://creativecommons.org/licenses/by/4.0/).

MDPI
St. Alban-Anlage 66
4052 Basel
Switzerland
Tel. +41 61 683 77 34
Fax +41 61 302 89 18
www.mdpi.com

International Journal of Environmental Research and Public Health Editorial Office
E-mail: ijerph@mdpi.com
www.mdpi.com/journal/ijerph

www.ingramcontent.com/pod-product-compliance
Lightning Source LLC
LaVergne TN
LVHW070448100526
838202LV00014B/1683